ADVANCES IN

Vascular Surgery

VOLUME 3

ADVANCES IN

Vascular Surgery

VOLUME 1

VOLUME 2

ADVANCES IN
Vascular Surgery

VOLUME 3

Editor-in-Chief
Anthony D. Whittemore, M.D.
Professor Surgery, Harvard University Medical School; Chief, Division of
Vascular Surgery, Brigham and Women's Hospital, Boston, Massachusetts

Associate Editors
Dennis F. Bandyk, M.D.
Professor of Surgery, Director, Vascular Surgery Division, University of South
Florida College of Medicine, Tampa, Florida

Jack L. Cronenwett, M.D.
Professor of Surgery, Dartmouth Medical School; Chief, Section of Vascular
Surgery, Dartmouth–Hitchcock Medical Center, Lebanon, New Hampshire

Norman R. Hertzer, M.D.
Chairman, Department of Vascular Surgery, Cleveland Clinic Foundation,
Cleveland, Ohio

Rodney A. White, M.D.
Professor of Surgery, University of California at Los Angeles School of
Medicine; Chief of Vascular Surgery, Associate Chairman, Department of
Surgery, Harbor–University of California at Los Angeles Medical Center,
Torrance, California

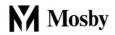 **Mosby**

St. Louis Baltimore Boston Chicago London Madrid Philadelphia Sydney Toronto

ℕ Mosby

Vice President and Publisher, Continuity Publishing: Kenneth H. Killion
Director, Editorial Development: Gretchen C. Murphy
Developmental Editor: Kris Baumgartner
Acquisitions Editor: Jennifer Roche
Manager, Continuity–EDP: Maria Nevinger
Project Manager: Jill C. Waite
Assistant Project Supervisor: Sandra Rogers
Proofreading Supervisor: Barbara M. Kelly
Vice President, Professional Sales and Marketing: George M. Parker
Senior Marketing Manager: Eileen M. Lynch
Marketing Specialist: Lynn D. Stevenson

Printed in the United States of America
Composition by The Clarinda Company
Printing/binding by The Maple-Vail Book Manufacturing Company

Mosby–Year Book, Inc.
11830 Westline Industrial Drive
St. Louis, Missouri 63146

Editorial Office:
Mosby–Year Book, Inc.
200 North LaSalle Street
Chicago, Illinois 60601

International Standard Serial Number: 1069-7292
International Standard Book Number: 0-8151-9407-2

Contributors

Joseph Patrick Archie, Jr., M.D., Ph.D.
Clinical Professor of Surgery, University of North Carolina at Chapel Hill
School of Medicine, Chapel Hill, North Carolina; Adjunct Professor of
Mechanical and Aerospace Engineering, North Carolina State University,
Raleigh, North Carolina

William H. Baker, M.D.
Professor and Chief, Section of Peripheral Vascular Surgery, Loyola University
of Chicago Stritch School of Medicine, Maywood, Illinois

Michael Belkin, M.D.
Assistant Professor of Surgery, Division of Vascular Surgery, Department of
Surgery, Brigham and Women's Hospital, Harvard Medical School, Boston,
Massachusetts

Denis D. Bensard, M.D.
Instructor in Surgery, Ohio State University School of Medicine, Columbus,
Ohio

F. William Blaisdell, M.D.
Professor and Chairman, Department of Surgery, University of California, Davis,
Medical Center, Sacramento, California

Edi Brogi, M.D.
Department of Pathology, Massachusetts General Hospital, Boston,
Massachusetts

Lawrence B. Cohen, M.D.
Associate Professor, Department of Plastic and Reconstructive Surgery, Eastern
Virginia Medical School, Norfolk, Virginia

Enrique Criado, M.D.
Assistant Professor of Vascular Surgery, University of North Carolina, Chapel
Hill, North Carolina

Jack Cronenwett, M.D.
Professor of Surgery, Chief, Section of Vascular Surgery, Dartmouth Medical
School, Dartmouth-Hitchcock Medical Center, Lebanon, New Hampshire

Gian Luca Faggioli, M.D.
Research Physician, University of Bologna, Bologna, Italy

Jerry Goldstone, M.D.
Professor of Surgery, Division of Vascular Surgery, University of California, San
Francisco, California

Richard J. Gusberg, M.D.
Professor and Chief, Vascular Surgery, Yale-New Haven Hospital, Yale
University School of Medicine, Director, Yale Vascular Center, New Haven,
Connecticut

Ziv J. Haskal, M.D.
Assistant Professor of Radiology, University of Pennsylvania School of Medicine, Philadelphia, Pennsylvania

K. Wayne Johnston, M.D., F.R.C.S.(C.)
Division of Vascular Surgery, The Toronto Hospital, Toronto, Ontario, Canada; Professor of Surgery and Chairman, Division of Vascular Surgery, University of Toronto, Toronto, Ontario, Canada

Blair A. Keagy, M.D.
Professor and Chief, Division of Vascular Surgery, University of North Carolina, Chapel Hill, North Carolina

Georg Kretschmer, M.D.
Associate Professor of Surgery, Department of Surgery, Division of Vascular Surgery, University of Vienna, Vienna, Austria

William C. Krupski, M.D.
Professor and Chief, Vascular Surgery, University of Colorado Health Sciences Center, Denver, Colorado

Peter Libby, M.D.
Vascular Medicine and Atherosclerosis Unit, Cardiovascular Division, Department of Medicine and Department of Pathology, Brigham and Women's Hospital, Boston, Massachusetts

Thomas F. Lindsay, M.D., F.R.C.S.(C.)
Division of Vascular Surgery, The Toronto Hospital, Toronto, Ontario, Canada; Assistant Professor of Surgery, University of Toronto, Toronto, Ontario, Canada

Arnold Miller, M.B., Ch.B., F.R.C.S., F.R.C.S.(C.), F.A.C.S.
Assistant Clinical Professor of Surgery, Harvard Medical School, Boston Massachusetts; Attending Surgeon, MetroWest Medical Center, Framingham, Massachusetts, and New England Deaconess Hospital, Boston, Massachusetts

Gregory L. Moneta, M.D.
Professor of Surgery, Division of Vascular Surgery, Oregon Health Sciences University School of Medicine, Portland, Oregon

Bruno Niederle, M.D.
Associate Professor of Surgery, Department of Surgery, Division of General Surgery, University of Vienna, Vienna, Austria

Marc A. Passman, M.D.
Research Fellow, Division of Vascular Surgery, Oregon Health Sciences University School of Medicine, Portland, Oregon

John M. Porter, M.D.
Professor of Surgery and Chief, Division of Vascular Surgery, Oregon Health Sciences University School of Medicine, Portland, Oregon

John J. Ricotta, M.D.
Professor of Surgery, Director, Division of Vascular Surgery, SUNY at Buffalo, Millard Fillmore Hospital, Buffalo, New York

Craig Rubinstein, M.B.M.S. (Melb.), F.R.A.C.S.
Department of Plastic and Reconstructive Surgery, Eastern Virginia Medical School, Norfolk, Virginia

Juha P. Salenius, M.D., Ph.D.

Vascular Research Fellow, Harvard Medical School, MetroWest Medical Center, Framingham and New England Deaconess Hospital, Boston, Massachusetts; Assistant Professor of Vascular Surgery, Tampere University, Tampere, Finland; Attending Vascular Surgeon, University Hospital, Tampere, Finland

Steven M. Santilli, M.D., Ph.D.

Assistant Professor, Department of Surgery, University of Minnesota; Section of Vascular Surgery, University of Minnesota Hospital and Clinic, VA Medical Center, Minneapolis, Minnesota

Thomas Sautner, M.D.

Department of Surgery, Division of General Surgery, University of Vienna, Vienna, Austria

Frederick J. Schoen, M.D., Ph.D.

Department of Pathology, Brigham and Women's Hospital, Boston, Massachusetts

Lewis B. Schwartz, M.D.

Vascular Fellow, Division of Vascular Surgery, Department of Surgery, Brigham and Women's Hospital, Harvard Medical School, Boston, Massachusetts

Galina Sukhova, Ph.D.

Vascular Medicine and Atherosclerosis Unit, Cardiovascular Division, Department of Medicine and Department of Pathology, Brigham and Women's Hospital, Boston, Massachusetts

Hiroyuki Tanaka, M.D., Ph.D.

Department of Cardiothoracic Surgery, Tokyo Medical and Dental University, Tokyo, Japan

Lloyd M. Taylor, Jr., M.D.

Professor of Surgery, Division of Vascular Surgery, Oregon Health Sciences University School of Medicine, Portland, Oregon

M. R. Tyrrell, F.R.C.S., F.R.C.S.(Ed.)

Senior Registrar, Department of Surgery, Guy's Hospital, London, England

John H. N. Wolfe, M.S., F.R.C.S.

Consultant Vascular Surgeon, St. Mary's Hospital, London, England

Preface

The Editorial Board is pleased to dedicate the initial portion of this third volume of *Advances in Vascular Surgery* to extra-anatomic arterial reconstruction, and we are fortunate to have one of the initial pioneers in this field, Dr. F. William Blaisdell, provide his historical perspective. The section includes a thorough technical description of thoracofemoral reconstruction from Dr. Blair Keagy's experience at the University of North Carolina and a practical guide to obturator bypass provided by Dr. Bruno Niederle and his group from Geneva.

In the section on carotid disease, we have included a thought-provoking contribution from Dr. Joseph Archie, outlining his approach to the stroke in the recovery room immediately following carotid endarterectomy. Dr. K. Wayne Johnston has reviewed the Canadian experience with management of the ruptured aortic aneurysm, a significant experience derived from the variety of clinical settings inherent in the Canadian health system. The technique of endoscopic sympathectomy has been improved, as noted in Dr. William Krupski's timely update. With sclerotherapy well established and transjugular intrahepatic portosystemic shunt (TIPS) evolving, the vascular surgeon is no longer regularly confronted with bleeding esophageal varices; yet, a thorough understanding of portal decompression with both conventional shunts and TIPS is required. Dr. Richard Gusberg has provided his approach to portal hypertension derived from his experience at Yale University.

The section on infrainguinal reconstruction includes an update on cryopreserved vein grafts and a chapter on the role of free-flap transfer for extensive ischemic ulcerations, an option that has become a practical reality. Finally, the basic science section presents current theory underlying the pathogenesis of intimal hyperplasia.

It is our hope that this volume will prove helpful for those clinicians responsible for the management of patients with vascular disease.

Anthony D. Whittemore, M.D.
Editor-in-Chief

Contents

Mosby Document Express

    Copies of the full text of journal articles referenced in this book are available by calling Mosby Document Express, toll-free, at 1-800-55-MOSBY.

    With Mosby Document Express, you have convenient 24-hour-a-day access to literally every journal reference within this book. In fact, through Mosby Document Express, virtually any medical or scientific article can be located and delivered by FAX, overnight delivery service, international airmail, electronic transmission of bit-mapped images (via Internet), or regular mail. The average cost of a complete delivered copy of an article, including copyright clearance charges and first-class mail delivery, is $12.

    For inquiries and pricing information, please call the toll-free number shown above.

PART I

Extra-Anatomic
Reconstruction

History of Extra-Anatomic Bypass Graft Procedures

F. William Blaisdell, M.D.

Professor and Chairman, Department of Surgery, University of California, Davis, Medical Center, Sacramento, California

V ascular reconstructive surgery was first attempted in the 1950s. There were sufficient difficulties with technical procedures and with graft replacements that complications such as graft infections, graft thromboses, and graft disruptions were relatively common. In most instances, the patients either did not survive the complication or lost the limb or limbs being revascularized. There was no real experience with long-term graft results, but it was believed that the more anatomic the graft replacement, the better the results, and that extra-anatomic bypass seemed ill-conceived.

As far as can be determined, credit for initiating extra-anatomic bypass should go to Drs. Norman Freeman and Frank Leeds of San Francisco, who were the first to carry out *femorofemoral bypass*. In the early 1950s, a satisfactory arterial prosthesis had not been developed, although there had been several cautious trials of homografts for arterial replacement. Freeman and Leeds,[1] in a 1952 issue of *California Medicine*, described using the splenic artery to bypass an abdominal aneurysm. The aneurysm in this instance was divided distally so that it thrombosed proximally. Circulation was maintained to the left iliac artery using the splenic artery. Apparently there was enough cross-circulation from one limb to the other to maintain viability through iliac collaterals.

Although the article by Freeman and Leeds emphasized the use of splenic artery bypass of the abdominal aorta (perhaps not a true extra-anatomic procedure), it also presented a case of common femoral to common femoral bypass using the superficial femoral artery (Fig 1), which was an extra-anatomic procedure. The procedure was said to have worked well, although the definitive case report was not included and information regarding this procedure was presented as a throw-away for the splenic artery bypass of the abdominal aneurysm.

Vetto[2] published ten cases of femorofemoral bypass in 1962 for treatment of unilateral iliac artery obstruction and was responsible for popularizing the procedure. In two of his cases the procedure was performed "to relieve complications of aortic surgery"; in one case it was used to treat thrombosis of a femoral aneurysm, in another it was used to bypass a common femoral embolus, and in the remainder it was used to treat unilateral atherosclerotic iliac artery obstructions. All operations but one were successful in establishing lower extremity blood flow. At the time

Advances in Vascular Surgery®, vol. 3
© 1995, Mosby–Year Book, Inc.

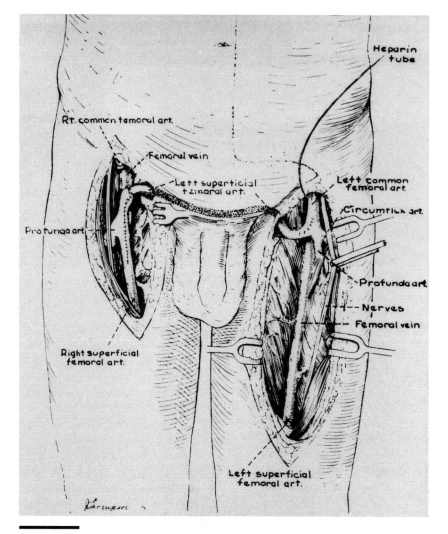

Labels in figure:
Heparin tube
Rt. common femoral art.
Femoral vein
Left superficial femoral art.
Left common femoral art.
Circumflex art.
Profunda art.
Profunda art.
Nerves
Femoral vein
Right superficial femoral art.
Left superficial femoral art.

FIGURE 1.

Femorofemoral bypass. (From Freeman NE, Leeds FH: *Calif Med* 77:229, 1952. Used by permission.)

of manuscript submission, four cases had been followed for 13 to 16 months, indicating that the first procedures were carried out in 1960. Vetto's use of a subcutaneous tunnel is well shown in the illustration from his original article (Fig 2). In the article he emphasized the operation's utility in aged and high-risk patients with unilateral iliac artery stenosis or occlusion.

McCaughan and Kahn[3] described two cases of *iliocontralateral/popliteal artery bypass* carried out in 1958. A crossover graft from one iliac artery to the opposite popliteal artery was used as an alternative to aortopopliteal graft in two high-risk patients with unilateral iliofemoral thrombosis (Fig 3). In one, the profunda femoris artery was anastomosed to the side of the graft before being carried down to the popliteal artery.

Lewis[4] described managing a type III dissection of the descending aorta in 1959 by *subclavian to external iliac artery bypass*. The left

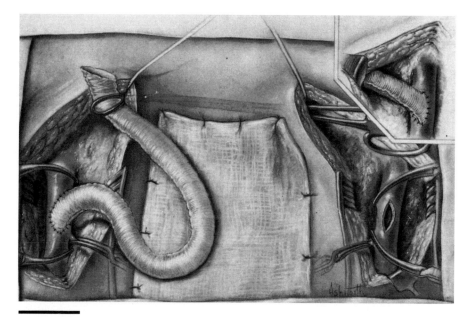

FIGURE 2.

Femorofemoral bypass. (From Vetto RM: *Surgery* 52:342, 1962. Used by permission.)

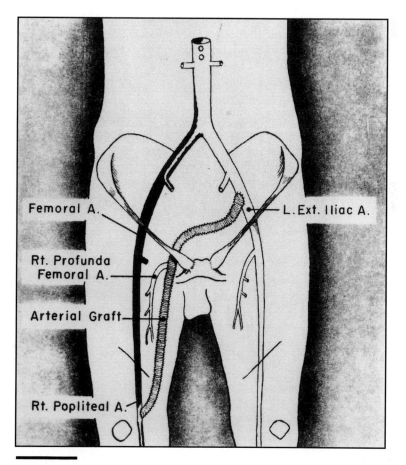

Femoral A.

L. Ext. Iliac A.

Rt. Profunda Femoral A.

Arterial Graft

Rt. Popliteal A.

FIGURE 3.

The iliolateral popliteal bypass. (From McCaughan JJ Jr, Kahn SF: *Ann Surg* 151:26, 1960. Used by permission.)

clavicle was removed, the subclavian artery divided, the distal end ligated, and a nylon graft 3/8 of an inch in diameter anastomosed end-to-end to the proximal vessel. The graft was brought down the anterior chest wall subcutaneously and paraxiphoid into the abdomen where it was anastomosed to an intra-abdominal bifurcated homograft. The aorta was ligated distal to the renal arteries, and the distal end of the homograft was anastomosed to the external iliac arteries (Fig 4). The patient was still alive and the graft functioning well 2 months later.

Thoracic aorta to femoral bypass rose out of a desperate clinical situation: we were confronted with a patient who presented with a proximal suture line disruption 1 month after repair of a ruptured abdominal aneurysm. The suture line disruption was resutured, although the aorta was extremely friable. Cultures from around the graft showed heavy growth of *Escherichia coli,* and the only treatment then available was multiple antibiotics and prayer. One month after the first operation, following continuing sepsis, the patient once again developed abdominal pain and shock. We found re-rupture of the proximal suture line and gross sepsis. After the aorta was cross-clamped above the renal arteries, the only alternative at that time (1960) appeared to be removal of the original graft. The proximal aortic stump was oversewn at a level just below the renal arteries. The common iliac arteries were then ligated and the abdomen closed. Next, the chest was opened by a small lateral intercostal incision.

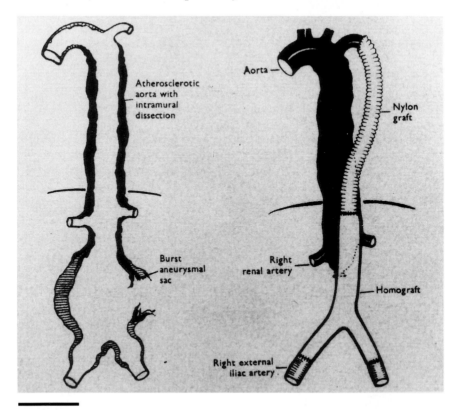

FIGURE 4.
Subclavian to abdominal aorta bypass. (From Lewis CD: *B-J Surg* 48:574, 1961. Used by permission.)

A 14-mm Dacron graft was anastomosed to the descending aorta, passed under the 12th rib, and a plane developed in the abdominal wall musculature to the left groin, where anastomosis to the common femoral artery was carried out. A 10-mm Dacron graft was anastomosed to the first and brought subcutaneously over the pubis to the contralateral femoral artery. The patient survived the procedure but died 1 month later of inanition and persistent abdominal sepsis (intravenous feeding was not yet available). At autopsy, the graft was patent and the patient had manifested no problems of perfusion of the lower half of the body (Fig 5).[5] It was obvious to us, however, that thoracotomy was a major procedure in a sick patient, and we explored alternatives to revascularize the lower extremities.

One of the problems to resolve was whether a small artery such as the axillary artery or the subclavian artery could supply sufficient blood to nourish the lower half of the body. We had previously carried out experiments measuring flows in the superficial femoral artery after placement of an arteriovenous fistula. We found that an artery the size of a superficial femoral artery could accommodate the entire resting cardiac output, so it appeared that the axillary artery of equivalent size could supply sufficient blood flow to both the arm and the leg to avoid a steal phenomenon (which was widely believed to be the result of any procedure

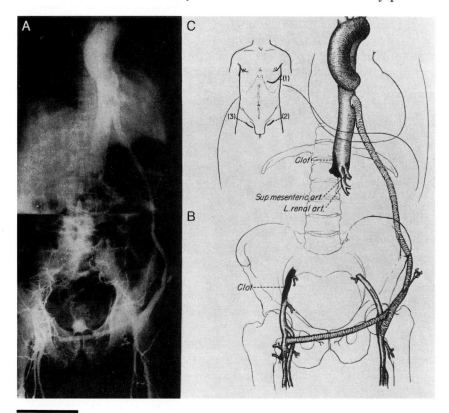

FIGURE 5.

A, B, and **C,** thoracic aorta to femoral bypass. (From Blaisdell FW, DeMattei GA, Gauder PJ: *Am J Surg* 102:583, 1961. Used by permission.)

of the type we proposed to carry out). Moreover, our belief was given credence by the experience of Freeman and Leeds, who had used the splenic artery to bypass an aortic aneurysm, although we were not aware of their experience at the time.

The next issue to resolve was the optimal location for the anastomosis. The first portion of the axillary artery as it emerges from under the clavicle has no major branches. The only branch is the highest thoracic. John Hunter advocated ligation of the axillary artery at this level for distal aneurysms because the collateral about the shoulder was excellent and ligation at this level rarely resulted in severe ischemia of the extremity.[6] Most important, the first portion of the artery moves very little with elevation of the shoulder, whereas more lateral placement at the level of the pectoralis minor or distal to the pectoralis minor results in considerable stress on the graft with any type of upper extremity exercise.

We were prepared to use an *axillofemoral graft* on the next aortic graft infection that we encountered. However, our first opportunity came when a patient developed acute arterial ischemia. He had previously suffered an above-the-knee amputation of the left leg and manifested acute ischemia of the right leg secondary to thrombosis of an aortofemoral graft. General anesthesia was being induced in preparation for carrying out an aortofemoral bypass when the patient developed a cardiac arrest. CPR was initiated and the patient was resuscitated; however, he had ischemic changes on his ECG. Therefore, our operative strategy changed, and, under local anesthesia, we carried out an axillofemoral bypass.[7] We had no preoperative arteriogram of the distal circulation of the leg. Subsequent arteriography showed that the outflow consisted of two large collaterals from a common femoral artery, and both profunda femoris and superficial femoral arteries were occluded (Fig 6). Fortunately, the patient maintained patency of his graft until his death 3 years later in the hospital men's rest room at the time of a follow-up visit. His wife recognized her husband's celebrity status and permitted autopsy verification of arterial patency. Of interest, Louw[8] carried out an identical procedure in South Africa a month following our initial procedure.

Subsequently, we had multiple opportunities to use the axillofemoral bypass, a primary indication being infection of abdominal aortic grafts. We found early, as others did, that use of cross-femoral bypass increased flow in the axillofemoral bypass and resulted in significantly better long-term patency than did unilateral axillofemoral grafts,[9] and we have since modified this by using a double-outflow technique.[10] LoGerfo et al.[11] in 1977 demonstrated that flows of 300^+ cc/min are optimal for graft patency; this is equivalent to the average blood flow in one extremity with patent circulation. When the bypass is performed to treat some complication of aneurysmal disease, a patent distal circulation is common and long-term patency is excellent. However, when the indications are occlusive disease, the distal circulation is not often fully patent, and blood flows in unilateral grafts are often in the range of 50–150 ml/min. Another important aspect regarding maximizing blood flow through the graft is the avoidance of parallel flow in native vessels. If the common iliac artery is occluded on one side, end-to-side anastomoses are used for the limb in-

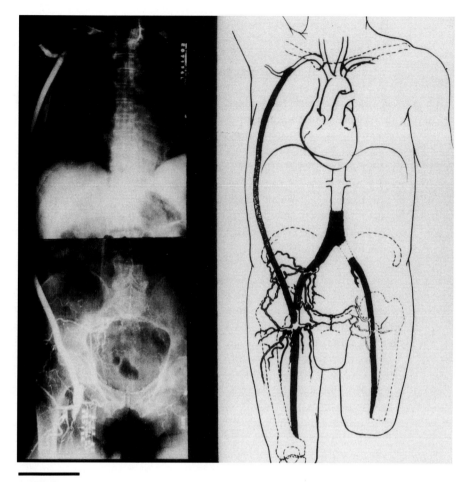

FIGURE 6.

Axillofemoral bypass. (From Blaisdell FW, Hall AD: Surg 54:563, 1963. Used by permission.)

flow to permit retrograde pelvic perfusion. Conversely, if iliac arteries are stenosed rather than occluded, both common femoral arteries should be divided for placement of the axillofemoral and femorofemoral grafts, and end-to-end anastomosis should be carried out.

Another technical point we felt was important in performing axillofemoral bypass was placement of the graft in the axis of the flexion of the body. This required a second incision in the mid- or posterior axillary line (none of the long tunnelers are satisfactory in this regard) for adequate lateral placement of the graft. This avoids kinking of the graft with flexion of the body and avoids stress on the proximal and distal anastomoses with exercise of the limbs.

Initially, to avoid an inadvertent compression of the graft in our patients, we asked them to avoid using belts and to convert to suspenders, and we advocated putting thumbtacks in their dressings during the acute postoperative period so that whenever they rolled over on their sides they were given a sharp message. These latter two forms of protection did not prove necessary, because the development of the externally supported graft as advocated by Sauvage[12] accomplished the equivalent and has markedly improved long-term results.

In 1963, Shaw and Baue[13] described three successful cases of *obturator foramen bypass* in which the circulation was rerouted through the obturator foramen to bypass groin graft infections. In this first article, they described their technique for carrying out this procedure. The proximal anastomosis is made to one of the iliac arteries or to the lower abdominal aorta using a retroperitoneal suprainguinal incision. The graft is then tunneled through the upper medial portion of the obturator foramen, carefully avoiding the obturator nerve and artery that pass through the medial anterior corner of that foramen. A hole is made sufficiently large to pass an index finger through, and a tunneler then is easily passed down the plane of the adductor musculature, ideally to the level of the adductor canal in the lower two thirds of the thigh, where the natural cleavage plane leads to the distal superficial femoral artery. The course of the graft so placed is well away from the infected groin incision (Fig 7). The advantage of this procedure is that the graft passes in the axis of flexion of the body, so there is no tendency for it to stretch or kink when the patient assumes a sitting position. The authors believed that either autogenous vein or a synthetic graft could be used for the procedure.

The final development in extra-anatomic bypass to the lower extremities was *ascending aorta–abdominal aorta bypass* or *ascending aorta–femoral bypass*. The concept of using the ascending aorta as a source for the proximal anastomosis should be credited to Schumaker,[14] who carried out ascending aorta to infrarenal abdominal aortic bypass and reported the case in 1968. The bypass was carried out for a mycotic aneurysm involving coarctation repair of the proximal descending aorta. Al-

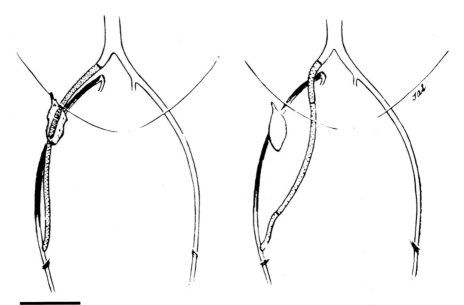

FIGURE 7.

Obturator bypass. (From Shaw RS, Baue AE: *Surgery* 53:75, 1963. Used by permission.)

though the operation was temporarily successful, the patient died several weeks later of his primary infection.[15]

Robinson et al.[16] performed the first successful ascending to infrarenal aortic bypass in 1968. This followed a recurrent dissection of the descending thoracic aorta and false aneurysm that developed after initial segmental graft replacement. Through a midline sternotomy and a left flank incision, a 14-mm Dacron graft was placed from the ascending aorta through the anterior part of the diaphragm extraperitoneally to the abdominal aorta near its bifurcation. A left thoracotomy was then used to

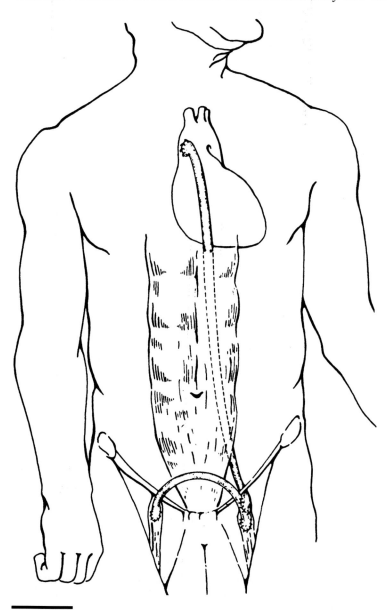

FIGURE 8.

Ascending aorta–femoral bypass. (From Frantz, et al: Surgery 75:471, 1974. Used by permission.)

remove the infected graft from the descending thoracic aorta after proximal and distal aortic ligation. The graft was said to be functioning well 1 year later.

Frantz et al.[17] performed ascending aorta to bilateral common femoral bypass for infrarenal aortic occlusion. A midline sternotomy was used to expose the ascending thoracic aorta after a midline abdominal incision confirmed extensive pathology involving the entire intra-abdominal aorta. Following side-to-end ascending aorta graft anastomosis, a bifurcation graft was brought subxiphoid and retroperitoneally to both common femoral arteries (Fig 8). Although the date of the operation was not given, at the time of the report in 1973 the graft was said to have been patent for 1 year.[17]

Many other "extra-anatomic" procedures have been used over the years. Femoroaxillary artery bypass was used by us in 1964. The graft thrombosed within a month of placement and our case was never reported. Others have reported using similar retrograde grafts, but no long-term results have been published, suggesting that the experience of other authors was similar to ours. The reason for this undoubtedly is that flow in the retrograde direction is much less than flow in the antegrade direction because of the smaller volume of tissue supplied. As a result, there is a greater tendency for grafts to thrombose.

Other anatomic procedures have included axillary-axillary bypass, ascending aorta to axillary bypass, subclavian-carotid and carotid-subclavian bypass, and carotid-carotid bypass. These smaller grafts have functioned quite well but are not the subject of this paper.

REFERENCES

1. Freeman NE, Leeds FH: Operations on large arteries. *Calif Med* 77:229, 1952.
2. Vetto RM: The treatment of unilateral iliac artery obstruction utilizing femoro-femoral graft. *Surgery* 52:342, 1962.
3. McCaughan JJ Jr, Kahn SF: Cross-over graft for unilateral occlusive disease of the iliofemoral arteries. *Ann Surg* 151:26, 1960.
4. Lewis CD: A subclavian artery as a means of blood supply to lower half of the body. *Br J Surg* 48:574, 1961.
5. Blaisdell FW, DeMattei GA, Gauder PJ: Extraperitoneal thoracic aorta to femoral by-pass graft as replacement for an infected aortic bifurcation prosthesis. *Am J Surg* 102:583, 1961.
6. Beekman R: Studies in aneurysm, by William and John Hunter. *Ann Med Hist* 8:124, 1936.
7. Blaisdell FW, Hall AD: Axillary-femoral artery bypass for lower extremity ischemia. *Surgery* 54:563, 1963.
8. Louw JH: Splenic to femoral and axillary to femoral bypass. *Lancet* 2:1401, 1963.
9. Blaisdell FW, Hall AD, Lim RC Jr: Aorto-iliac arterial substitution utilizing subcutaneous grafts. *Ann Surg* 172:775, 1970.
10. Ward RE, Holcroft JW, Conti S, et al: New concepts in the use of axillofemoral bypass grafts. *Arch Surg* 118:573, 1983.
11. LoGerfo FW, Johnson WC, Corson JD, et al: A comparison of the late patency rates of axillobilateral femoral and axillounilateral femoral grafts. *Surgery* 81:33, 1977.
12. El-Massry S, Saad E, Sauvage LR: Axillofemoral bypass with externally sup-

ported knitted Dacron grafts: A follow-up through twelve years. *J Vasc Surg* 13:107, 1933.

13. Shaw RS, Baue AE: Management of sepsis complicating arterial reconstructive surgery. *Surgery* 53:75, 1963.

14. Shumaker HB Jr, King H, Nahrwold DL: Coarctation of the aorta. *Curr Probl Surg* 5:16, 1968.

15. Wukasch DC, Codey DA, Saniford FM, et al: Ascending aorta–abdominal aorta bypass: Indications, techniques, and report of 12 patients. *Ann Thorac Surg* 23:442, 1977.

16. Robinson G, Siegelman S, Attai L: Recurrent dissecting aneurysms of aorta. *NY State J Med* 72:2328, 1972.

17. Frantz SL, Kaplitt MJ, Beil AR Jr, et al: Ascending aorta–bilateral femoral artery bypass for the totally occluded infrarenal abdominal aorta. *Surgery* 75:471, 1974.

Axillofemoral Bypass

Marc A. Passman, M.D.

Research Fellow, Division of Vascular Surgery, Oregon Health Sciences
University School of Medicine, Portland, Oregon

Lloyd M. Taylor, Jr., M.D.

Professor of Surgery, Division of Vascular Surgery, Oregon Health Sciences
University School of Medicine, Portland, Oregon

Gregory L. Moneta, M.D.

Professor of Surgery, Division of Vascular Surgery, Oregon Health Sciences
University School of Medicine, Portland, Oregon

John M. Porter, M.D.

Professor of Surgery and Chief, Division of Vascular Surgery, Oregon Health
Sciences University School of Medicine, Portland, Oregon

H istorically, axillofemoral bypass was introduced as an alternative
procedure to standard aortofemoral revascularization for patients
with severe perioperative risk factors or clinical situations in which anatomic reconstruction was not feasible. Because of early disappointing primary patency rates, axillofemoral bypass was perceived as a compromised
procedure with a limited clinical role. However, in the past decade, patency rates achieved with axillofemoral bypass have improved dramatically, temporally associated with use of the externally supported graft.
Results achieved with modern axillofemoral bypass approach or equal
those achieved with conventional aortofemoral bypass. This alone more
than justifies a careful reevaluation of the role of axillofemoral bypass in
the treatment of aortoiliac occlusive disease.

HISTORICAL BACKGROUND

Freeman and Leeds[1] reported what is widely regarded as the first extra-
anatomic bypass in 1952. They placed an endarterectomized superficial
femoral artery subcutaneously over the pubis to carry blood from one
femoral artery to the other. In 1959, Lewis of Perth,[2] during resection of
a ruptured abdominal aneurysm, was unable to anastomose an arterial
homograft to the proximal aorta because of extensive rupture and dissection. He sutured a crimped nylon graft to the left subclavian artery and
tunneled it subcutaneously across the chest and into the abdomen at the
level of the xiphoid process for anastomosis to the proximal aortic homograft, demonstrating for the first time that an upper extremity artery
could provide inflow to the lower half of the body. In 1960, Blaisdell and
associates[3] placed an extraperitoneal thoracic aorta to left femoral bypass
graft for treatment of an infected infrarenal aortic prosthetic graft. A sec-

Advances in Vascular Surgery®, vol. 3
© 1995, Mosby–Year Book, Inc.

ond graft was then tunneled suprapubically to the right common femoral artery. In 1962, Vetto[4] reported the first clinical series of transabdominal, subcutaneous femorofemoral graft operations to bypass unilateral iliac artery obstruction in poor-risk patients.

In 1963, Blaisdell[5] and Louw[6] independently reported use of a bypass between the axillary and ipsilateral femoral arteries for unilateral lower extremity ischemia. Blaisdell's original axillounifemoral bypass was in a patient resuscitated from a cardiac arrest that occurred during induction of anesthesia for repair of an acutely thrombosed aortic graft. Louw used an axillounifemoral saphenous vein bypass to revascularize the right leg and a splenic artery–femoral artery Teflon bypass for the left leg in a high-risk patient with limb-threatening infrarenal aortic occlusive disease. To avoid separate bilateral axillofemoral bypasses in patients with bilateral iliac occlusive disease, Sauvage and associates, in 1966,[7] added the femorofemoral extension to the axillofemoral graft, thereby introducing the axillobifemoral procedure.

INDICATIONS

Originally, axillofemoral bypass was restricted to situations in which aortofemoral bypass was judged impossible or inadvisable because of local conditions precluding its use. The early enthusiasm for axillofemoral bypass as an alternative to revascularization in the presence of infected aortofemoral grafts soon expanded to include high-risk patients requiring revascularization for limb-threatening ischemia.[8–12] However, as experience began to accumulate, it became apparent that the rate of thrombosis of axillofemoral grafts was relatively high.[13–17] Moore and colleagues[17] reviewed an 8-year series of 52 axillofemoral bypasses, which included the original bypasses performed by Blaisdell and Hall,[5] and reported a primary patency of 60% at 1 year and 10% at 5 years. Eugene and associates[18] reported a 50% thrombosis rate of axillofemoral grafts at 2 years. These reports concluded that axillofemoral bypass was indicated only for poor-risk patients whose poor medical condition rendered conventional anatomic vascular reconstruction unacceptable.

Contrasting results were reported by others. In 1977, Johnson and coworkers[19] reviewed their 10-year experience of aortic and axillobifemoral grafts, reporting operative mortalities of 5.5% and 1.8%, respectively, and a 5-year patency rate of 76% for both groups. In 1979, Ray and associates[20] reported a secondary patency of 72% for axillofemoral bypass, compared with a primary patency of 91% for aortofemoral bypass at 9 years. These authors concluded that for patients with an increased operative risk, axillofemoral bypass was a reasonable alternative to aortofemoral bypass.

These conflicting results have caused controversy regarding specific indications for use of axillofemoral bypass grafts. There is currently widespread acceptance of the procedure for treatment of limb-threatening aortoiliac disease in patients who have a high risk for intra-abdominal vascular reconstruction, but there are no universally accepted criteria placing patients into this high-risk category. In general, prohibitive factors include advanced age, debilitation, severe cardiac disease, severe pulmonary disease, short life expectancy, and sepsis.[21–23]

A persistent perception of poor patency of axillofemoral bypass has been in part the impetus for recent reports challenging the previously held principle of extra-anatomic bypass and removal of infected prosthetic for aortic graft sepsis with or without aortoenteric fistula. Several authors have suggested in situ graft replacement with antibiotic treatment,[24, 25] percutaneous drainage,[26] or muscle flap coverage[27] as an alternative. These approaches are controversial, and the principle of axillofemoral bypass and removal of the infected graft remains the standard treatment.[28–30]

Axillofemoral bypass combined with induced aneurysmal thrombosis has also been used for treatment of abdominal aortic aneurysms. In 1965, Blaisdell and colleagues[31] performed an initial right axillofemoral and femorofemoral bypass combined with interruption of the left femoral artery proximal to the bypass, followed 1 month later by ligation of both common iliac arteries and the infrarenal aorta proximal to the aneurysm. Leather and co-workers,[32] in 1979, reported using simultaneous axillobifemoral bypass and aneurysmal thrombosis induced by interruption of the external and internal iliac arteries with metal clips and intra-arterial bucrylate in cases of persistent aneurysmal flow. They concluded that use of combined extra-anatomic bypass and induced aneurysmal thrombosis was a reasonable alternative for poor-risk patients. Although various groups reported favorable results with this nonresective approach,[33–35] others found an unacceptably high rate of complications, including failure of induced aneurysmal thrombosis and aneurysm rupture.[36–39] Schwartz and associates[39] reported an operative mortality rate of 31% for a nonresective approach as compared with less than 3% for elective conventional aortic graft replacement. The excessive morbidity and mortality of axillofemoral grafting with induced thrombosis of abdominal aortic aneurysms has led to the general abandonment of this procedure, although use of axillofemoral grafting with aneurysm neck ligation remains an option in selected patients.

Other acknowledged indications for axillofemoral bypass have included mycotic aneurysms,[40, 41] inflammatory aneurysms,[42] aortic coarctation,[43] arterial trauma,[44] embolism from degenerative atherosclerosis of the aorta,[45] and acute aortic occlusion.[46–49] Local "hostile" factors, such as prior irradiation, extensive adhesions, severe aortic calcification, malignancy, and previous enteric contamination, are also indications for its use.[50]

TECHNICAL CONSIDERATIONS

The modern operative approach for axillofemoral bypass is a variation of the technique described by Blaisdell and Hall.[5] Patients are positioned supine with the arm abducted to 90° to maximize the distance between the axillary and femoral arteries. Wide preparation and draping of the supra- and infraclavicular areas, axilla, chest, abdomen, and femoral regions are then performed.

A two-team approach is preferred to shorten operative time. The axillary artery is exposed through an infraclavicular incision. The fibers of the pectoralis major muscle are separated. The first portion of the axillary artery between the chest wall and the medial border of the pectoralis minor is used for anastomosis, as recommended by Blaisdell and Hall,[5] because of its relatively fixed position and single collateral branch. The femoral vessels are exposed in the usual manner by use of vertical groin incisions. The common femoral artery at its bifurcation is preferred for the anastomosis; however, if there is significant atherosclerotic disease,

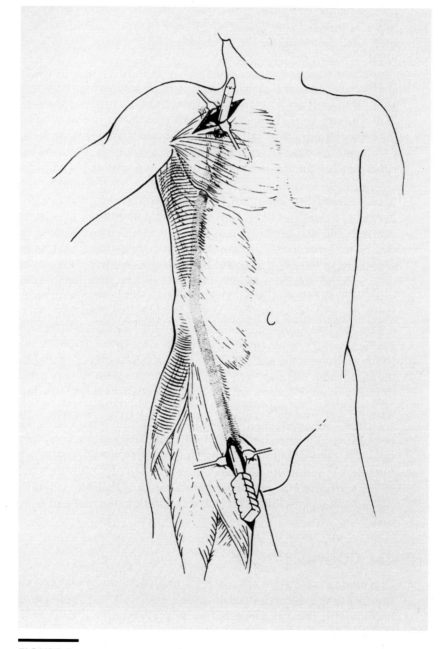

FIGURE 1.

The use of the Oregon tunneler between axillary and femoral exposures. The route is from the femoral incision, medial to the anterior iliac spine, subcutaneous to the inferior border of the pectoralis major, then submuscular to the axillary artery. (From Taylor LM Jr, Moneta GL, McConnell DB, et al: *Arch Surg* 129:588–595, 1994. Used by permission.)

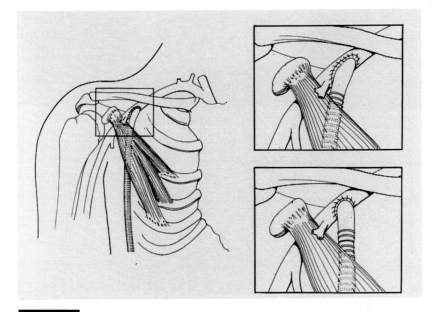

FIGURE 2.

Standard technique of axillofemoral proximal anastomosis. Graft is placed beneath the plane of the transsected pectoralis minor and anastomosed to the first portion of the axillary artery, medial to the pectoralis minor and origin of the thoracoacromial artery. *Upper insert,* standard end-to-end anastomosis. *Lower insert,* anastomosis as recommended by graft manufacturer. Note the minimal bevel, which equalizes pulling force around the suture line. (From Taylor LM Jr, Park TC, Edwards JM, et al: *J Vasc Surg* 20:520–528, 1994. Used by permission.)

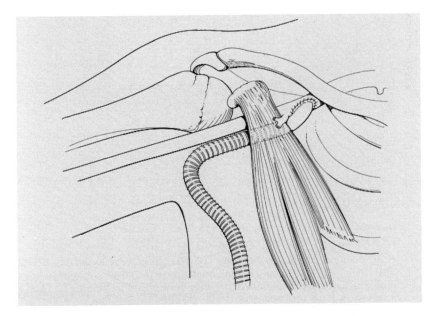

FIGURE 3.

Modified technique of axillofemoral proximal anastomosis. Graft is anastomosed in an end-to-side fashion to the first portion of the axillary artery and routed parallel and adjacent to the artery beneath the pectoralis minor for 8 to 10 cm before being directed in a gentle and redundant curve in the axilla to lie against the chest wall in the subcutaneous position. (From Taylor LM Jr, Park TC, Edwards JM, et al: *J Vasc Surg* 20:520–528, 1994. Used by permission.)

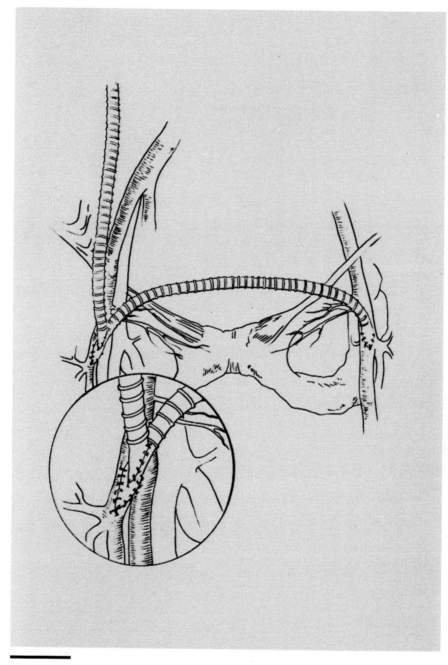

FIGURE 4.

Axillofemoral bypass technique. The femorofemoral bypass is performed first, with the distal axillofemoral limb anastomosed to the "cobra head" of the ipsilateral femoral anastomosis *(insert)*. (From Taylor LM Jr, Moneta GL, McConnell DB, et al: *Arch Surg* 129:588–595, 1994. Used by permission.)

the profunda femoris artery can be used instead. A subcutaneous tunnel is formed from the ipsilateral femoral incision, medial to the anterior iliac spine, along the lateral aspect of the abdomen at the mid-axillary line, to the inferior border of the pectoralis major, and then submuscular to the axillary artery. Use of the Oregon tunneler allows passage of the graft without the need for additional counterincisions (Fig 1). For an infected groin wound, the distal graft is tunneled laterally for anastomosis to the deep or superficial femoral artery. A second subcutaneous suprapubic tunnel is formed between femoral exposures.

Axillary anastomosis is performed in an end-to-side fashion to a longitudinal arteriotomy on the anterior surface of the first portion of the axillary artery, medial to the pectoralis minor and to the origin of the thoracoacromial artery (Fig 2). The graft is routed parallel and adjacent to the axillary artery for 8 to 10 cm before forming a gentle curve in the axilla to its inferior course. This redundancy allows for arm extension, distributing any potential tension across the curve of the graft rather than at the proximal anastomosis (Fig 3). This technique of proximal anastomosis is intended to prevent anastomotic disruption.[85] The femorofemoral limb is anastomosed to the respective femoral arteries first, and then the distal end of the axillofemoral component is anastomosed in an end-to-side fashion to the "cobra head" of the ipsilateral femoral limb (Fig 4). This configuration maximizes flow along the entire length of the axillofemoral component.

RESULTS

Despite relatively low operative mortality rates, patency rates reported for axillofemoral grafting have been quite variable, as summarized in Table 1. Factors suggested as influencing patency rates have included graft configuration (axillounifemoral vs. axillobifemoral), adequacy of distal runoff, severity of aortoiliac occlusive disease (limb-threatening ischemia vs. claudication), unsuspected inflow disease, graft material (Dacron vs. polytetrafluoroethylene), and the use of externally supported grafts.

Increasing opinion has favored the axillobifemoral configuration over the axillounifemoral graft because of the significantly lower primary patency rate of 19% to 37% at 5 years for single limb grafts.[20, 50–53] The presumed physiologic basis is that the femorofemoral limb significantly increases flow through the axillofemoral limb, thereby improving patency of the graft. LoGerfo and colleagues[51] found that axillobifemoral bypass had superior long-term patency when compared with axillounifemoral bypass, achieving five-year secondary patency rates of 74% versus 37%, respectively. This higher patency was attributed to increased flow through the axillobifemoral grafts, averaging 621 mL/min compared with 273 mL/min for the axillounifemoral grafts. These results were supported by Kalman and associates[54] who reported a 3-year patency of 77% for axillobifemoral and 58% for axillounifemoral bypass. In contrast, Ascer and coworkers[55] found no significant difference between axillounifemoral and axillobifemoral grafting. In their 5-year review, primary patency rates were 44% for the axillounifemoral group and 50% for the axillobifemoral group. There was also no difference in the 5-year secondary patency and limb salvage rates. Until a well-controlled randomized study is conducted, the preference of axillobifemoral grafting over axillounifemoral grafting will remain theoretical.

Adequacy of runoff has been considered a major factor contributing to the long-term patency of the axillofemoral bypass. Ray and colleagues[20] reported a secondary patency for axillobifemoral bypass of 95% at 9 years

TABLE 1.
Cumulative Patency Rates of Axillofemoral Bypass

Author	Year	No.	Mortality Rate (%)	Patency Rate (%)			Graft Configuration*	Primary vs. Secondary
				1 yr	3 yrs	5 yrs		
Mannick, Williams, Nasbeth[14]	1970	43	7.0	78	—	—	Axillounifemoral	Primary
Moore, Hall, Blaisdell[17]	1971	44	9.0	60	26	10	Both	Primary
Johnson, LoGerfo, Vollman, et al.[19]	1977	56	1.8	84	—	76	Axillobifemoral	Secondary
Eugene, Goldstone, Moore[18]	1977	35	8.0	60	40	30	Axillounifemoral	Primary
LoGerfo, Johnson, Corson, et al.[51]		24	—	60	36	36	Axillobifemoral	Primary
	1977	64	8.0	56	37	37	Axillounifemoral	Secondary
		66		87	74	74	Axillobifemoral	Secondary
DeLaurentis, Sala, Russell, et al.[56]	1978	42	7.1	69	—	—	Both	Primary
Ray, O'Connor, Davis, et al.[20]	1979	33	3.7	75	75	67	Axillounifemoral	Secondary
Burrell, Wheeler, Gregory, et al.[64]	1982	21	—	90	85	77	Axillobifemoral	Secondary
		36	8.0	72	66†		Axillounifemoral	Secondary
Kenney, Sauvage, Wood, et al.[60]	1982	38		97	97†		Axillobifemoral	Secondary
		92	—	85	78‡	66	Axillounifemoral	Secondary
		22		100	100‡		Axillounifemoral§	Secondary

Author	Year	No.						Graft	
Ascer, Veith, Gupta, et al.[55]	1984	34	5.3	95	90	71	Axillounifemoral	Secondary
Donaldson, Louras, Buckman, et al.[61]	1986	22	8.0	90	77	77	Axillobifemoral	Secondary
		100		88	72	72	Both	Secondary
Schultz, Sauvage, Mathisen, et al.[70]	1986	56	—	95	88	75	Axillounifemoral§	Primary
Rutherford, Patt, Pearce[50]	1987	15	0	—	—	97	Axillounifemoral§	Secondary
				—	—	37	Axillounifemoral	Secondary
Kalman, Hosang, Cina, et al.[54]	1987	27	8.8	74	58	81	Axillobifemoral	Secondary
		31				—	Axillounifemoral	Primary
Cina, Ameli, Kalman, et al.[21]	1988	59	4.9	90	77	—	Axillobifemoral	Primary
		41		80	72	72	Both	Secondary
Mason, Smirnov, Newton, et al.[74]	1989	37	2.7	87	81	—	Both	Primary
Harris, Taylor, McConnell, et al.[72]	1990	76	4.5	93	85	85	Axillobifemoral§	Primary
El-Massry, Saad, Sauvage, et al.[71]	1993	79	5.1	97	92	87	Both§	Secondary
Taylor, Moneta, McConnell, et al.[73]	1994	184	4.9	95	86	79	Both§	Secondary

*Axillounifemoral, axillobifemoral, or both
†2.7 years
‡4 years
§Externally supported graft

when both superficial femoral vessels were patent, compared with 79% at 5 years when only the deep femoral was patent. Rutherford and associates[50] found that occlusion of the superficial femoral artery markedly affected long-term patency, reducing the 5-year primary patency of the axillobifemoral bypass from 92% to 41% and that of the axillounifemoral bypass from 54% to 0%. This observation has led some authors to recommend femoral artery endarterectomy, profundaplasty, or distal segmental grafting to improve axillofemoral outflow.[51, 56, 57]

In patients with limb-threatening ischemia and severe atherosclerotic disease of the common, superficial, and deep femoral arteries, axillopopliteal bypass has also been advocated when other standard operations are not feasible.[58, 59] Overall 1-, 3-, and 5-year cumulative primary patency rates of axillopopliteal bypass have been reported at 58%, 45%, and 40%, with comparable limb salvage rates of 83%, 68%, and 58%, respectively.[59]

Although most published reports have suggested restricting axillofemoral bypass to poor-risk patients with limb-threatening ischemia, some have also used it for claudication. In the series by Eugene and associates[18] and Rutherford and co-workers,[50] 12% of axillofemoral bypasses were performed for claudication, whereas in the series by Kenney and colleagues,[60] 68% were performed for claudication. When results were analyzed on the basis of indications, a trend toward improved long-term patency in grafts performed for claudication as compared with limb salvage was noted. Donaldson and associates[61] reported a 3-year primary patency of 46% for patients with claudication compared with 28% for those with limb-threatening ischemia. Similarly, Ray and co-workers[20] found long-term patency rates of 81% and 50% for claudication and limb salvage, respectively.

Unsuspected occlusive disease proximal to the axillary artery can significantly influence patency. Calligaro and colleagues[62] used arteriography to prospectively determine the incidence of unsuspected inflow stenosis in 40 consecutive patients undergoing axillofemoral grafting. A 25% prevalence of stenosis greater than 50% luminal diameter was demonstrated by arteriography; only one fourth of these were predicted by pressure measurements. The authors concluded that upper-extremity noninvasive measurements were unreliable in predicting underlying inflow stenosis and recommended routine arteriographic assessment prior to axillofemoral bypass. We have not identified a problem with asymptomatic critical inflow stenoses. We routinely use noninvasive pressure measurements, reserving angiography for patients with abnormal tests results. When pressures are equal, the right arm is preferred for inflow because of the increased prevalence of left subclavian atherosclerotic disease.[63]

The role of prosthetic graft material in axillofemoral bypass patency is uncertain. Two nonrandomized studies suggested improved patency for knitted Dacron rather than woven grafts.[17, 18] Burrell and associates[64] compared patencies of Dacron and polytetrafluoroethylene (PTFE) and found no significant difference. Nitzberg and co-workers[65] reported a 4-year primary cumulative patency rate of 66% for axillofemoral grafts performed with PTFE, in contrast to 24% for those performed with Dacron. This discrepancy probably represents evolution of technique, because Dacron was used in all grafts prior to 1978, and PTFE was used between 1978 and 1989. Others have observed lower infection rates with PTFE compared with Dacron.[30, 66] This has been supported experimentally by decreased bacterial colonization with PTFE.[67] Nevertheless, without the benefit of a randomized trial, no prosthetic material is clearly superior.

Numerous reports have suggested an association between graft occlusion and the subcutaneous location of axillofemoral grafts. Clinically, most axillofemoral graft occlusions are noted as patients arise from sleep.[14, 51] One proposed mechanism has been decreased blood flow secondary to the normal decrease in cardiac output associated with sleep. Another possibility is external compression with graft deformation due to body weight. Detailed investigation of external graft compression has produced conflicting results. Jarowenko and colleagues[68] noted no significant change in pulse-volume recordings of ankle-brachial indices with external compression by body weight in six patients 2 to 7 months after axillobifemoral bypass. Cavallaro and associates[69] on the other hand, found a statistically significant decrease of approximately 50% in ankle-brachial indices and pulse-volume amplitudes at 5 minutes of external body weight compression.

In an effort to resist the graft deformation produced by external compression and to control kinking, the externally supported Dacron prosthesis was introduced by Sauvage and associates in 1978, with markedly improved patency rates for grafts in the axillofemoral position.[60] From 1978 to 1984, 56 externally supported Dacron axillofemoral grafts were implanted with a 5-year primary patency of 75% and secondary patency of 97%.[70] El-Massry and co-workers[71] recently reported a long-term follow-up of this series. During a 12-year period, axillofemoral bypass grafts were performed on 77 patients, with a primary patency of 78% at 5 years and 73% at 7 years, and no change thereafter.

Externally supported PTFE became available in 1981, and we began using this prosthesis at the Oregon Health Sciences University in Portland, Oregon, exclusively in 1983. Before 1983, our experience with axillofemoral bypass using nonsupported prostheses was disappointing, with a 1-year patency of 51% (unpublished data), leading to limited use of the procedure except when absolutely indicated.[72] Since 1983, patency with the externally supported PTFE has improved. Between January 1984 and November 1993, 184 axillofemoral graft procedures were performed in 164 patients, 91% of which involved axillobifemoral grafts. Life-table primary patency, secondary patency, limb salvage, and survival at 5 years were 71%, 79%, 92%, and 52%, respectively (Figs 5 through 7).[73]

Previous published comparisons of axillofemoral and aortofemoral bypass procedures have been retrospective and anecdotal. Mason and colleagues[74] found that aortofemoral bypass had a slightly higher 3-year cumulative patency of 89%, and alternative procedures, including axillofemoral bypass, had 81% patency, which was not significantly different. Schneider and associates[75] found primary and secondary patency rates of 63% and 76% for axillofemoral bypass, compared with 85% and 91% for aortofemoral bypass, respectively. Similarly, Bunt[76] reported a life-table patency of 94% at 2 years for patients undergoing aortofemoral grafting, compared with 83% at 2 years for axillofemoral procedures. Aor-

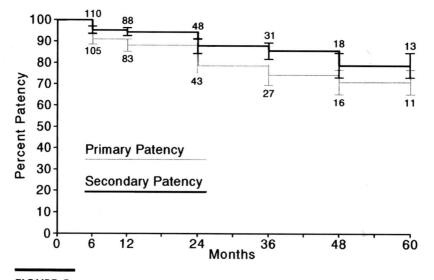

FIGURE 5.

Life-table primary and secondary patency rates of the axillofemoral procedures (N = 184). (From Taylor LM Jr, Moneta GL, McConnell DB, et al: *Arch Surg* 129:588–595, 1994. Used by permission.)

tofemoral procedures had a complication rate of 12% and a mortality rate of 1.8%, as compared with negligible morbidity and mortality rates for axillofemoral bypass. They concluded that restricting aortofemoral bypass to better-risk patients and liberalizing the use of extra-anatomic bypass might decrease overall patient morbidity and mortality without jeopardizing limb preservation.

Aortobifemoral bypass remains standard treatment for symptomatic aortoiliac occlusive disease because of excellent long-term patency, ex-

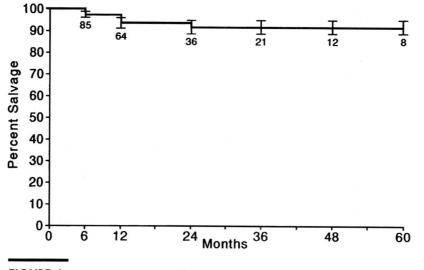

FIGURE 6.

Life-table limb salvage rates for 149 limbs at risk for loss treated by 127 axillofemoral bypass procedures. (From Taylor LM Jr, Moneta GL, McConnell DB, et al: *Arch Surg* 129:588–595, 1994. Used by permission.)

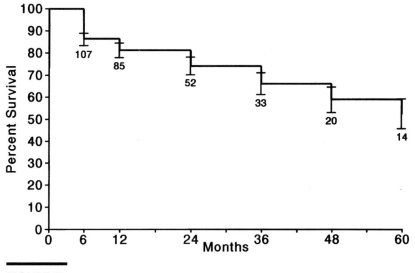

FIGURE 7.
Life-table survival for axillofemoral bypass (N [n] = 167).

ceeding 85%.[77–79] However, these historic patency figures must be viewed in perspective. Today, patients undergoing revascularization for aortoiliac disease are characterized by more advanced age and a higher prevalence of limb-threatening ischemia and multilevel disease than patients undergoing aortofemoral bypass several decades ago. Many patients treated operatively in the past for claudication would be managed today by nonoperative measures or by less invasive procedures. In fact, contemporary patency rates of aortofemoral bypass grafts performed for lower extremity revascularization, assessed by modern reporting standards, are largely unknown.

COMPLICATIONS

In a recent literature review by Bunt and Moore[80] of 917 axillofemoral bypasses, the incidence of graft-related complications was 1.6%. Operative mortality has ranged between 2%, reported by Johnson and co-workers,[19] and 9%, reported by Kalman and colleagues.[54] Five-year survival has ranged from a low of 26%, reported by Eugene and associates,[18] to 66% reported by Johnson and co-workers.[19]

Disruption of axillary anastomoses was first reported by Daar and Finch, in 1978.[81] In their case, a Dacron graft became detached from the axillary artery when the sutures pulled through the artery early in the postoperative period. Since then, multiple authors have described axillary arterial anastomotic ruptures, presenting as infraclavicular pain, swelling, hematoma, compression of brachial nerves, graft occlusion, or lower extremity ischemia.[82–84]

Disruption occurred in 5% of our patient population, 1 to 46 days postoperatively (mean, 21 days).[85] Operative findings suggested two patterns of graft disruption in response to the force produced by arm elevation: an initial tear at the "heel" of the graft with suture pullout at the "toe," and complete graft disruption adjacent to the anastomosis (Fig 8). Factors contributing to this complication are the technical placement of the proximal anastomosis, the angle between the graft and the axillary artery, and the variable distance between the axillary and femoral arteries, depending on body position. The presence of graft disruption with an intact anastomosis in two of our ten cases may represent structural failure of PTFE, rather than an inherent risk of axillofemoral grafting. Because PTFE vascular grafts are formed as an extruded polymer, rather than woven or knitted fabric, they may be prone to alteration of structure by clamping or penetration with needles, producing weakness and subsequent disruption.

Multiple recommendations have been made to avoid disruption, including placing the anastomosis on the first part of the axillary artery; draping to allow full arm and shoulder movement and testing the graft for tension prior to determining the final length; cutting the graft slightly longer than necessary; creating a gentle redundant curve of the graft along the axillary artery at the proximal anastomosis, as outlined previously; and postoperatively avoiding motion that places tension on the graft. The treatment of disruption involves placement of a new interposition graft between the previous axillofemoral graft and the axillary artery.

Early or late thrombosis of the axillary artery, which may or may not be associated with distal upper extremity embolization, has also been an infrequent complication.[86-89] Although some patients with axillary ar-

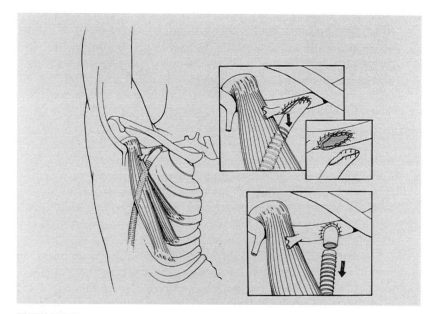

FIGURE 8.

Operative findings in cases of graft disruption. Force producing disruption occurs with arm abduction/shoulder elevation as illustrated. *Upper insert,* combined disruption with tear at "heel" and suture pullout at "toe." *Lower insert,* complete circumferential graft disruption adjacent to anastomosis. (From Taylor LM Jr, Park TC, Edwards JM, et al: *J Vasc Surg* 20:520–528, 1994. Used by permission.)

tery thrombotic occlusion remain asymptomatic, affected patients can experience a wide variety of symptoms, from moderate exercise-induced to limb-threatening ischemia. The development of axillary artery thrombosis has been attributed to traction on the standard "T" anastomosis, secondary to an excessive increase of body weight or too short a graft. This produces a "Y" deformity and thus limits flow in the axillary artery. Reducing the angle between the graft and the axillary artery and increasing proximal graft redundancy have both been recommended to avoid this traction effect.

Upper extremity thromboembolic complications require prompt diagnosis. A high index of suspicion should exist in any patient seen with upper extremity ischemia in the presence of an ipsilateral axillofemoral graft. Treatment options include thrombolytic therapy and surgical correction. We recommend proximal graft disconnection, exploration of the axillary graft anastomosis with extension or vein patch, and embolectomy through a distal arm incision.

Other described, but less frequent, complications have included graft infection, brachial plexus injury,[90] arterial steal,[90] perigraft seroma,[91] and structural graft failure with pseudoaneurysm formation.[92]

CONCLUSION

Primary patency of axillofemoral grafts in excess of 70% at 3 to 5 years has now been reported by a number of investigators.[60, 70–73, 93] Current results are not significantly different from those reported for other treatment modalities, including aortofemoral grafting and transluminal angioplasty. On the basis of this contemporary trend, the role of axillofemoral bypass as an alternative to aortofemoral bypass in the management of aortoiliac disease requires re-evaluation. Axillofemoral bypass grafting should no longer be considered a "disadvantaged" or "compromised" procedure for infrequent use only; rather, it should be regarded as an acceptable procedure with specifically defined advantages and disadvantages for the treatment of patients requiring inflow reconstruction to the lower extremity.

REFERENCES

1. Freeman NE, Leeds FH: Operations on large arteries: Application of recent advances. *Calif Med* 77:229–233, 1952.
2. Lewis CD: A subclavian artery as the means of blood-supply to the lower half of the body. *Br J Surg* 48:574–575, 1961.
3. Blaisdell FW, DeMattei GA, Gauder PJ: Extraperitoneal thoracic aorta to femoral bypass graft as replacement for an infected aortic bifurcation prosthesis. *Am J Surg* 102:583–585, 1961.
4. Vetto RM: The treatment of unilateral iliac artery obstruction with a transabdominal, subcutaneous, femorofemoral graft. *Surgery* 52:342–345, 1962.
5. Blaisdell FW, Hall AD: Axillary-femoral artery bypass for lower extremity ischemia. *Surgery* 54:563–568, 1963.
6. Louw JH: Splenic-to-femoral and axillary-to-femoral bypass grafts in diffuse atherosclerotic occlusive disease. *Lancet* 29:1401–1402, 1963.

7. Sauvage LR, Wood SJ: Unilateral axillary bilateral femoral bifurcation graft: A procedure for the poor risk patient with aortoiliac disease. Surgery 60:573–577, 1966.

8. Gorman JF, Douglas FM: Axillary-femoral artery bypass. Arch Surg 91:509–512, 1965.

9. Jackson BB, Ward WW: Contralateral axillofemoral bypass graft. Am J Surg 110:926–928, 1965.

10. Alpert J, Brief DK, Parsonnet V: Vascular restoration for aortoiliac occlusion and an alternative approach to the poor risk patient. J Newark Beth Israel Hosp 18:4–7, 1967.

11. Pierangeli A, Guernilli N: The axillo-femoral bypass as a treatment of the obstruction of the aorto-iliac junction in the poor risk patient. J Cardiovasc Surg 8:353–360, 1967.

12. Mannick JA, Nabseth DC: Axillofemoral bypass graft—A safe alternative to aortoiliac reconstruction, N Engl J Med 278:460–466, 1968.

13. Blaisdell FW, Hall AD, Lim RC, et al: Aorto-iliac arterial substitution utilizing subcutaneous grafts. Ann Surg 172:775–780, 1970.

14. Mannick JA, Williams LE, Nasbeth DC: The late results of axillofemoral grafts. Surgery 68:1038–1043, 1970.

15. Parsonnet V, Alpert J, Brief DK: Femorofemoral and axillofemoral grafts—Compromise or preference. Surgery 67:26–33, 1970.

16. Pollock AV: Axillary-femoral bypass grafts in the treatment of aorto-iliac occlusive disease. Br J Surg 59:704–706, 1972.

17. Moore WA, Hall AD, Blaisdell FW: Late results of axillary-femoral bypass grafting. Am J Surg 122:148–154, 1971.

18. Eugene J, Goldstone J, Moore WA: Fifteen year experience with subcutaneous bypass grafts for lower extremity ischemia. Ann Surg 186:177–183, 1977.

19. Johnson WC, LoGerfo FW, Vollman RW, et al: Is axillo-bilateral femoral graft an effective substitute for aortic-bilateral iliac/femoral graft? Ann Surg 186:123–129, 1977.

20. Ray LI, O'Connor JB, Davis CC, et al: Axillofemoral bypass: A critical reappraisal of its role in the management of aortoiliac occlusive disease. Am J Surg 138:117–128, 1979.

21. Cina C, Ameli FM, Kalman P, et al: Indications and role of axillofemoral bypass in high risk patients. Ann Vasc Surg 2:237–241, 1988.

22. Naylor AR, Ah-See AK, Engeset J: Axillofemoral bypass for salvage procedure in high risk patients with aortoiliac disease. Br J Surg 77:659–661, 1990.

23. Calligaro KD, Azurin DJ, Dougherty MJ, et al: Pulmonary risk factors of elective abdominal aortic surgery. J Vasc Surg 18:914–920, 1993.

24. Walker WE, Cooley DA, Duncan JM, et al: The management of aortoduodenal fistula by in situ replacement of the infected abdominal aortic graft. Ann Surg 205:727–732, 1987.

25. Robinson JA, Johansen K: Aortic sepsis: Is there a role for in situ graft reconstruction? J Vasc Surg 13:677–684, 1991.

26. Tobin KD: Aortobifemoral perigraft abscess: Treatment by percutaneous catheter drainage. J Vasc Surg 8:339–343, 1988.

27. Cosselli JS, Crawford ES, Williams TW Jr, et al: Treatment of postoperative infection of ascending aorta and transverse aortic arch, including use of viable omentum and muscle flaps. Ann Thorac Surg 50:868–881, 1990.

28. O'Hara PJ, Hertzer NR, Beven EF, et al: Surgical management of infected abdominal aortic grafts: Review of a 25 year experience. J Vasc Surg 3:725–731, 1986.

29. Olah A, Vogt M, Laske A, et al: Axillo-femoral bypass and simultaneous removal of the aorto-femoral vascular infection site: Is the procedure safe? Eur J Vasc Surg 6:252–254, 1992.

30. Bacourt F, Koskas F: Axillobifemoral bypass and aortic exclusion for vascular septic lesions: A multicenter retrospective study of 98 cases. *Ann Vasc Surg* 6:119–126, 1992.
31. Blaisdell FW, Hall AD, Thomas AN: Induced thrombosis of an abdominal aortic aneurysm. *Am J Surg* 109:560–565, 1965.
32. Leather RP, Shah D, Goldman M, et al: Nonresective treatment of abdominal aortic aneurysms: Use of acute thrombosis and axillofemoral bypass. *Arch Surg* 114:1402–1408, 1979.
33. Savarese RP, Rosenfield JC, DeLaurentis DA: Alternatives in the treatment of abdominal aortic aneurysms. *Am J Surg* 142:226–230, 1981.
34. Kwaan JH, Khan RJ, Connolly JE: Total exclusion for the management of abdominal aortic aneurysms. *Am J Surg* 146:93–97, 1983.
35. Karmody AM, Leather RP, Goldman M, et al: The current position of nonresective treatment for abdominal aortic aneurysm. *Surgery* 94:591–597, 1983.
36. Cho SI, Johnson WC, Bush HL Jr, et al: Lethal complications associated with nonrestrictive treatment of abdominal aortic aneurysms. *Arch Surg* 117:1214–1217, 1982.
37. Corbett CR, Chilvers AS: Ruptured abdominal aortic aneurysm treated by ligation of the aorta and an axillobifemoral bypass. *J Cardiovasc Surg* 25:510–512, 1984.
38. Inahara T, Geary GL, Mukherjee D, et al: The contrary position to the nonresective treatment for abdominal aortic aneurysm. *J Vasc Surg* 2:42–48, 1985.
39. Schwartz RA, Nichols K, Silver D: Is thrombosis of the infrarenal abdominal aortic aneurysm an acceptable alternative? *J Vasc Surg* 3:448–455, 1986.
40. Scher LA, Brener BJ, Goldenkranz RJ, et al: Infected aneurysms of the abdominal aorta. *Arch Surg* 115:975–978, 1980.
41. Taylor LM Jr, Deitz DM, McConnell DB, et al: Treatment of infected abdominal aneurysms by extraanatomic bypass, aneurysm excision, and drainage. *Am J Surg* 155:655–658, 1988.
42. Hill J, Charlesworth D: Inflammatory abdominal aortic aneurysms: A report of thirty-seven cases. *Ann Vasc Surg* 2:352–357, 1988.
43. Connery CP, DeWeese JA, Eisenberg BK, et al: Treatment of aortic coarctation by axillofemoral bypass grafting in the high-risk patient. *Ann Thorac Surg* 52:1281–1284, 1991.
44. Feliciano DV, Accola KD, Burch JM: Extraanatomic bypass for peripheral arterial injuries. *Am J Surg* 158:506–510, 1989.
45. Kaufman JL, Stark K, Brolin RE: Disseminated atheroembolism from extensive degenerative atherosclerosis of the aorta. *Surgery* 102:63–70, 1987.
46. Drager SB, Riles TS, Imparato AM: Management of acute aortic occlusion. *Am J Surg* 138:293–295, 1979.
47. McCullough JL Jr, Mackey WC, O'Donnell TF Jr, et al: Infrarenal aortic occlusion: A reassessment of surgical indications. *Am J Surg* 146:178–182, 1983.
48. Webb KH, Jacocks MA: Acute aortic occlusion. *Am J Surg* 155:405–407, 1988.
49. Agee JM, Kron IL, Flanagan R, et al: The risk of axillofemoral bypass grafting for acute vascular occlusion. *J Vasc Surg* 14:190–194, 1991.
50. Rutherford RB, Patt A, Pearce WH: Extra-anatomic bypass: A closer view. *J Vasc Surg* 6:437–446, 1987.
51. LoGerfo FW, Johnson WC, Corson JD, et al: A comparison of the late patency rates of axillobilateral femoral and axillounilateral femoral grafts. *Surgery* 81:33–40, 1977.
52. Hepp W, de Jonge K, Pallua N: The late results following extra-anatomic bypass procedures for chronic aortoiliac occlusive disease. *J Cardiovasc Surg* 29:181–184, 1988.

53. Harris JP, Niesobska V, Carroll SE, et al: Extra-anatomic bypass grafting. *Can J Surg* 32:113–118, 1989.

54. Kalman PG, Hosang M, Cina C, et al: Current indications for axillounifemoral and axillobifemoral bypass grafts. *J Vasc Surg* 5:828–832, 1987.

55. Ascer E, Veith FJ, Gupta SK, et al: Comparison of axillounifemoral and axillobifemoral bypass operations. *Surgery* 97:169–174, 1984.

56. DeLaurentis DA, Sala LE, Russell E, et al: A twelve year experience with axillofemoral and femorofemoral bypass operations. *Surgery* 147:881–887, 1978.

57. Dalman RL, Taylor LM Jr, Moneta GL, et al: Simultaneous operative repair of multilevel lower extremity occlusive disease. *J Vasc Surg* 13:211–221, 1991.

58. Gupta SK, Veith FL, Ascer E, et al: Five year experience with axillopopliteal bypasses for limb salvage. *J Cardiovasc Surg* 26:321–324, 1985.

59. Ascer E, Veith FJ, Gupta SK: Axillopopliteal bypass grafting: Indications, late results, and detrminants of long-term patency. *J Vasc Surg* 10:285–291, 1989.

60. Kenney DA, Sauvage LR, Wood SJ, et al: Comparison of noncrimped, externally supported (EXS) and crimped, nonsupported Dacron prostheses for axillofemoral and above-knee femoropopliteal bypass. *Surgery* 92:931–946, 1982.

61. Donaldson MC, Louras JC, Bucknam CA: Axillofemoral bypass: A tool with a limited role. *J Vasc Surg* 3:757–763, 1986.

62. Calligaro KD, Ascer E, Veith FJ, et al: Unsuspected inflow disease in candidates for axillofemoral bypass operations: A prospective study. *J Vasc Surg* 11:832–837, 1990.

63. Gross WS, Glannigan DP, Kraft RO, et al: Chronic upper extremity ischemia: Etiology, manifestations and operative management. *Arch Surg* 113:419–423, 1978.

64. Burrell MJ, Wheeler JR, Gregory RT, et al: Axillofemoral bypass: A ten-year review. *Ann Surg* 195:796–799, 1982.

65. Nitzberg RS, Welch HJ, O'Donnell TF, et al: The influence of graft material on patency of axillofemoral grafts. In Veith FJ, editor, *Current critical problems in vascular surgery*. St. Louis, 1991, Quality Medical Publishing, pp 270–283.

66. Yeager RA, McConnell DB, Sasaki TM, et al: Aortic and peripheral prosthetic graft infection: Differential management and causes of mortality. *Ann J Surg* 150:36–43, 1985.

67. Goeau-Brissoniere O, Leport C, Guidoin R, et al: Experimental colonization of a PTFE vascular graft with Staphylococcus aureus: A quantitative and morphologic study. *J Vasc Surg* 5:743–748, 1987.

68. Jarowenko MV, Buchbinder D, Shah DM: Effect of external pressure on axillofemoral bypass grafts. *Ann Surg* 3:274–276, 1981.

69. Cavallaro A, Sciacca V, de Marzo L, et al: The effect of body weight compression on axillo-femoral by-pass patency. *J Cardiovasc Surg* 29:476–479, 1988.

70. Schultz GA, Sauvage LR, Mathisen SR, et al: A five- to seven-year experience with externally-supported Dacron prostheses in axillofemoral and femoropopliteal bypass. *Ann Vasc Surg* 1:214–223, 1986.

71. El-Massry S, Saad E, Sauvage LR, et al: Axillofemoral bypass with externally supported, knitted Dacron grafts: A follow-up through twelve years. *J Vasc Surg* 17:107–115, 1993.

72. Harris EJ, Taylor LM Jr, McConnell DB, et al: Clinical results of axillobifemoral bypass using externally supported polytetrafluoroethylene. *J Vasc Surg* 12:416–421, 1990.

73. Taylor LM Jr, Moneta GL, McConnell DB, et al: Axillofemoral grafting with externally supported polytetrafluoroethylene. *Arch Surg* 129:588–595, 1994.
74. Mason RA, Smirnov VB, Newton B, et al: Alternative procedures to aorto-bifemoral grafting. *J Cardiovasc Surg* 30:192–197, 1989.
75. Schneider JR, McDaniel MD, Walsh DB, et al: Axillofemoral bypass: Outcome and hemodynamic results in high-risk patients. *J Vasc Surg* 15:952–963, 1992.
76. Bunt TJ: Aortic reconstruction vs extra-anatomic bypass and angioplasty. *Arch Surg* 121:1166–1170, 1986.
77. Malone JM, Moore WS, Goldstone J: The natural history of bilateral aortofemoral bypass grafts for ischemia of the lower extremities. *Arch Surg* 110:1300–1306, 1975.
78. Jones AF, Kempczinski RF: Aortofemoral bypass grafting: A reappraisal. *Arch Surg* 116:301–305, 1981.
79. Szilagyi DE, Elliot JP, Smith RF, et al: A thirty-year survey of the reconstructive surgical treatment of aortoiliac occlusive disease. *J Vasc Surg* 3:421–436, 1986.
80. Bunt TJ, Moore W: Optimal proximal anastomosis/tunnel for axillofemoral grafts. *J Vasc Surg* 3:673–676, 1986.
81. Daar AS, Finch DRA: Graft avulsion: An unreported complication of axillofemoral bypass grafts. *Br J Surg* 65:442–446, 1978.
82. Alexander RH, Selby JH: Axillofemoral bypass grafts using polytetrafluoroethylene. *South Med J* 73:1325–1329, 1980.
83. White GH, Donayre CE, Williams RA, et al: Exertional disruption of axillofemoral graft anastomosis: "The axillary pullout syndrome." *Arch Surg* 125:625–627, 1990.
84. Brophy CM, Quist WC, Kwolek C, et al: Disruption of proximal axillobifemoral bypass anastomosis. *J Vasc Surg* 15:218–220, 1992.
85. Taylor LM Jr, Park TC, Edwards JM, et al: Acute disruption of polytetrafluoroethylene grafts adjacent to axillary anastomoses: A complication of axillofemoral grafting. *J Vasc Surg* 20:520–528, 1994.
86. Bandyk DF, Thiele BL, Radke HM: Upper-extremity emboli secondary to axillofemoral graft thrombosis. *Arch Surg* 116:393–395, 1981.
87. Hartman AR, Fried KS, Khalil I, et al: Late axillary artery thrombosis in patients with occluded axillo-femoral bypass grafts. *J Vasc Surg* 2:285–287, 1985.
88. Farina C, Schultz RD, Feldhaus RJ: Late upper limb acute ischemia in a patient with an occluded axillo-femoral bypass graft. *J Cardiovasc Surg* 31:178–181, 1990.
89. McLafferty RB, Porter JM: Upper extremity thromboembolism secondary to axillary-femoral bypass thrombosis. *Perspect Vasc Surg* 6:121–126, 1993.
90. Kempczinski R, Penn I: Upper extremity complications of axillofemoral grafts. *Am J Surg* 136:209–212, 1978.
91. Buche M, Schoevaerdts JC, Jaumin P, et al: Perigraft seroma following axillofemoral bypass: Report of three cases. *Ann Vasc Surg* 1:374–377, 1986.
92. Piazza D, Ameli FM, von Schroeder HP, et al: Nonanastomotic pseudoaneurysm of expanded polytetrafluoroethylene axillofemoral bypass graft. *J Vasc Surg* 17:777–779, 1993.
93. Whittens CHA, VanHoutte HJKP, VanUrk H: European prospective randomized multicentre axillo-bifemoral trial. *Eur J Vasc Surg* 6:115–123, 1992.

Descending Thoracic Aorta to Femoral Artery Bypass

Blair A. Keagy, M.D.

Professor and Chief, Division of Vascular Surgery, University of North Carolina, Chapel Hill, North Carolina

Enrique Criado, M.D.

Assistant Professor of Vascular Surgery, University of North Carolina, Chapel Hill, North Carolina

HISTORICAL PERSPECTIVE

Since the inception of reconstructive aortic surgery in the 1950s, surgeons have been challenged to find alternative ways to revascularize the lower extremities while avoiding the abdominal aorta in patients with aortic graft infections or intra-abdominal catastrophes, and in other situations where avoidance of the abdominal cavity was preferable. The first experiences with bypass from the descending thoracic aorta to the femoral arteries were reported in 1961 by Stevenson and Sauvage,[1] followed by a report from Blaisdell[2] during that same year. Other attempts to bypass the abdominal aorta were made by obtaining inflow from the ascending aorta and routing a graft anteriorly through the chest and abdomen to the iliac or femoral arteries. This procedure requires a very long graft and difficult tunneling. It is an operation that involves both the thoracic and the abdominal cavity to a greater extent than in conventional transabdominal aortic surgery. Therefore, and understandably, bypasses originating in the ascending aorta were not often used.

In 1963, shortly after the first reports on thoracofemoral bypass, Blaisdell[3] described the new technique of axillofemoral bypass. The technical ease and minimal invasiveness of axillofemoral bypass made it popular as the extra-anatomic procedure of choice for lower extremity revascularization, and dissipated interest in the use of alternative extra-anatomic reconstructions. For this reason, the experience with bypass from the descending thoracic aorta to the femoral arteries has remained mainly anecdotal until recent years when a few centers were able to accrue a sizable number of cases.[4-7] In our review of the world literature, we found 193 cases reported up to 1993 (Table 1).[7] Since then, our experience has increased to a total of 41 cases.

For the last 12 years we have used the descending thoracic aorta as a source of inflow in selected patients. During our early experience until 1990, the ratio of thoracofemoral bypasses to conventional aortofemoral/iliac bypasses was 16:78 for a period of 8½ years.[8] During that same period, the ratio of thoracofemoral to axillofemoral bypasses was 16:36. The

Advances in Vascular Surgery®, vol. 3
© 1995, Mosby–Year Book, Inc.

TABLE 1.

Published Experience With Descending Thoracic Aorta to Iliofemoral
Artery Bypass*

Author	Year	Number of Patients
Stevenson, Sauvage, Harkins[1]	1961	1
Blaisdell, DeMattei, Gauder[2]	1961	1
Robicsek, McCall, Sanger, et al.[8]	1967	1
Reichle, Tyson, Soloff, et al.[9]	1970	1
Nunn and Kamal[10]	1972	3
Froysaker, Skagseth, Dundas, et al.[11]	1973	6
Finseth and Abbot[12]	1974	1
Jarrett, Darling, Mundth[13]	1975	2
Cevese and Gallucci[14]	1975	6
Buxton, Simpson, Johnson, et al.[15]	1976	1
Lakner and Lukacs[16]	1983	2
Reilly, Ehrenfeld, Stoney[17]	1984	5
Enon, Chevalier, Moreau, et al.[18]	1985	3
Feldhaus, Sterpetti, Schultz, et al.[19]	1985	18
Haas, Moulder, Kerstein[20]	1985	3
DeLaurentis[21]	1986	10
Hussain[22]	1988	8
Schellack, Fulenwider, Smith[23]	1988	3
Bradham, Locklair, Grimball[24]	1989	2
Bowes, Youkey, Pharr, et al.[4]	1990	26
O'Brien, Waldron, McCabe, et al.[25]	1991	1
Kalman, Johnston, Walker[26]	1991	6
Branchereau, Magnan, Moracchini, et al.[5]	1992	30
McCarthy, Mesh, McMillan, et al.[6]	1993	21
Criado and Keagy[7]	1994	32
TOTAL		193

*From Criado E, Keagy BA: *Ann Vasc Surg* 8:38–47, 1994. Used by permission.

updated ratios through September 1994 are 41:115 for aortofemoral bypass and 41:60 for axillofemoral bypass. These ratios indicate that in addition to our recent increase in the use of thoracofemoral bypass, we have
also increased, although to a lesser extent, our volume of aortofemoral
and axillofemoral bypasses. In our practice we continue to use standard
aortobifemoral bypass as the procedure of choice for primary aortoiliac
reconstruction. However, our positive experience with thoracofemoral bypass has made us liberalize its use not only for patients in whom extra-
anatomic bypass is mandatory but also for some selected patients in
whom a primary conventional reconstruction is judged less than optimal.

INDICATIONS

In the past, thoracofemoral bypass was used sporadically as a remedial
aortic reconstruction mostly in patients with aortic graft infections or

other intra-abdominal catastrophes. Despite the challenging indications of its early use, the results were satisfactory. During the last decade, a significant experience with thoracofemoral bypass has been accumulated, and the indications and results of the procedure have been defined. Our review of the world's experience from 1983 to 1993 comprised 146 patients collected from ten different institutions (Table 2).[7] In a metanalysis of that collective experience, over one half of the operations were secondary aortic reconstructions; two thirds of these were performed in patients with at least one previous standard aortic graft thrombosis and one third were performed after removal of infected grafts from the abdominal aorta. Forty-two percent of the thoracofemoral bypasses consisted of primary aortic reconstructions; roughly one half of these were performed because of the presence of adverse conditions in the abdomen and one half because of a variety of reasons (Table 3).

Although the indication to use thoracofemoral bypass as a secondary reconstruction after abdominal aortic graft thrombosis or infection is straightforward, its use as a primary procedure may be controversial and

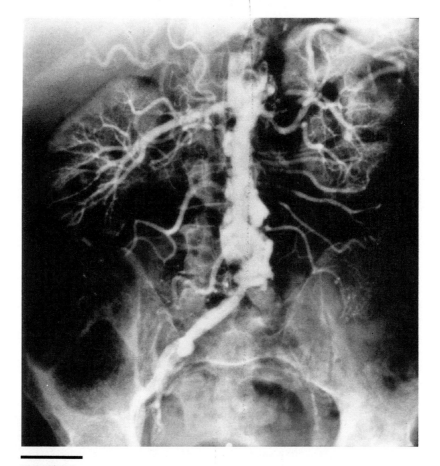

FIGURE 1.

Aortogram of a patient with disabling lower extremity claudication who underwent a bypass from the descending thoracic aorta to the femoral arteries. The figure illustrates a very severely diseased infrarenal aorta, judged to be a lesser option as a source of inflow compared with a healthy descending thoracic aorta.

TABLE 2.

Collective Experience With 146 Patients With Bypass From the Descending Thoracic Aorta for Aortoiliac Reconstruction 1983–1993*

Author/Year	No. of Cases	Primary Reconstruction	Secondary Reconstruction	Indication				Operative Deaths
				Failed Aortic Graft	Infected Aortic Graft	Hostile Abdomen	Other	
Lackner and Lukacs/1983[16]	2	2	0	0	0	0	2	0
Feldhaus, Sterpetti, Schultz, et al./1985[19]	18	3	15	12	3	3	0	1
Haas, Moulder, Kerstein/1985[20]	3	3	0	0	0	2	1	1
Enon, Chevalier, Moreau, et al./1985[18]	3	3	0	0	0	3	0	0

Schellack, Fulenwider, Smith/1988[23]	3	0	3	3	0	0	0	0
Hussain/1988[22]	8	6	2	2	0	3	3	0
Bowes, Youkey, Pharr/1990[4]	26	16	10	9	1	6	10	1
McCarthy, Mesh, McMillan, et al./1993[6]	21	3	18	5	12	4	0	0
Branchereau, Magnan, Moracchini, et al./1992[5]	30	7	23	13	9	5	3	3
Criado and Keagy/1994[7]	32	19	13	12	1	4	15	2
TOTAL	146	62(42%)	84(58%)	56(38%)	26(18%)	30(21%)	34(23%)	8(5.5%)

*From Criado E, Keagy BA: Ann Vasc Surg 8:38–47, 1994. Used by permission.

TABLE 3.

Indications for Bypass From the Descending
Thoracic Aorta to the Femoral Arteries*

Abdominal aortic graft infection
Multiple abdominal aortic graft failures
Axillofemoral bypass failure
Previous abdominal sepsis
Pancreatitis
Abdominal radiation therapy
Multiple abdominal operations
Large ventral hernias
Abdominal stomas
Heavily diseased infrarenal aorta
Hypoplastic abdominal aorta
Horseshoe kidney
Fear of impotence
Simultaneous visceral revascularization

---

*From Criado E, Keagy BA: *Ann Vasc Surg* 8:38–47,
1994. Used by permission.

---

requires further discussion. There are situations, generally referred to as
"hostile abdomen," in which pre-existing abdominal conditions, such as
septic or inflammatory disease or previous radiation therapy, make the
placement of a transabdominal infrarenal aortic graft ill advised. Other
indications for the use of thoracofemoral bypass as a primary aortic reconstruction are patients with unusual problems, such as horseshoe kidney or hypoplastic abdominal aorta, in whom dissection and graft anastomosis at the level of the infrarenal aorta can be difficult, hazardous, or
suboptimal. A heavily diseased infrarenal aorta in some cases can be unsuitable for a proximal anastomosis and can be a genuine reason to perform a thoracofemoral bypass (Fig 1).

Although a severely calcified and stenotic infrarenal aorta can be endarterectomized and safely used for anastomosis of an aortofemoral graft,
there is little merit in doing so when a potentially better alternative is
available. There is evidence that the aortic segment proximal to the celiac
artery is seldom affected by atherosclerosis,[28] and the most distal descending thoracic aorta falls within this region. Therefore, it is our argument that
an anastomosis placed at this level should provide better long-term patency than a heavily diseased infrarenal aorta. Patients requiring simultaneous aortofemoral and splanchnic revascularization can benefit from a
bypass from the descending thoracic aorta performed through a retroperitoneal thoracoabdominal approach. This provides simultaneous access to
the celiac, mesenteric, and renal arteries and allows a means of antegrade
bypass to these vessels with an excellent anatomic configuration.[29]

RESULTS

The results revealed in our metanalysis of the recent collective experience with thoracofemoral bypass are quite encouraging, considering that

TABLE 4.
Life Table Analysis. Primary Patency of 146 Grafts Originating in the Descending Thoracic Aorta. Collective Experience Metanalysis, 1983–1993*

Interval (mos)	No. of Grafts at Risk	No. of Failed Grafts	No. Withdrawn Patent Because of			Interval Patency (%)	Cumulative Patency (%)	Standard Error (%)
			Death	Duration of Follow-up	Incomplete Follow-up			
In hospital	146	5	7	0	0	96	96.5	1.5
6	134	6	2	11	5	95	91.9	2.3
12	110	4	0	9	2	96	88.3	2.9
24	95	4	5	17	3	95	84.1	3.4
36	66	2	4	17	2	96	81.0	4.3
48	41	1	2	8	0	97	78.7	5.7
60	30	2	2	6	0	92	72.7	6.9
72	20	0	2	4	0	100	72.7	8.5
84	14	0	1	2	0	100	72.7	10.2
96	11	0	1	0	0	100	72.7	11.5

*From Criado E, Keagy BA: *Ann Vasc Surg* 8:38–47, 1994. Used by permission.
Patients withdrawn from life table analysis because of graft failure as a result of thrombosis (20) or infection (4), death, duration of follow-up, or incomplete follow-up.

TABLE 5.
Life Table Analysis. Secondary Patency of 146 Grafts Originating in the Descending Thoracic Aorta. Collective Experience Metanalysis, 1983–1993*

Interval (mos)	No. of Grafts at Risk	No. of Failed Grafts	No. Withdrawn Patent Because of			Interval Patency (%)	Cumulative Patency (%)	Standard Error (%)
			Death	Duration of Follow-up	Incomplete Follow-up			
In hospital	146	4	7	0	0	97	97.2	1.3
6	135	3	2	13	5	98	94.9	1.9
12	112	2	0	9	2	98	93.1	2.3
24	99	3	5	20	3	96	89.8	2.9
36	68	1	4	18	2	98	88.2	3.7
48	43	1	2	9	0	97	85.8	4.9
60	31	1	2	6	0	96	82.7	6.2
72	22	0	2	5	0	100	82.7	7.3
84	15	0	1	2	0	100	82.7	8.9
96	12	0	1	1	0	100	82.7	9.9

*From Criado E, Keagy BA: Ann Vasc Surg 8:38–47, 1994. Used by permission.
Patients withdrawn from life table analysis because of graft failure due to thrombosis or infection, death, duration of follow-up, or incomplete follow-up.

a majority of cases were secondary reconstructions and that many of the primary procedures were performed in patients presenting with unusual challenges. The overall operative mortality was 5.5%, similar to that in comparable series of conventional aortofemoral bypass. In our experience, we had two deaths, both at the beginning of our series (4.8% mortality), and currently we have performed 35 consecutive cases without any deaths. Although axillofemoral bypass is an acceptable extra-anatomic reconstruction, its durability makes it unsuitable for patients with long life expectancies.[30] In this regard, thoracofemoral bypass offers a superior alternative; a 5-year primary graft patency rate of 72.7% was found in our metanalysis, which remained unchanged into the eighth year of follow-up (Table 4). With a few graft limb revisions, the secondary graft patency rate increased to 82.7% at 8 years (Table 5). It is important to note that the majority of graft limb failures found with this procedure occurred in patients with multiple previous failed reconstructions at the femoral level. Therefore, better results are to be expected in patients without previous bypass failures.

PREOPERATIVE EVALUATION

Because the condition of the abdominal aorta is generally unknown during the initial patient encounter, the preoperative assessment is the same as with any patient having lower extremity ischemia. A good history and physical examination is performed, followed by evaluation in the peripheral vascular laboratory. Noninvasive tests include segmental arterial pressures, waveform analysis, and recording of femoral artery acceleration times. If the patient's symptoms warrant intervention, an aortogram with runoff is obtained. This shows the condition of the abdominal aorta as well as the status of the iliac and lower extremity vessels.

Early in our experience we obtained routine angiography or CT scan of the descending thoracic aorta in all patients in whom a thoracobifemoral bypass operation was contemplated. This generally necessitated additional contrast injection with increased risk of renal toxicity. However, because there was no instance in which the thoracic aorta was found to be of poor quality in regard to supporting an anastomosis, we no longer require thoracic arteriography prior to performing the operation. The preoperative cardiopulmonary evaluation is identical to that used for a transabdominal aortofemoral bypass. Pulmonary function tests are advisable in any patient with suspected limited pulmonary reserve. A severely decreased forced expiratory volume (FEV_1) is a relative contraindication for the procedure.

SURGICAL TECHNIQUE

POSITIONING

Patient positioning on the operating table is crucial to the overall success of the procedure. A double-lumen endotracheal tube is used so that the left lung can be deflated to facilitate exposure of the aorta. The left arm is elevated over the head on a splint, and the drapes are placed so that the left hemithorax (including the scapula), abdomen, and both groins are exposed. The pelvis is placed as flat as possible so that both groins are easily accessible. By sequentially rotating the table, the surgeon can alternately work in the chest and in the iliofemoral region (Fig 2). To decrease the operative time, a double team approach is desirable for this procedure. We generally start by the simultaneous dissection of both femoral (or iliac) arteries.

THORACOTOMY

A small posterolateral left thoracotomy incision is made overlying the eighth or ninth intercostal space. The posterior end of the incision ends just behind the tip of the scapula. Skin flaps are developed superiorly and inferiorly, and the latissimus dorsi muscle is not divided but rather mobilized and retracted posteriorly. The thoracic cavity is entered through the eighth or ninth intercostal space. The intercostal muscles are divided as far posteriorly as possible to facilitate rib spreading. Early in our series, a standard rib spreader was used, whereas more recently the Omni retractor has been used to retract the ribs, hold the latissimus dorsi muscle posteriorly, retract the deflated lung in a superior direction, and retract the left diaphragm inferiorly.

The inferior pulmonary ligament is divided to the level of the inferior pulmonary vein and the deflated lung is retracted superiorly. The descending thoracic aorta is mobilized and optionally encircled with an umbilical tape. The intercostal arteries are carefully preserved during dissection of the aorta. The posterior portion of the diaphragm is separated from the chest wall for a distance of about 5 cm for later tunneling.

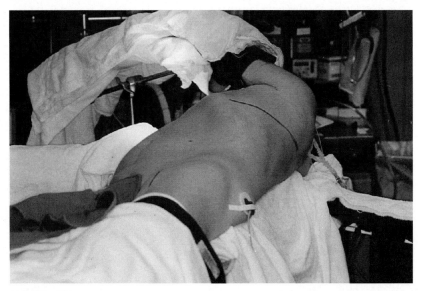

FIGURE 2.
Patient positioning is of extreme importance for the success of bypass from the descending thoracic aorta to the femoral arteries. The patient is placed on a bean bag with a right axillary roll. The left scapula has to be exposed as well as the proximal spine. The pelvis is placed as flat as possible to allow access to the femoral arteries. The posterior extent of the thoracotomy incision is placed just medial to the tip of the left scapula.

GROIN INCISIONS

The site of the distal anastomosis depends on the condition of the iliofemoral segments. We favor anastomosis to the external iliac artery if the vessel is adequate; otherwise, the femoral vessels are used. This decision is based on the preoperative angiogram and the condition of the vessels at the time of operation.

When the external iliac arteries are selected for the distal anastomoses, oblique groin incisions are made two fingerbreadths above the inguinal ligaments. After exposure of the left external iliac artery, a hand is inserted over the psoas muscle, and behind the left kidney during the tunneling procedure. When the femoral artery is chosen for a distal anastomosis, it is exposed through a vertical incision in a fashion similar to that used in a conventional aortofemoral bypass. On the left side, however, the vertical groin incision is extended 2 to 3 inches above the ligament, and the oblique muscles are divided in the direction of the fibers to enter the left suprainguinal retroperitoneal space, overlying the external iliac artery. This space is used to direct tunneling of the graft from the chest to both groins.

TUNNELING

Tunneling is quite easy. Three fingers are inserted from the chest into the retroperitoneum posterior to the left kidney, at the site of detachment of the posterior portion of the diaphragm. The opposite hand is inserted from the suprainguinal retroperitoneal incision along the psoas muscle and behind the kidney until the two hands meet (Fig 3).

A tunnel is then made from the left retroperitoneal suprainguinal space to the right side. This tunnel can be placed in the subcutaneous tissue if a straight tube graft is used from the aorta to the left femoral artery, and from there a side graft is taken to the right femoral region, as in a standard femorofemoral bypass. We favor left-to-right tunneling posterior to the rectus muscle, and cephalad to the bladder, because it offers better graft protection and a gentler curve for the right limb of the prosthesis. This tunnel must be created very carefully to avoid the bladder and peritoneal contents. In patients with previous laparotomies this tunneling occasionally can be difficult because of scarring and therefore requires extra caution. Although we have never experienced any complications during this part of the procedure, bladder perforation has been mentioned by others as a possible problem. Figure 4 shows the limbs of the standard bifurcation graft after it has been tunneled from the chest; the right limb is placed behind the rectus muscle.

PROXIMAL ANASTOMOSES

We routinely use bifurcated collagen-impregnated Dacron grafts to avoid preclotting. When a unilateral thoracofemoral or iliac bypass is planned, we use an 8- or 10-mm straight Dacron graft. The proximal anastomosis is constructed before the graft is tunneled. The entire length of the graft is preserved, and the proximal end is beveled to tailor an end-to-side anastomosis. After systemic heparinization, a side-biting clamp is placed on the descending thoracic aorta while the proximal anastomosis is per-

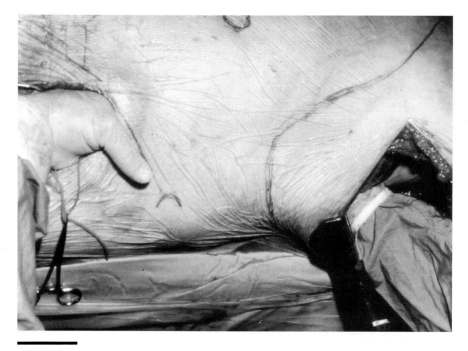

FIGURE 3.
After exposure of the descending thoracic aorta and femoral or iliac arteries is completed, a left retroperitoneal tunnel is created by placing one hand through the incision in the left posteromedial diaphragm and bluntly pushing the fingers posterior to the left kidney. The opposite hand is introduced over the left psoas muscle, posterior to the left kidney, until the fingers of both hands meet. An umbilical tape is placed in the tunnel for later routing of the graft. The chest incision is on the right side of this figure. (From Criado E, Keagy B: *Contemp Surg* 39:15–19, 1991. Used by permission.)

formed. The Beck clamp is ideal for this because it is constructed to prevent slippage. By using a partial occlusion clamp, strain on the left ventricle is minimized and flow to the spinal cord and visceral vessels is maintained while the proximal anastomosis is completed. A continuous-wave Doppler is used to confirm distal aortic flow after the clamp is applied. The proximal anastomosis is performed with 2-0 or 3-0 polypropylene suture. A running suture is generally used, although interrupted sutures may be used if the aortic wall appears thin (Fig 5). Figure 6 shows the completed anastomosis. The graft has been tunneled through the detached posterior portion of the diaphragm. In this picture, pledgets were used to reinforce the suture line, a technique preferred by one of the members of our group.

DISTAL ANASTOMOSES

The right limb of the graft is placed behind the rectus muscle into the right suprainguinal region. The appropriate distal anastomoses are performed depending on the condition of the outflow vessels. When the femoral artery (or arteries) is to be used, the graft is tunneled under the appropriate inguinal ligament.

With the older knitted and with woven Dacron prostheses, the uncut

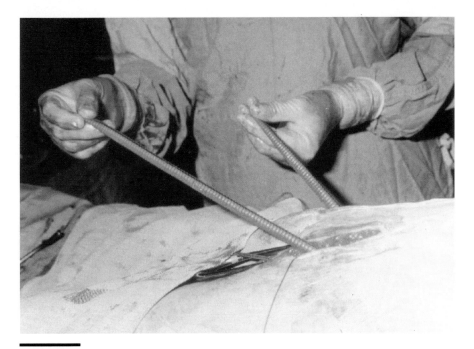

FIGURE 4.

This figure illustrates placement of a bifurcated graft from the descending thoracic aorta to the femoral arteries after appropriate tunneling. Impregnated Dacron grafts may not be long enough to reach the right femoral artery and occasionally require graft limb extension by cutting the redundant segment of the left limb and anastomosing it to the right limb in an end-to-end fashion.

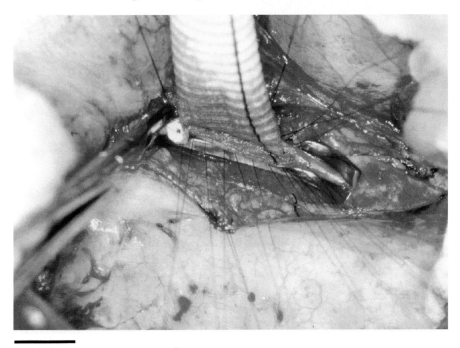

FIGURE 5.

Close-up of the proximal stenosis being completed with interrupted pledgeted 3-0 polypropylene sutures. Note that a partially occluding clamp is being used to avoid cross-clamping of the descending thoracic aorta.

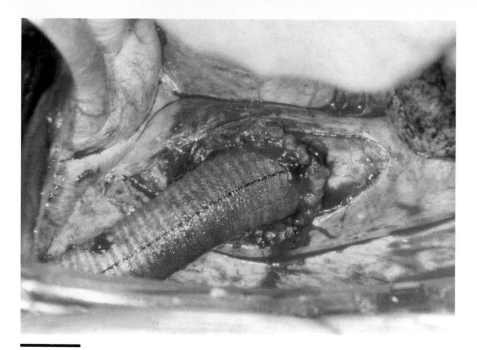

FIGURE 6.

Completed proximal anastomosis with interrupted pledgeted polypropylene sutures. Note the smooth angle of the takeoff of the graft directed posteriorly and distally into the retroperitoneal tunnel.

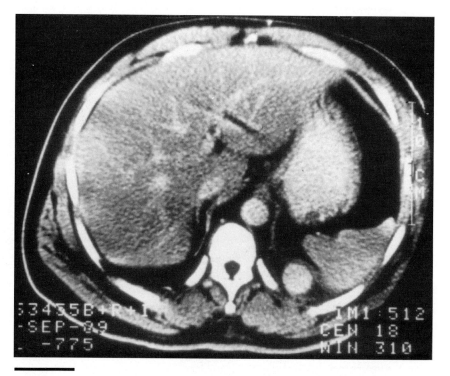

FIGURE 7.

Postoperative CT scan of a patient with a bifurcated graft from the descending thoracic aorta to the femoral arteries. This cross section shows the body of a bifurcated graft located in the posterior retroperitoneum, medial to the spleen. (From Criado E, Keagy B: *Contemp Surg* 39:15–19, 1991. Used by permission.)

bifurcation graft is long enough to complete the operation. Some of the currently available coated grafts are shorter, and in most instances an extension must be placed on the right limb of the graft to reach the right femoral artery. This is easily solved by cutting the redundant segment of the left limb of the graft and anastomosing it end-to-end to the right limb.

CLOSURE

A 32F chest tube is inserted and connected to underwater seal drainage. The ribs are approximated with subperiosteal sutures to prevent compression of the intercostal nerves. The intercostal muscle is approximated with absorbable running suture. The latissimus dorsi muscle is not divided, but it is generally sutured anteriorly to help isolate the subcutaneous area from the chest cavity. A closed-suction catheter is inserted to prevent accumulation of fluid under the skin flaps.

GRAFT POSITION

The CT scan in Figure 7 shows the body of the graft in the posterior portion of the retroperitoneum, medial to the spleen. Figure 8 shows the mid-abdominal portion of the same CT scan, with the two limbs of the bifurcated graft seen posterior to the left kidney. Although the body of the graft is longer than in a standard aortobifemoral graft, the prosthesis is

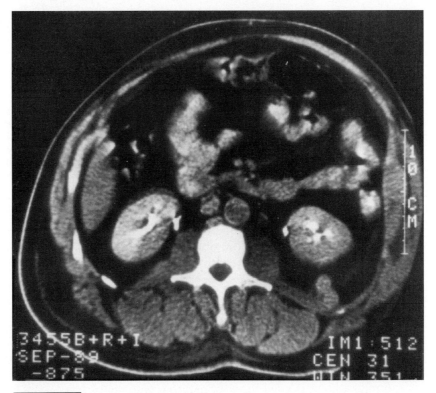

FIGURE 8.
CT scan of the same patient as in Figure 9, at a lower level, showing both limbs of a bifurcated graft in the posterior retroperitoneum behind the left kidney. (From Criado E, Keagy B: *Contemp Surg* 39:15–19, 1991. Used by permission.)

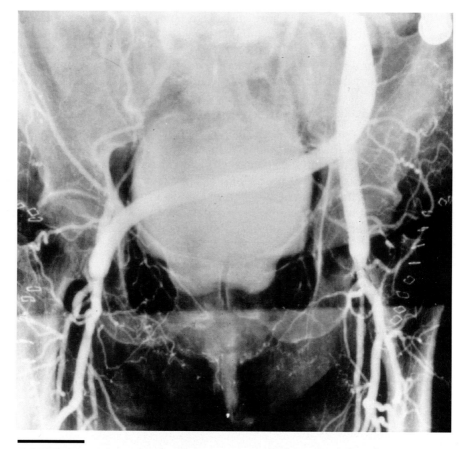

FIGURE 9.

Postoperative angiogram of a patient with a bypass from the descending thoracic aorta to the femoral arteries. A bifurcated Dacron graft has been tunneled to the left femoral artery, retroperitoneally and posterior to the rectus muscle. Note the smooth angulation of the right limb of the graft entering the right groin. (From Criado E, in T.J. Bunt (ed.) *Vascular Graft Infections*, Armonk, Futura Publishing Co., Inc., 1994, pp 341–349. Used by permission.)

well protected inside the chest and abdomen, and remote from the gastrointestinal tract. A postoperative angiogram (Fig 9) shows the gentle curve of the right limb of the graft as well as distal anastomoses that were performed to the femoral arteries.

POSTOPERATIVE CARE

The chest tube is removed on the second or third postoperative day. The patient may be fed on the first or second day after operation in most cases, and early ambulation is encouraged. With the muscle-sparing thoracotomy, pain and morbidity from the thoracotomy are minimized. An epidural catheter is used for perioperative pain control.

DISCUSSION

The decision of when to perform a thoracobifemoral bypass has undergone an evolution as more experience is gained with the operation. A "hostile abdomen," previous abdominal aortic graft infection, and thrombosis are generally accepted reasons to perform this procedure. A more controversial indication is the presence of a severely diseased abdominal aorta as defined by angiography. As we have become more experienced in performing a thoracobifemoral bypass, we have increasingly favored this source of inflow over a heavily calcified and stenotic atherosclerotic abdominal aorta.

We believe that the thoracobifemoral bypass offers a certain margin of safety over an abdominal aortic bypass in some circumstances. The thoracic aorta is almost always of good quality despite generalized atherosclerosis. The thoracic approach avoids temporary occlusion of renal blood flow, which may be necessary when the abdominal aorta is occluded at the level of the renal arteries and a suprarenal clamp is applied. In addition, abdominal aortic endarterectomy is avoided, and dissection in the area of the iliac arteries is not necessary, which may decrease the incidence of impotence in the male. Furthermore, placement of the proximal anastomosis in the chest eliminates the risk of aortoenteric fistula formation.

Some surgeons have suggested that the axillobifemoral bypass is an acceptable alternative to an abdominal aortic bypass operation. We have generally reserved the axillobifemoral bypass for emergency situations in which rapid lower extremity revascularization is mandatory, for cases in which infection of a traditional aortobifemoral bypass requires its removal, or for patients whose general medical condition is such that an operation on a major body cavity would carry undue risk. The long-term success of the axillobifemoral bypass is not optimum, so it is sometimes necessary to convert an emergently performed axillobifemoral bypass to a thoracobifemoral bypass. It has been our practice to do this conversion in those patients who are young and represent good operative risk.

One objection to the thoracobifemoral bypass graft cited by some authors has been the possibility of proximal progression of the aortic thrombus in patients with an occluded abdominal aorta, producing occlusion of the renal arteries and renal failure. This potential problem has not been observed in our patients, nor has it been noted in a survey of the world's literature.[7]

One of the potential advantages of this operation is a decrease in postoperative morbidity. Because the peritoneal cavity is not entered, prolonged postoperative ileus is avoided, and the patient may be fed in the early postoperative period. Incisional hernia is rare, and the use of a muscle-sparing thoracotomy seems to decrease the severity of postthoracotomy pain. Tunneling is a simple procedure, provided the proper routes are used. It is important to stay behind the left kidney and on the psoas muscle when the prosthesis is brought from the chest to the suprainguinal regions. The right limb of the graft is placed behind the rectus muscle to avoid kinking and to provide additional protection.

In summary, thoracofemoral bypass is indicated in those patients in whom the abdominal aorta must be avoided as a source of bypass and who have life expectancies long enough to warrant a durable bypass procedure. Our experience and that reported in the literature reflect that bypass from the descending thoracic aorta to the femoral arteries is currently underused and that the results available justify its more liberal use.

REFERENCES

1. Stevenson JK, Sauvage LR, Harkins HN: A bypass homograft from thoracic aorta to femoral arteries for occlusive vascular disease. *Am Surg* 27:632–637, 1961.
2. Blaisdell FW, DeMattei GA, Gauder PJ: Extraperitoneal thoracic aorta to femoral bypass. *Am J Surg* 102:583–585, 1961.
3. Blaisdell FW, Hall AD: Axillary-femoral artery bypass for lower extremity ischemia. *Surgery* 54:563, 1963.
4. Bowes DE, Youkey JR, Pharr WP, et al: Long term follow-up of descending thoracic aorto-iliac/femoral bypass. *J Cardiovasc Surg* 31:430–437, 1990.
5. Branchereau A, Magnan P-E, Moracchini P, et al: Use of descending thoracic aorta for lower limb revascularisation. *Eur J Vasc Surg* 6:255–262, 1992.
6. McCarthy WJ, Mesh CL, McMillan WD, et al: Descending thoracic aorta-to-femoral artery bypass: Ten years' experience with a durable procedure. *J Vasc Surg* 17:336–348, 1993.
7. Criado E, Keagy BA: Use of the descending thoracic aorta as an inflow source in aortoiliac reconstruction: Indications and long term results. *Ann Vasc Surg* 8:38–47, 1994.
8. Robicsek F, McCall MM, Sanger PW, et al: Recurrent aneurysm of the abdominal aorta: Insertion of a vascular prosthesis from the distal aortic arch to the femoral arteries. *Ann Thorac Surg* 3:549–552, 1967.
9. Reichle FA, Tyson RR, Soloff LA, et al: Salmonellosis and aneurysm of the distal abdominal aorta; Case report with a review. *Ann Surg* 171:219–228, 1970.
10. Nunn DB, Kamal MA: Bypass grafting from the thoracic aorta to femoral arteries for high aortoiliac occlusive disease. *Surgery* 72:749–755, 1972.
11. Froysaker T, Skagseth E, Dundas P, et al: Bypass procedures in the treatment of obstructions of the abdominal aorta. *J Cardiovasc Surg* 14:317–321, 1973.
12. Finseth F, Abbot WM: One-stage operative therapy for *Salmonella* mycotic abdominal aortic aneurysm. *Ann Surg* 179:8–11, 1974.
13. Jarrett F, Darling RC, Mundth ED, et al: Experience with infected aneurysms of the abdominal aorta. *Arch Surg* 110:1281–1286, 1975.
14. Cevese PG, Gallucci V: Thoracic aorta-to-femoral artery bypass. *J Cardiovasc Surg* 16:432–438, 1975.
15. Buxton B, Simpson L, Johnson N, et al: Descending thoracic aortofemoral bypass for distal aortic reconstruction after removal of an infected Dacron prosthesis. *Med J Aust* 2:133–136, 1976.
16. Lakner G, Lukacs L: High aortoiliac occlusion: Treatment with thoracic aorta to femoral arterial bypass. *J Cardiovasc Surg* 4:532–534, 1983.
17. Reilly LM, Ehrenfeld WK, Stoney RJ: Delayed aortic prosthetic reconstruction after removal of an infected graft. *Am J Surg* 148:234–239, 1984.
18. Enon B, Chevalier JM, Moreau P, et al: Revascularisation des membres inferieurs a partir de l'aorte thoracique descendante. *J Chir (Paris)* 122:539–543, 1985.
19. Feldhaus RJ, Sterpetti AV, Schultz RD, et al: Thoracic aorta-femoral artery bypass: Indications, technique, and late results. *Ann Thorac Surg* 40:588–592, 1985.
20. Haas KL, Moulder PV, Kerstein MD: Use of thoracic aortobifemoral artery bypass grafting as an alternative procedure for occlusive aortoiliac disease. *Am Surg* 51:573–576, 1985.
21. DeLaurentis DA: The descending thoracic aorta in reoperative surgery, in Bergan JJ, Yao JST (eds): *Reoperative Arterial Surgery.* Orlando, Grune & Stratton, 1986, pp 195–203.

22. Hussain SA: Descending thoracic aorta to bifemoral bypass graft without laparotomy. *Int Surg* 73:263–266, 1988.

23. Schellack J, Fulenwider JT, Smith RBI: Descending thoracic aortofemoral-femoral bypass: A remedial alternative for the failed aortobifemoral bypass. *J Cardiovasc Surg* 29:201–204, 1988.

24. Bradham RR, Locklair PRJ, Grimball A: Descending thoracic aorta to femoral artery bypass. *J S C Med Assoc* 85:283–286, 1989.

25. O'Brien DP, Waldron RP, McCabe JP, et al: Descending thoracic aorto-bifemoral bypass graft: A safe alternative in the high risk patients. *Ir Med J* 84:58–59, 1991.

26. Kalman PG, Johnston KW, Walker PM: Descending thoracic aortofemoral bypass as an alternative for aortoiliac revascularization. *J Cardiovasc Surg* 32:443–446, 1991.

27. Reference deleted in galleys.

28. Frazier OH, Oalmann MC, Strong JP, et al: Clinical applications of the supraceliac aorta: Anatomical and pathologic observations. *J Thorac Cardiovasc Surg* 93:631–633, 1987.

29. Criado E, Keagy BA: Descending thoracic aorta to femoral artery bypass. *Contemp Surg* 39:15–19, 1991.

30. Blaisdell FW: Axillofemoral bypass: Long-term results, in Yao JST, Pearce WH editors: *Long-Term Results in Vascular Surgery.* Norwalk Connecticut, 1993. Appleton & Lange, pp 395–399.

Femorofemoral Bypass for Limb Ischemia During Intra-Aortic Balloon Pump Therapy

Lewis B. Schwartz, M.D.
Vascular Fellow, Division of Vascular Surgery, Department of Surgery, Brigham and Women's Hospital, Harvard Medical School, Boston, Massachusetts

Michael Belkin, M.D.
Assistant Professor of Surgery, Division of Vascular Surgery, Department of Surgery, Brigham and Women's Hospital, Harvard Medical School, Boston, Massachusetts

C linical use of the intra-aortic balloon pump (IABP) was introduced in 1966 for myocardial support during cardiogenic shock.[1] Its indications have since broadened and now include unstable angina, pump failure after cardiopulmonary bypass, and stabilization of patients with critical left main coronary artery stenosis or planned cardiac transplantation. Innovations in IABP design and insertion technique have accompanied its widespread application. Catheter size has been significantly reduced from its original size of 14F to the currently available 9.5F and 8.5F systems. Simpler and safer insertion techniques have also evolved, including use of percutaneous puncture and the more recent development of sheathless catheters.

Despite these advances, the significant morbidity and mortality associated with IABP use have been remarkably constant (Figs 1 and 2). This constancy has been preserved despite a more critically ill patient population, but it also reflects the continued expectation that patients requiring IABP support are likely to have concomitant peripheral vascular atherosclerosis. The purpose of this review is to discuss the diagnosis and management of vascular complications of IABPs with special reference to the technique of femorofemoral bypass for lower-extremity ischemia.

LIMB ISCHEMIA

By far the most common complication of IABP use is lower-extremity ischemia, which has been reported in 13% of patients in a collected series of over 10,000 cases (Table 1). Ischemia usually occurs as a result of luminal encroachment when the sizable IABP catheter is inserted into an iliac or femoral artery already narrowed by pre-existing atherosclerosis.

Advances in Vascular Surgery®, vol. 3
© 1995, Mosby–Year Book, Inc.

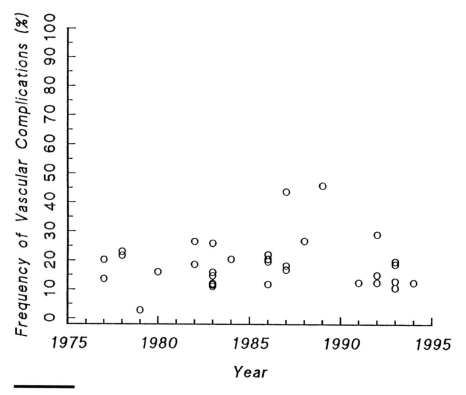

FIGURE 1.

Risk of vascular complications of IABP placement by year. Data collected from review of literature for series from 1977 to 1994, reporting on ≥100 patients.[2−11, 13−20, 22, 23, 25, 28, 31, 34, 35, 37−41, 47−49]

Other causes involve pericatheter thrombosis and arterial dissection at the time of insertion. The association of peripheral vascular disease with complications of IABPs is well established,[2−11] and the status of the peripheral circulation should always be carefully assessed prior to the initiation of IABP therapy. Just as cardiac disease is a major risk factor in patients undergoing peripheral vascular surgery, peripheral vascular disease is among the strongest predictors of mortality in patients undergoing cardiac surgery and/or requiring IABP support.[12] Other purported risk factors for the development of ischemia during IABP use include advanced age,[13] smoking,[8, 11] female gender,[4, 6, 11, 14, 15] obesity,[9] diabetes,[2, 4, 6, 9] protracted duration of support,[5, 16, 17] and inadvertent insertion distal to the femoral bifurcation.[18] Whether percutaneous insertion results in more frequent complications continues to be debated,[3, 5, 13, 15, 17, 19−24] although most centers use the percutaneous route in routine cases.

Because of the high risk of the development of vascular compromise, the extremities should be carefully monitored during IABP use in all cases. Patients typically present with serious comorbid conditions, are frequently being treated with α-adrenergic agents, and are often noncommunicative, so it is important to remain vigilant for the development of ischemia. Any complaints of extremity pain or paresthesia, or a change in the peripheral pulse exam, should prompt timely evaluation by a vascular specialist. Examination of flow velocity with ultrasound is invalu-

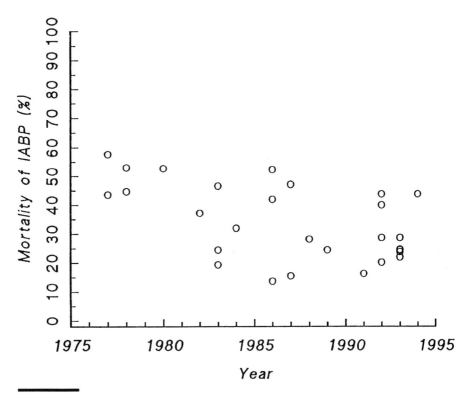

FIGURE 2.

Mortality of IABP placement by year. Data collected from review of literature for series from 1977 to 1994, reporting on ≥100 patients.[2–11, 14–18, 23, 25, 28, 34, 35, 37, 38, 40, 42, 45, 47, 48]

able in this setting because the presence of signals in one or more distal vessels usually indicates viability of the foot. The absence of audible signals along with extremity pallor, coolness, and poor or absent capillary refill usually indicates impending limb loss, and irreversible ischemic damage may be expected within 6 to 8 hours. It is during this time period that intervention may be life- or limb-saving.

If the limb is threatened, the first step should be evaluation of the adequacy of heparinization and placement of the patient in the reverse Trendelenburg position, which may augment flow enough to preserve viability. If these measures fail to improve perfusion, the relative value of continued IABP therapy must be assessed. In many cases, the myocardium has recovered sufficiently to allow for IABP removal; adequate reperfusion of the extremity usually follows. If the patient cannot tolerate weaning of the IABP, then the outer balloon sheath may be gently retracted from around the balloon catheter, allowing for a larger intraluminal area for blood flow. Assuming a flow velocity of 200 cm/sec for a 1-cm-inner-diameter femoral artery, an asymptomatic 50% stenosis would reduce resting blood flow from 157 to 39 mL/min. Insertion of a 9.5F (3.2-mm-diameter) sheath over an 8.5F catheter could be expected to further reduce flow to 23 mL/min. The simple maneuver of retracting the sheath and leaving the catheter in place would augment flow by 17% (to 27 mL/min), which may be enough to preserve the extremity.

TABLE 1.
Vascular Complications of the IABP

First Author Year	No.	Vascular Complications (% of total)	Extremity Ischemia (% of total)	Number Requiring Local Surgical Therapy (% of ischemia)	Number Requiring Bypass (% of ischemia)	Major Amputation (% of ischemia)	Overall Mortality (% of total)
Lefemine[36] 1977	86	14 (16)	10 (12)	NR	NR	1 (10)	NR
Beckman[40] 1977	273	37 (14)	16 (6)	NR	NR	2 (12)	119 (44)
Pace[16] 1977	104	21 (20)	15 (14)	NR	NR	NR	60 (58)
McEnany[34] 1978	747	162 (22)	49 (7)	49 (100)	0 (0)	0 (0)	334 (45)
McCabe[37] 1978	100	23 (23)	10 (10)	2 (20)	1 (20)	0 (0)	53 (53)
Sutorius[41] 1979	109	3 (3)	NR	NR	NR	NR	NR
Bregman[42] 1980	27	0 (0)	NR	NR	NR	NR	6 (22)
Alpert[28] 1980	332	53 (16)	37 (11)	36 (97)	NR	9 (0)	175 (53)
Harvey[26] 1981	77	2 (30)	12 (16)	NR	NR	NR	NR
Vignola[43] 1981	65	5 (9)	5 (7)	4 (80)	0 (0)	0 (0)	15 (28)
Hauser[35] 1982	113	21 (19)	13 (11)	3 (23)	0 (0)	1 (8)	42 (37)
Goldman[19] 1982	389	103 (26)	42 (11)	NR	NR	NR	NR
Alcan[20] 1983	151	24 (16)	16 (11)	10 (63)	0 (0)	0 (0)	NR
Perler[39] 1983	794	87 (11)	50 (6)	20 (40)	1 (2)	0 (0)	NR
Shahian[14] 1983	108	28 (26)	16 (15)	NR	NR	0 (0)	21 (19)
Martin[21] 1983	100	12 (12)	8 (8)	8 (100)	0 (0)	2 (25)	NR
Todd[18] 1983	102	15 (15)	12 (12)	6 (50)	0 (0)	0 (0)	25 (24)
Pennington[31] 1983	378	44 (12)	24 (6)	NR	NR	1 (4)	176 (47)

Study							
Gottlieb[3] 1984	206	42 [20]	22 [11]	NR	NR	2 (9)	66 (32)
Palletier[17] 1986	102	20 [20]	15 [15]	13 [87]	0 (0)	2 (13)	14 (14)
Goldberger[13] 1986	112	23 [20]	12 [11]	NR	NR	0 (0)	NR
Kantrowitz[25] 1986	733	161 [22]	161 [22]	86 [53]	15 (9)	4 (2)	308 (42)
Sanfelippo[15] 1986	637	75 [12]	66 [10]	NR	NR	2 (3)	333 (52)
Alderman[4] 1987	103	45 [44]	45 [44]	14 [31]	1 (2)	0 (0)	16 (16)
Goldberg[22] 1987	101	17 [17]	12 [12]	11 [92]	0 (0)	0 (0)	NR
Iverson[5] 1987	395	72 [18]	63 [16]	NR	NR	6 (10)	186 (47)
Hedenmark[24] 1988	90	24 [27]	18 [20]	9 [50]	1 (6)	1 (6)	44 (49)
Curtis[23] 1988	202	54 [27]	49 [24]	14 [29]	2 (4)	1 (2)	57 (28)
Funk[6] 1989	249	114 [46]	114 [46]	28 [25]	1 (1)	1 (1)	61 (24)
Kvilekval[7] 1991	153	19 [12]	12 [8]	11 [92]	4 (33)	0 (0)	25 (16)
Yuen[44] 1991	91	18 [20]	14 [15]	8 [57]	1 (7)	0 (0)	38 (42)
Creswell[45] 1992	672	NR	NR	NR	NR	NR	193 (29)
Miller[9] 1992	367	55 [15]	44 [12]	31 [70]	9 (20)	6 (14)	74 (20)
Mackenzie[8] 1992	100	29 [29]	25 [25]	18 [72]	2 (8)	1 (4)	40 (40)
Naunheim[38] 1992	580	72 [12]	69 [12]	34 [49]	0 (0)	4 (6)	254 (44)
Eltchaninoff[2,46] 1993	240	31 [13]	21 [9]	9 [43]	0 (0)	1 (5)	57 (24)
Makhoul[10] 1993	436	46 [11]	40 [9]	28 [70]	5 (12)	5 (12)	125 (29)
Pinkard[47] 1993	123	23 [19]	9 [7]	NR	NR	NR	27 (22)
Tatar[48] 1993	122	24 [20]	20 [16]	11 [55]	0 (0)	0 (0)	30 (25)
Barnett[11] 1994	580	72 [12]	69 [12]	29 [42]	5 (7)	4 (6)	254 (44)
Totals*	10438	1711 [18]	1235 [13]	492 [53]	49 (6)	47 (4)	3228 (38)

*Percentages are weighted.
NR = not reported.

If retracting the sheath fails to return viability, or if a sheathless catheter is already in place, alternate routes of catheter entry should be considered. The IABP may be placed via the opposite femoral artery if a strong pulse is present or, in selected cases, via the axillary or subclavian arteries. If these sites are unavailable or not technically feasible, then the best strategy for limb salvage is femorofemoral bypass from the nonaffected limb to the affected limb distal to the balloon insertion site.

OPERATIVE TECHNIQUE FOR FEMOROFEMORAL BYPASS

Patients who require extra-anatomic bypass for limb ischemia secondary to an indwelling intraaortic balloon pump are often hemodynamically unstable, and transportation to the operating room may be hazardous. In these cases, extremity revascularization may be performed in the intensive care unit in the patient's hospital bed. Operating in the intensive care unit requires adequate lighting, suction, and the same assistance and instruments that are available in the operating room. Portable operative lights and headlights are particularly useful. Femorofemoral bypass is generally performed under local anesthesia, supplemented with intravenous sedation as needed.

The operative approach in the donor groin is a standard longitudinal incision with control of the common, superficial, and deep femoral arteries. Exposure in the recipient groin is more difficult, complicated by the presence of the balloon catheter. Once the common femoral artery and its branches are exposed, the route of the bypass graft is determined by the location of the balloon catheter. If the balloon catheter enters the common femoral artery well above the femoral artery bifurcation, a medial approach to the profunda femoris artery beneath the balloon catheter is used (Fig 3,A). However, if the balloon catheter enters the common femoral artery at or below the bifurcation, it is usually preferable to place the bypass graft over the balloon catheter (Fig 3,B). Patients requiring urgent extra-anatomic bypass typically have superficial femoral artery occlusion; therefore, the anastomosis in the recipient groin is usually placed at the profunda femoris origin. In most cases, the patient is systemically anticoagulated with heparin and the anastomoses are performed with standard vascular surgical techniques. Polytetrafluoroethylene grafts are preferable in this setting because of their purported decreased propensity for late graft infections. A subcutaneous tunnel is fashioned as an elongated loop well above the pubic rami to allow the donor and recipient ends of the graft to ascend and descend gradually and avoid kinking. This is especially important where the graft is crossing over or under the intraaortic balloon pump catheter. Because those patients who develop ischemic complications from intra-aortic balloon pump insertion generally have severe systemic peripheral vascular disease, the inflow on the side of the donor limb is often suboptimal. The goal of this surgery is short-term restoration of perfusion to the ischemic limb for salvage, so this compromised inflow is usually adequate. Occasionally, however, the donor limb may have such severe iliac disease that a femorofemoral bypass is not a suitable alternative. In these cases, unilateral axillofemoral bypass

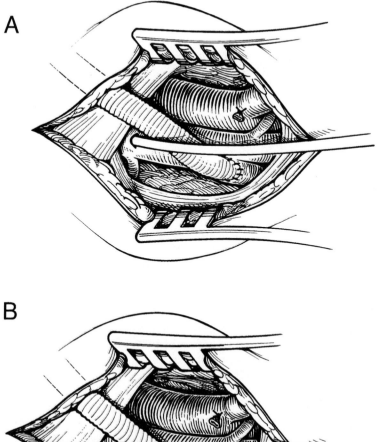

FIGURE 3.

The recipient limb of femorofemoral bypass grafting for IABP-induced extremity ischemia. **A,** bypass graft passes beneath IABP catheter inserting onto the profunda femoris artery. **B,** bypass graft positioned above low-lying IABP catheter.

may be performed with the same general operative approach and techniques in the recipient groin.

After completion of the bypass, the wounds are closed with deep absorbable sutures and skin staples. Restoration of Doppler signals at the pedal level is indicative of a successful bypass with probable short-term limb salvage. Fasciotomies are usually unnecessary in this setting because ischemic intervals are generally less than 6 to 8 hours, and the intensity of reperfusion has been modest. Nonetheless, patients should be closely examined for evidence of calf swelling and the development of a compartment syndrome.

After the patient has been weaned from balloon pump support, it is preferable to remove the balloon surgically under direct vision. Occasionally, when excellent flow is recovered in a native vessel after balloon extraction, the femorofemoral bypass graft may also be removed at that time. More often, however, inflow in the native groin remains compromised, and the extra-anatomic bypass graft should be allowed to remain intact. For those patients who suffer ischemic complications due to insertion of the intra-aortic balloon pump catheter directly into the femoral bifurcation, it is often possible to repair the bifurcation with endarterectomy and patch angioplasty with removal of the extra-anatomic bypass. After balloon pump removal and recovery, the patient's peripheral vascular status may be more completely evaluated by noninvasive studies and, if necessary, arteriography. In a minority of cases, a more definitive reconstructive procedure may be appropriate at that time.

RESULTS

Most cases of extremity ischemia after IABP insertion can be managed by sheath retraction and/or catheter removal. Roughly 50% of patients with extremity ischemia will require additional local surgical therapy, such as thrombectomy, endarterectomy, or patch angioplasty (see Table 1). Fortunately, only about 5% of cases will require formal revascularization for preservation of the extremity. Outcome has generally been favorable, with major amputation occurring in less than 5% of ischemic complications and less than 0.01% of IABP insertions overall. Even though amputation is infrequent, prolonged ischemia may result in painful postischemic neuropathy or persistent neurologic deficit,[3, 5, 11, 13, 25, 26] underscoring the importance of prompt intervention.

Patients in whom the IABP cannot be removed, necessitating femorofemoral bypass, represent an especially challenging group. Over 120 such patients have been reported in the literature, with an overall mortality of 48%.[7, 9-11, 23, 24, 27-30] Patients who do survive generally recover completely, however, because only five major amputations have been reported after successful femorofemoral bypass for IABP-induced ischemia. This technique thus remains efficacious when other options have been exhausted.

OTHER COMPLICATIONS

Nonischemic complications of IABP counterpulsation are infrequent. The second most common complication is major bleeding, occurring in about 2% of cases in the collected series. Hematoma can usually be managed with blood transfusions only, although active bleeding and/or pseudoaneurysm formation may require local surgical repair. Local or systemic infection is also surprisingly rare, with a similar incidence of about 2%. Other reported complications include spinal cord ischemia with paralysis,[31-33] pseudoaneurysm formation,[2, 5, 9, 14, 16-18, 21, 24, 26, 34] arteriovenous fistula (AVF) formation,[8] deep venous thrombosis,[13] persistent lymphatic drainage,[8] cerebrovascular accident,[3, 35] renal failure or embolism,[3, 26] and pericardial tamponade.[36]

Although uncommon, death as a direct consequence of IABP use has been repeatedly documented. The most common mechanism is aortoiliac dissection and/or perforation, which has been responsible for over 30 deaths in the combined series.[10, 11, 13, 14, 16, 17, 20, 21, 26, 31, 34, 37, 38] Its occurrence can be avoided by extreme care in wire advancement with abortion of the procedure if any resistance is encountered. Surprisingly, the second most common mechanism of IABP-induced mortality is visceral ischemia and infarction, which has been reported by at least four different investigators.[3, 9, 16, 39]

REFERENCES

1. Kantrowitz A: Origins of intraaortic balloon pumping. *Ann Thorac Surg* 50:672–674, 1990.
2. Eltchaninoff H, Dimas AP, Whitlow PL: Complications associated with percutaneous placement and use of intraaortic balloon counterpulsation. *Am J Cardiol* 71:328–332, 1993.
3. Gottlieb SO, Brinker JA, Borkon AM, et al: Identification of patients at high risk for complications of intraaortic balloon counterpulsation: A multivariate risk factor analysis. *Am J Cardiol* 53:1135–1139, 1984.
4. Alderman JD, Gibliani GI, McCabe CH, et al: Incidence and management of limb ischemia with percutaneous wire-guided intraaortic balloon catheters. *J Am Coll Cardiol* 9:524–530, 1987.
5. Iverson LIG, Herfindahl G, Ecker RR, et al: Vascular complications of intraaortic balloon counterpulsation. *Am J Surg* 154:99–103, 1987.
6. Funk M, Gleason J, Foell D: Lower limb ischemia related to the use of the intraaortic balloon pump. *Heart Lung* 18:542–552, 1989.
7. Kvilekval KHV, Mason RA, Newton B, et al: Complications of percutaneous intra-aortic balloon pump use in patients with peripheral vascular disease. *Arch Surg* 126:621–623, 1991.
8. Mackenzie DJ, Wagner WH, Kulber DA, et al: Vascular complications of the intra-aortic balloon pump. *Am J Surg* 164:517–521, 1992.
9. Miller JS, Dodson TF, Salam AA, et al: Vascular complications following intra-aortic balloon pump insertion. *Am Surg* 58:232–238, 1992.
10. Makhoul RG, Cole CW, McCann RL: Vascular complications of the intra-aortic balloon pump: An analysis of 436 patients. *Am Surg* 59:564–568, 1993.
11. Barnett MG, Swartz MT, Peterson GJ, et al: Vascular complications from intraaortic balloons: Risk analysis. *J Vasc Surg* 19:81–89, 1994.
12. Gersh BJ, Rihal CS, Rooke TW, et al: Evaluation and management of patients with both peripheral vascular and coronary artery disease. *J Am Coll Cardiol* 18:203–214, 1991.
13. Goldberger M, Tabak SW, Shah PK: Clinical experience with intra-aortic balloon counterpulsation in 112 consecutive patients. *Am Heart J* 111:497–502, 1986.
14. Shahian DM, Neptune WB, Ellis FH Jr, et al: Intraaortic balloon pump morbidity: A comparative analysis of risk factors between percutaneous and surgical techniques. *Ann Thorac Surg* 36:644–653, 1983.
15. Sanfelippo PM, Baker NH, Ewy HG, et al: Experience with intraaortic balloon counterpulsation. *Ann Thorac Surg* 41:36–41, 1986.
16. Pace PD, Tilney NL, Lesch M, et al: Peripheral arterial complications of intra-aortic balloon counterpulsation. *Surgery* 82:685–688, 1977.

17. Pelletier LC, Pomar JL, Bosch X, et al: Complications of circulatory assistance with intra-aortic balloon pumping: A comparison of surgical and percutaneous techniques. *J Heart Transplant* 5:138–142, 1986.

18. Todd GJ, Bregman D, Voorhees AB, et al: Vascular complications associated with percutaneous intraaortic balloon pumping. *Arch Surg* 118:963–964, 1983.

19. Goldman BS, Hill TJ, Rosenthal GA, et al: Complications associated with the use of the intra-aortic balloon pump. *Can J Surg* 25:153–156, 1982.

20. Alcan KE, Stertzer SH, Wallsh E, et al: Comparison of wire-guided percutaneous insertion and conventional surgical insertion of intra-aortic balloon pumps in 151 patients. *Am J Med* 75:24–28, 1983.

21. Martin RS III, Moncure AC, Buckley MJ, et al: Complications of percutaneous intra-aortic balloon insertion. *J Thorac Cardiovasc Surg* 85:186–190, 1983.

22. Goldberg MJ, Rubenfire M, Kantrowitz A, et al: Intraaortic balloon pump insertion techniques: A randomized study comparing percutaneous and surgical techniques. *J Am Coll Cardiol* 9:515–523, 1987.

23. Curtis JJ, Boland M, Bliss D, et al: Intra-aortic balloon cardiac assist: Complication rates for the surgical and percutaneous insertion techniques. *Am Surg* 54:142–147, 1988.

24. Hedenmark J, Ahn H, Henze A, et al: Complications of intra-aortic balloon counterpulsation with special reference to limb ischemia. *Scand J Thorac Cardiovasc Surg* 22:123–125, 1988.

25. Kantrowitz A, Wasfie T, Freed PS, et al: Intraaortic balloon pumping, 1967 through 1982: Analysis of complications in 733 patients. *Am J Cardiol* 57:976–983, 1986.

26. Harvey JC, Goldstein JE, McCabe JC, et al: Complications of percutaneous intraaortic balloon pumping. *Circulation* 64(suppl II):II114–II117, 1981.

27. Barsamian EM, Goldman M, Crane C, et al: Femorofemoral bypass graft in intra-aortic balloon counterpulsation. *Arch Surg* 111:1070–1072, 1976.

28. Alpert J, Parsonnet V, Goldenkranz RJ, et al: Limb ischemia during intra-aortic balloon pumping: Indications for femoro-femoral crossover graft. *J Thorac Cardiovasc Surg* 79:729–734, 1980.

29. Gold JP, Cohen J, Shemin RJ, et al: Femorofemoral bypass to relieve acute leg ischemia during intra-aortic balloon pump cardiac support. *J Vasc Surg* 3:351–354, 1986.

30. Friedell ML, Alpert J, Parsonnet V, et al: Femorofemoral grafts for lower limb ischemia caused by intra-aortic balloon pump. *J Vasc Surg* 5:180–186, 1987.

31. Pennington DG, Swatz M, Codd JE, et al: Intraaortic balloon pumping in cardiac surgical patients: A nine-year experience. *Ann Thorac Surg* 36:125–131, 1983.

32. Riggle KP, Oddi MA: Spinal cord necrosis and paraplegia as complications of the intra-aortic balloon. *Crit Care Med* 17:475–476, 1989.

33. Orr E, McKittrick J, D'Agnostino R, et al: Paraplegia following intra-aortic balloon support. *J Cardiovasc Surg* 30:1013–1014, 1989.

34. McEnany MT, Kay HR, Buckley MJ, et al: Clinical experience with intraaortic balloon pump support in 728 patients. *Circulation* 58(suppl I):I124–I132, 1978.

35. Hauser AM, Gordon S, Gangadharan V, et al: Percutaneous intraaortic balloon counterpulsation: Clinical effectiveness and hazards. *Chest* 82:422–425, 1982.

36. Lefemine AA, Kosowsky B, Madoff I, et al: Results and complications of intraaortic balloon pumping in surgical and medical patients. *Am J Cardiol* 40:416–420, 1977.

37. McCabe JC, Abel RM, Subramanian VA, et al: Complications of intra-aortic balloon insertion and counterpulsation. *Circulation* 57:769–773, 1978.
38. Naunheim KS, Swartz MT, Pennington DG, et al: Intraaortic balloon pumping in patients requiring cardiac operations: Risk analysis and long term follow-up. *J Thorac Cardiovasc Surg* 104:1661, 1992.
39. Perler BA, McCabe CJ, Abbott WM, et al: Vascular complications of intra-aortic balloon counterpulsation. *Arch Surg* 118:957–962, 1983.
40. Beckman CB, Geha AS, Hammond GL, et al: Results and complications of intraaortic balloon counterpulsation. *Ann Thorac Surg* 24:550–559, 1977.
41. Sutorius DJ, Majeski JA, Miller SF: Vascular complications as a result of intra-aortic balloon pumping. *Am Surg* 45:512–516, 1979.
42. Bregman D, Nichols AB, Weiss MB, et al: Percutaneous intraaortic balloon insertion. *Am J Cardiol* 46:261–264, 1980.
43. Vignola PA, Swaye PS, Gosselin AJ: Guidelines for effective and safe percutaneous intraaortic balloon pump insertion and removal. *Am J Cardiol* 48:660–664, 1981.
44. Yuen JC: Percutaneous intra-aortic balloon pump: Emphasis on complications. *South Med J* 84:956–960, 1991.
45. Creswell LL, Rosenbloom M, Cox JL, et al: Intraaortic balloon counterpulsation: Patterns of usage and outcome in cardiac surgery patients. *Ann Thorac Surg* 54:11–20, 1992.
46. Eltchaninoff H, Whitlow PL: Complications immédiates et à distance du ballon de contrepulsion intra-aortique percuatené: Données récentes à propos d'une série de 200 patients consécutifs. *Arch Mal Coeur* 86:1465–1470, 1993.
47. Pinkard J, Utley JR, Leyland SA, et al: Relative risk of aortic and femoral insertion of intraaortic balloon pump after coronary artery bypass grafting procedures. *J Thorac Cardiovasc Surg* 105:721–728X, 1993.
48. Tatar H, Cicek S, Demirkilic U, et al: Vascular complications of intraaortic balloon pumping: Unsheathed versus sheathed insertion. *Ann Thorac Surg* 55:1518–1521, 1993.
49. Kantrowitz A, Phillips SJ, Butner AN, et al: Technique of femoral artery cannulation for phase. *J Thorac Cardiovasc Surg* 56:219–220, 1968.

Obturator Canal Bypass

Thomas Sautner, M.D.

Department of Surgery, Division of General Surgery, University of Vienna, Vienna, Austria

Bruno Niederle, M.D.

Associate Professor of Surgery, Department of Surgery, Division of General Surgery, University of Vienna, Vienna, Austria

Georg Kretschmer, M.D.

Associate Professor of Surgery, Department of Surgery, Division of Vascular Surgery, University of Vienna, Vienna, Austria

O bturator bypass is one of several extra-anatomic techniques available for vascular reconstruction. The term extra-anatomic applies to those procedures in which vascular grafts are implanted through non-physiologic planes remote from the normal anatomic pathway. The basic objective is the maintenance of blood supply to limbs or organs in situations where orthotopic reconstruction is not feasible.[1-3] It is generally understood that such techniques imply a reduction in long-term patency to maximize patient survival.[4]

Deep infection in the groin constitutes a life- and limb-threatening complication that may result from direct vascular surgery, vascular access, tumor, or trauma with concomitant compromised circulation to the limb.[5] These difficult situations, which preclude orthotopic restoration of lower limb perfusion, have led to a number of extra-anatomic vascular reconstructions designed to circumvent the groin.[1, 6, 7]

The obturator bypass represents one such approach in which the graft is tunneled through the obturator canal mediodorsal to the femoral neck and the hip joint, thus circumventing the femoral triangle. This primary procedure maintains arterial supply to the limb yet allows aggressive treatment of various lesions in the groin.

HISTORY

Shaw and Baue[8] in 1963 were the first to direct a vascular graft through the obturator foramen. Since their initial report, roughly 280 cases have been reported and, in part, reviewed by subsequent authors.[9-29] Table 1 provides an overview of series and reviews published during the last decade.

Although the obturator canal bypass is considered a standardized procedure, it is rarely mentioned in articles covering current methods of extra-anatomic vascular reconstructions.[1-3] As Blaisdell[1] has emphasized, this is partially explained by the lack of experience with this type

Advances in Vascular Surgery®, vol. 3

© 1995, Mosby–Year Book, Inc.

TABLE 1.

Publications on the Obturator Canal Bypass During the Last Decade

Author, Year	No. Patients Reported	Median Patency, (mo) (Reported Patients Only)
Prenner, Rendl, 1982[9]	5	3
Cotton, 1982[10]	10	18
Buchardt, Hansen, Holstein, Krogh Christoffersen, et al, 1982[11]	7	12
Wood, 1982[12]	3	12
Cockburn, Bains, Whitmore, et al, 1982[13]	1	*
Erath, Gale, Smith, et al, 1982[14]	8	18
Pearce, Ricco, Yao, et al, 1983[15]	9	3
Calvelo, Garcia, Rospide, Sanchez, et al, 1985[16]	7	*
Joffe, Lankovsky, Mordechay, et al, 1985[17]	1	6†
Rawson, 1986[18]	5	30
Pietri, Pancrazio, Adovasio, et al, 1987[19]	7	*
Nevelsteen, Mees, Deleersnijder, et al, 1987[20]	55	*
Niederle, Polterauer, Kretschmer, et al, 1988[21]	27	*
Geroulakos, Parvin, Bell, et al, 1988[22]	8	5
Soots, Mikati, Warembourg, et al, 1988,[23]	1	18†
Sottiurai, Smith, Dial, et al, 1990[24]	3	*
Atnip, 1991[25]	1	14†
Stain, Weaver, Yellin, et al, 1991[26]	2	*
Cheng, Fok, Wong, et al, 1992[27]	2	*
Lai, Huber, Hogg, et al, 1993[28]	6	*
Sautner, Niederle, Herbst, et al, 1994[29]	34	62
Total	175‡	

*No median patency reported or deducible.
†Single case report.
‡Total number of patients reported is 175 instead of 202 because 27 of the 34 patients reported by us in 1994[29] had already been published elsewhere in 1988.[21]

of extra-anatomic bypass. Indeed, the largest patient cohorts available in the literature are limited to only two reports.[20, 21] In a recent publication we attempted to assess the efficacy of the obturator canal bypass based on our own experience in conjunction with an analysis of all available reports published during the last decade.[29]

OPERATIVE TECHNIQUE

The patient is placed in the supine position with slight hyperextension of the hip joints to avoid hindrance from the abdominal wall during the tunneling procedure, especially in obese patients.[30] In the case of an infected groin, special attention is paid to isolation of the femoral triangle and to meticulous antiseptic preparation of both abdomen and limb to prevent any contamination of the new anastomotic sites.

For initial exposure of the iliac vessels, we prefer the extraperitoneal approach to minimize intra-abdominal complications.[30] Because fatalities have been reported as a result of bowel perforation or intestinal obstruction, the transperitoneal route should be reserved for cases of reoperative surgery.[11] The site selected for the distal anastomosis is then prepared at the distal femoral or popliteal artery, either above or below the knee, or even more distally, depending on the local situation.[30]

The peritoneal sac and the lower pelvic organs are gently swept aside, and the obturator foramen is identified and exposed by blunt dissection.[30, 31] Identification of the obturator artery and vein before creating the tunnel is crucial to avoid serious bleeding from these vessels due to inadvertent laceration.[20] The membrane of the obturator foramen should be perforated in the anteromedial portion (Fig 1). Some authors advocate initiating the tunnel at the thigh and guiding the instrument proxi-

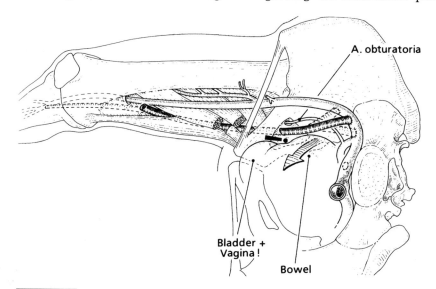

FIGURE 1.

The donor vessel is the external iliac artery which is prepared using an extraperitoneal approach. It should not undergo ligation to preserve maximum collateral circulation to the leg. The proximal anastomosis is constructed by using a side-to-end technique between the artery and the graft. Sweeping the peritoneal sac, ureter and bladder to the midline (*arrow*) gives access to the foramen obturatum. The membrana obturatoria is perforated in the anteromedial portion to leave the obturator vessels and the nerve unharmed. The tunnel is constructed from proximal to distal to minimize the trauma to organs (*exclamation mark*). The distal end-to-side anastomosis can be created with the superficial femoral, the popliteal or one of the crural arteries.

mally.[9, 15] We believe, however, that the tunnel should be constructed from proximal to distal, because this provides better anatomic visualization[10, 14, 18] and minimizes the risk of trauma to organs of the lower pelvis.[11, 29, 32] The tunneling procedure itself is carried out either with long, slim grasping forceps with blunt jaws[30] or with a special tunneling instrument.[20] Either the common iliac artery or the aorta may serve as the donor vessel, and the proximal anastomosis is constructed usually in a side-to-end manner.[17, 25, 29] Distal anastomotic sites include all segments of the superficial femoral artery,[29] the crural arteries, and even the deep femoral artery.[25] Whenever possible, perfusion of the iliac or deep femoral artery should be preserved to avoid compromising blood flow to the thigh.[11, 20, 29]

In cases of groin infection, the inguinal area must be debrided after completion of the obturator canal bypass. In accordance with the experience of most other authors, our own experience suggests that all prosthetic material from preceding operations should be completely removed to avoid persistent infection of the groin and the potential for recurrent bleeding.[29, 33]

BYPASS MATERIAL

The choice of the graft material has varied in different reports over time.[9, 29] Polyester fiber prostheses (Dacron) were used until the mid-seventies when the introduction of polytetrafluoroethylene (PTFE) provided the alternative most surgeons currently prefer.[29] Apart from these two alloplastic vascular substitutes, biologic grafts including autogenous saphenous vein or tanned human umbilical vein have been implanted.[12, 14, 18, 29] Although saphenous vein grafts naturally yield the most favorable patency rates,[12, 14, 18] the vein is often not available in adequate length and diameter. Therefore, alloplastic material is used for the majority of obturator bypass reconstructions.[29]

HEMODYNAMIC CONSIDERATIONS

The use of the obturator foramen allows a direct routing of the graft from the iliac to the femoral vessels with minimal kinking of the bypass during flexion of the hip joint.[1, 20] Pearce and colleagues[15] showed that even maximal flexion of the hip does not affect the ankle-brachial index in patients with an obturator bypass. Bypass kinking or compression may be further minimized by the use of externally reinforced grafts.[29, 30]

INDICATION

Since its initial report by Shaw and Baue[8] in 1963, obturator canal bypass has been most often indicated for infection of the groin after direct surgery (59%) or percutaneous vascular access (16%).[9, 29] Apart from infection, obturator canal bypass has been used in patients suffering from traumatic soft-tissue and skin loss,[18, 26, 29] aneurysm formation,[9, 10, 29] or neoplasm.[34] The more common indications for obturator canal bypass are summarized in Table 2. In 135 pooled cases published since 1982, infec-

TABLE 2.

Indications for the Application of the Obturator Canal Bypass, Since 1982

Indication	No. Patients	Percent
Infection		
After arterial surgery (with/without bleeding)	53	39
False aneurysm	8	6
Bleeding (no prior arterial surgery)	4	3
Aneurysm after infection	3	2
Abscess after drug injection	3	2
After coronary catheter	2	1.5
After dialysis shunt surgery	1	0.7
Groin infection with impending bleeding	1	0.7
Infected hematoma with impending bleeding	1	0.7
Septic embolism	1	0.7
Infection and bleeding after trauma	1	0.7
	78	58
Complications after arterial surgery		
Scarred groin after multiple procedures	22	16
False aneurysm	8	6
Femoral artery aneurysm	2	1.5
Anastomotic aneurysm	1	0.7
Bypass aneurysm	1	0.7
Occluded aortofemoral bypass	1	0.7
	35	26
Extensive occlusive disease of iliac/femoral vessels	15	11
Indications not related to infection or arterial surgery		
Scarred/necrotic groin after irradiation	3	2
Bleeding after irradiation	2	1.5
Tumor erosion bleeding	1	0.7
Scarred groin after trauma	1	0.7
	7	5
Total	135	100

tion remains the most frequent reason for extra-anatomic reconstruction through the foramen obturatum (58%), followed by such other complications of vascular surgery for atherosclerosis as aneurysm formation and scarring (26%). Application of the obturator bypass in patients without atherosclerotic disease of the iliac or femoral vessels (i.e., tissue loss or necrosis after trauma, radiotherapy, or tumor) accounts for roughly 5% of obturator canal bypass patients. Few patients with traumatic or oncologic lesions of the femoral vessels, therefore, require bypass through the obturator foramen, but when indicated, extra-anatomic reconstruction enables restitution of the blood supply to the limb while permitting extensive debridement or tumor resection.[13, 18, 26, 34]

Some authors[9, 20] have advocated the use of an obturator canal bypass as a primary reconstruction in patients with severe atherosclerosis of the iliac and femoral arteries in whom appropriate recipient vessels in the groin are not available. Superior patency and limb salvage rates when compared with conventional orthotopic bypass for this indication, however, have not been demonstrated.[20] The use of the obturator canal route should be considered after multiple surgical procedures in the femoral triangle because revascularization of the limb is possible without the hazards of repeated dissection and concomitant interruption of collateral vessels.[24]

RESULTS

Perioperative mortality of patients undergoing obturator canal bypass varies from negligible to 15% depending on the cohort of patients reported.[29] In our personal experience, generalized sepsis after local infection in the groin is the main cause of death, in accordance with the experience of other authors.[7, 26] Most lethal septic complications, however, occurred in patients operated on prior to 1980; improvement in supportive therapy during the past decade has reduced perioperative mortality substantially.

The majority of intraoperative complications occur in connection with preparation of the obturator foramen during creation of the tunnel. Trauma to the obturator vessels or nerve is reported in up to 3% of patients.[20, 29] Injury to lower pelvic organs can also occur during tunneling, and accidental perforation of the bladder,[32] sigmoid colon,[11] and vagina[29] has occurred. These injuries can best be avoided by tunneling from proximal to distal. In one case, erosion of the rectum by the graft occurred postoperatively.[20] Intra-abdominal complications are usually limited to patients operated on by way of the transperitoneal approach.[11, 20] Recurrent bleeding occurs primarily in patients whose initial operation is required for hemorrhage from an infected groin. Recurrent bleeding occurred in 30% of these patients in our series and was treated by debriding, oversewing, and providing additional coverage with a rotational muscle flap in two cases.[35] Complete excision of the infected prosthetic material is essential to avoid recurrent hemorrhage.

Several authors report tissue necrosis and ulceration of the thigh as a consequence of ligation of the iliac and/or the deep femoral artery during obturator bypass. This complication probably results from impaired blood flow in collaterals originating from these vessels.[11, 20] All patients in our series who subsequently required early above-knee amputation had undergone such ligation in conjunction with obturator reconstruction.[29]

Early bypass occlusion may occur in as many as 16% of patients, depending on the underlying disease.[12, 16] Early occlusion, as one would expect, occurs predominantly in patients operated on for occlusive vascular disease.[20] Long-term patency rates are available from two large series[20, 21] that demonstrate cumulative 3-year patency rates of 52% and

59% and 5-year rates of 37% and 59%, respectively. Respective limb salvage rates in these two series were 55% and 76% after 5 years.[20, 21] Because long-term results of obturator bypass are not available in large individual series, we attempted to achieve more reliable results by performing a joint analysis of all available and properly documented cases of obturator bypass. A review of the pertinent literature since 1982 revealed a total of 125 obturator bypasses.[29] Of these, 57 were sufficiently documented with regard to demographic data, indication, and secondary patency rates to be analyzed jointly with the results of our own series (Fig 2). The resulting analysis of 90 patients showed secondary patency rates of 56% at 3 and 5 years (Fig 3).[29]

This joint series consisted of patients suffering from occlusive arterial disease as well as from other nonatherosclerotic lesions such as infection and/or soft-tissue loss of the groin after drug injection, trauma, radiotherapy-induced scarring, or tumor surgery. When patency rates were reviewed according to indication, marked differences between patients with occlusive arterial disease and those operated on for nonatherosclerotic diseases became obvious (see Fig 2). Although only 52% of the grafts in patients with atherosclerosis were patent after 5 years, the patency rate for the nonatherosclerotic group was 84%. Nevelsteen and associates[20] also reported considerable differences in patency rates depending on the site of the distal anastomosis. Whereas patients with above-knee reconstructions had a 3-year patency rate of 71%, only 45% of patients with below-knee anastomoses remained patent for 3 years.[20]

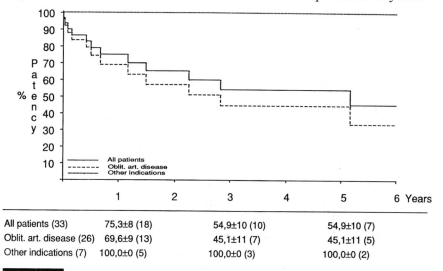

All patients (33)	75,3±8 (18)	54,9±10 (10)	54,9±10 (7)
Oblit. art. disease (26)	69,6±9 (13)	45,1±11 (7)	45,1±11 (5)
Other indications (7)	100,0±0 (5)	100,0±0 (3)	100,0±0 (2)

FIGURE 2.

Kaplan-Meier estimates of secondary patency rates of 33 obturator bypass reconstructions at the Department of Surgery, University of Vienna, Vienna, Austria.[29] The figures below the bottom line refer to percent patency (±SE) at 1, 3, and 5 years for the respective groups of patients. The figures added in parentheses refer to the numbers of patients at risk at the respective points in time. In five of these patients (15%), graft patency was re-established by thrombectomy at a median of 9 months (3, 6, 9, 13, and 21 months). Primary patency rates were 64±8% at 1 year and 46±9% at 3 and 5 years.

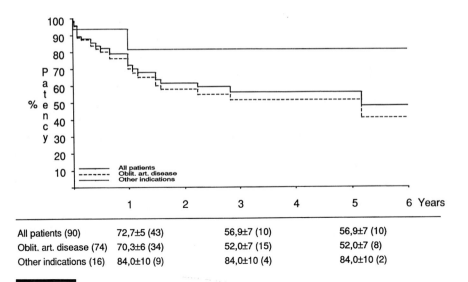

All patients (90)	72,7±5 (43)	56,9±7 (10)	56,9±7 (10)
Oblit. art. disease (74)	70,3±6 (34)	52,0±7 (15)	52,0±7 (8)
Other indications (16)	84,0±10 (9)	84,0±10 (4)	84,0±10 (2)

FIGURE 3.

Kaplan-Meier estimates of secondary patency rates of 90 obturator bypass reconstructions (joint analysis of cases reported in the literature and personal series at the Department of Surgery, University of Vienna, Vienna, Austria).[29] The figures below the bottom line refer to percent patency (±SE) at 1, 3, and 5 years for the respective groups of patients. The figures added in parentheses refer to the numbers of patients at risk at the respective points in time. Primary patency rates were 68±6% at 1 year and 53±7% at 3 and 5 years.

ALTERNATIVE APPROACHES TO GROIN INFECTION

The initial attempt to resolve a groin infection involving a vascular prosthesis is often limited to conservative measurements such as local antibiotic irrigation and drainage.[7, 28] In patients with advanced stage III infection, this therapeutic approach generally fails.[5, 7, 28] Some authors advocate simple ligation and excision of infected pseudoaneurysms, which reliably controls hemorrhage but leads to either major limb loss[7] or severe claudication in almost all patients.[27] Another frequently used technique to treat an infected alloplastic graft in the groin consists of "biologic coverage" by muscle flap or omental wrap.[24, 35] A comparative evaluation of both obturator bypass and biologic coverage of infected bypasses was carried out at our institution.[35] This analysis, derived from comparable patient cohorts, showed that obturator bypass and coverage of prostheses with biologic material appeared to be equally effective with regard to patency and limb salvage as long as hemorrhage had not occurred. In cases of septic hemorrhage, however, the obturator bypass yielded superior results. On the other hand, coverage of an infected vascular prosthesis allows preservation of the circulation to the deep femoral artery and its collaterals, an option that is not always available in patients treated with an obturator bypass.

CONCLUSIONS

Alternative extra-anatomic routes that have been used to bypass an infected groin include the axillofemoral approach,[6,26] the femorofemoral bypass using the perineal route,[6, 36] and the so-called "lateral route."[37, 38] These approaches certainly may provide valuable alternatives in selected cases, but none are uniformly applicable in all situations. Among extra-anatomic techniques, the obturator canal bypass is an elegant but infrequently used reconstruction. The primary advantage of this method lies in the barrier of healthy tissue that separates the bypass canal and the graft from the inguinal area. Because of the scarcity of reports describing long-term results, we evaluated our personal experience.

During three decades, fewer than 300 cases have been described in sufficient detail to define the indications of the obturator canal bypass. Infection involving the groin vessels after arterial or vascular access surgery remains the predominant indication, whereas the sequelae of tumor and/or radiotherapy, trauma, and various other rare problems form a much smaller, heterogeneous group. The extraperitoneal approach is clearly preferred and has been used to avoid intra-abdominal complications in two thirds of the patients reported.[29] Tunneling of the bypass from proximal to distal, or vice versa, remains controversial.[29] Injury to the neurovascular bundle in the obturator canal can best be avoided by appropriate anatomy-guided dissection.[30] Care should be taken to preserve the deep femoral arterial system during inguinal debridement to prevent ischemia of the thigh that may lead to tissue necrosis or amputation, irrespective of graft patency.[11, 20, 29] This pitfall is most likely to occur when exsanguinating hemorrhage from the femoral triangle requires prompt hemostasis. In our experience, as well as that of others, the obturator bypass has proved superior in preventing recurrent hemorrhage when compared with muscle flap coverage of the femoral vessels.[35]

In patients operated on for infection in the inguinal region, however, both the obturator bypass and coverage with biologic material seems to be equally effective.[35] Long-term patency rates of the obturator canal bypass equal those of orthotopic iliofemoral reconstructions, provided comparable groups of patients are assessed, because results depend largely on the underlying disease.[4, 29] As is true for most peripheral vascular procedures, distal runoff is one of the most crucial determinants of graft performance.[20, 29] Not surprisingly, then, results of the obturator canal bypass for peripheral arterial occlusive disease are substantially worse than they are in patients operated on for other indications. In patients with malignant disease or lesions of the pelvic or femoral arteries caused by radiotherapy, superb long-term patency rates may be expected.[29] The obturator bypass has proved a durable means with which to manage a variety of lesions in the femoral triangle that preclude in situ reconstruction.

REFERENCES

1. Blaisdell FW: Extraanatomical bypass procedures. *World J Surg* 12:798–804, 1988.
2. Porter JM, Harris EJ Jr, Taylor LM Jr, et al: Extra-anatomic bypass: A new look (supporting view). In *Advances in Surgery*, vol 26. St Louis, 1993, Mosby, pp 133–149.
3. Stoney RJ, Quingley TM: Extra-anatomic bypass: A new look (opposing view),

in Cameron JL (ed): *Advances in Surgery,* vol 26. St Louis, 1993, Mosby, pp 152–163.

4. Kretschmer G, Niederle B, Schemper M, et al: Extra-anatomic femorofemoral crossover bypass (FF) vs. unilateral orthotopic iliofemoral bypass (IF): An attempt to compare results based on data matching. *Eur J Vasc Surg* 5:75–82, 1991.

5. Szilagyi DE, Smith RF, Elliot JP, et al: Infection in arterial reconstruction with synthetic grafts. *Ann Surg* 176:321–333, 1972.

6. Cormier JM, Ward AS, Lagneau P, et al: Infection complicating aortoiliac surgery. *J Cardiovasc Surg* 21:303–314, 1980.

7. Casali RE, Tucker WE, Thompson BW, et al: Infected prostetic grafts. *Arch Surg* 115:577–580, 1980.

8. Shaw RS, Baue AE: Management of sepsis complicating arterial reconstructive procedures. *Surgery* 53:75–86, 1963.

9. Prenner KV, Rendl KH: Indications and technique of obturator bypass, in Greenhalgh RM (ed): *Extra-anatomic and secondary arterial reconstruction,* ed 1. London, 1982, Pitman Books, pp 201–221.

10. Cotton LT: Obturator canal bypass for aneurysm in the thigh, in Greenhalgh RM (ed): *Extra-anatomic and secondary arterial reconstruction,* ed 1. London, 1982, Pitman Books, pp 222–227.

11. Buchardt Hansen HJ, Holstein P, Krogh Christoffersen J: Obturator bypass to avoid an infected or scarred groin, in Greenhalgh RM (ed): *Extra-anatomic and secondary arterial reconstruction,* ed 1. London, 1982, Pitman Books, pp 228–236.

12. Wood RFM: Arterial grafting through the obturator foramen in secondary hemorrhage from the femoral vessels. *Angiology* 33:385–382, 1982.

13. Cockburn AG, Bains MS, Whitmore WF Jr: Bypass graft for femoral involvement by metastatic carcinoma of the penis. *J Urol* 127:1191–1193, 1982.

14. Erath HG Jr, Gale SS, Smith BM, et al: Obturator foramen grafts: The preferable alternate route? *Am Surg* 48:65–69, 1982.

15. Pearce WH, Ricco JB, Yao JST, et al: Modified technique of obturator bypass in failed or infected grafts. *Ann Surg* 197:344–347, 1983.

16. Calvelo A, Garcia Rospide V, Sanchez R, et al: Obturator foramen bypass. *J Cardiovasc Surg* 26:405–406, 1985.

17. Joffe B, Lankovsky Z, Mordechay I: Cross over ileo-popliteal bypass through the obturator foramen: An additional route for extra-anatomic limb blood supply. *Int Surg* 70:345–347, 1985.

18. Rawson HD: Arterial grafting through the obturator foramen. *Aust N Z J Surg* 56:127–130, 1981.

19. Pietri P, Pancrazio F, Adovasio R, et al: Long term results of extra anatomical bypasses. *Int Angiol* 6:429–433, 1987.

20. Nevelsteen A, Mees U, Deleersnijder J, et al: Obturator bypass: A sixteen year experience with 55 cases. *Ann Vasc Surg* 1:558–563, 1987.

21. Niederle B, Polterauer P, Kretschmer G, et al: Der Obturator bypass—Indikation und Ergebnisse bei 27 Patienten. *Angio Arch* 16:90–92, 1988.

22. Geroulakos G, Parvin SD, Bell PRF: Obturator bypass—The alternative route for sepsis in the femoral triangle. *Acta Chir Scand* 154:111,112, 1988.

23. Soots G, Mikati A, Warembourg H Jr, et al: Treatment of lymphorrhea with exposed or infected vascular prosthetic grafts in the groin using sartorius myoplasty. *J Cardiovasc Surg* 29:42–45, 1988.

24. Sottiurai VS, Smith B, Dial P: Aortobipopliteal bypass via the obturator foramina. *J Cardiovasc Surg* 31:121–123, 1990.

25. Atnip RG: Crossover ilioprofunda reconstruction: An expanded role for obturator foramen bypass. *Surgery* 110:106–108, 1991.

26. Stain SC, Weaver FA, Yellin AE: Extra-anatomic bypass of failed traumatic arterial repairs. *J Trauma* 31:575–578, 1991.
27. Cheng SWK, Fok M, Wong J: Infected femoral pseudoaneurysms in intravenous drug abusers. *Br J Surg* 79:510–512, 1992.
28. Lai DTM, Huber D, Hogg J: Obturator foramen bypass in the management of infected prosthetic vascular grafts. *Aust N Z J* 63:811–814, 1993.
29. Sautner T, Niederle B, Herbst F, et al: The value of obturator canal bypass. *Arch Surg* 129:718–722, 1994.
30. Kretschmer G, Niederle B, Wunderlich M: Obturator canal bypass, in Greenhalgh RM (ed): Vascular and Endovascular Surgical Techniques. An Atlas, London, 1994, Saunders, pp 260–265.
31. Brücke P, Piza F: Zur Indikation des Obturator-Bypass. *Zentralbl Chir* 93:489–493, 1968.
32. Sheiner NM, Sigman H, Stilman A: An unusual complication of obturator foramen arterial bypass. *J Cardiovasc Surg* 10:324–328, 1969.
33. Rudich M, Gutierrez IZ, Gage AA: Obturator foramen bypass in the management of infected vascular prostheses. *Am J Surg* 137:657–660, 1979.
34. Donahoe PK, Froio RA, Nabseth DC: Obturator bypass in radical excision of inguinal neoplasm. *Ann Surg* 166:147–149, 1967.
35. Kretschmer G, Niederle B, Huk I, et al: Groin infections following vascular surgery: Obturator bypass (BYP) versus "biologic coverage" (TRP)—A comparative analysis. *Eur J Vasc Surg* 3:25–29, 1989.
36. Lawrence PF, Albo D Jr: Femorofemoral bypass with an infrascrotal perineal approach for the patient with an infected groin wound. *J Vasc Surg* 3:485–487, 1985.
37. Trout HH, Smith CA: Lateral iliopopliteal arterial bypass as an alternative to obturator bypass. *Am Surg* 48:63–64, 1982.
38. Gyurko G: Laterally directed femoral bypass. *Acta Chir Hung* 24:59–65, 1983.

PART II

Carotid Disease

Carotid Endarterectomy for Acute Stroke

Steven M. Santilli, M.D., Ph.D.
Assistant Professor, Department of Surgery, University of Minnesota; Section of Vascular Surgery, University of Minnesota Hospital and Clinic, VA Medical Center, Minneapolis, Minnesota

Jerry Goldstone, M.D.
Professor of Surgery, Division of Vascular Surgery, University of California, San Francisco, California

C arotid endarterectomy has been used in the treatment of cerebral vascular disease since it was first performed successfully by Debakey and associates on August 7, 1953.[1] Since that time, the popularity of this procedure has waxed and waned, but recent prospective, randomized trials investigating carotid endarterectomy have firmly established the procedure as effective therapy[2, 3] for selected groups of patients with symptomatic and asymptomatic cerebral vascular disease.

In addition to a reduction in stroke risk, all of the contemporary randomized clinical trials have demonstrated that to derive benefit from the procedure, morbidity and mortality rates must be kept low, generally below 5%.[2, 3] Considerable variations in operative morbidity and mortality have been reported, but recent studies suggest that elective procedures can be done with a combined risk of 1% to 3%.[2, 3] Although the risks of operation are dependent on many factors, the patient's clinical condition at the time of the operation is perhaps the most important determinant of operative morbidity and mortality. The timing of carotid endarterectomy after the onset of an acute neurologic deficit remains controversial. Concern exists about the reportedly high operative morbidity and mortality in these conditions, possibly related to postoperative cerebral hemorrhage. Bruetman and colleagues[4] documented postoperative cerebral hemorrhage in 6 patients out of 900 undergoing surgical treatment of extracranial cerebrovascular disease. They postulated that the cause of this phenomenon was restoration of blood flow into the newly ischemic area, thereby converting an ischemic infarction into a hemorrhagic infarction. Other surgeons have reported similar results in small series of patients. Some experimental data support this hypothesis although contributing factors make extrapolation of these studies to the clinical experience difficult,[5–7] resulting in uncertainty about the role of surgery in preventing or limiting brain death in acute clinical syndromes.

This chapter reviews the natural history and results of treatment for acute and progressing stroke. Management options are discussed and recommendations are proposed based on our current understanding of these disease processes.

THE NATURAL HISTORY OF ACUTE ISCHEMIC STROKE

Many factors contribute to the ultimate outcome of patients after an acute ischemic stroke, including the patency or presence of collateral circulation, factors influencing cerebral perfusion, local factors at the site of injury, and the time course of ischemia. These factors make it difficult to predict the natural history of patients with acute stroke. The Joint Study of Extracranial Arterial Occlusion[8] reported on 237 patients with an acute stroke who were admitted to 24 institutions. One hundred eighty-seven patients who had coma or altered mental status were treated medically. These patients had a mortality of 20%, whereas 5% had a worsening of their neurologic deficit, 22% remained unchanged, and 53% demonstrated neurologic improvement at the time of discharge. Current data suggest that an initial ischemic stroke carries a 20% to 30% hospital mortality as well as significant and permanent morbidity.[9] In addition, once a stroke has occurred there is a high risk for recurrent stroke and an even higher related morbidity and mortality. Several studies have shown that patients who experienced an ischemic stroke and were treated nonoperatively had a subsequent incidence of recurrent stroke between 4.8% and 21% per year.[10–18] Approximately 30% of the recurrent cerebral ischemic episodes in these patients were fatal (Table 1). Because survivors of ischemic stroke are at high risk of recurrent strokes, which have an even

TABLE 1.
Natural History of Ischemic Stroke

Author	No. of Patients	% Fatal Strokes	% Recurrent Strokes	% Strokes per Year
Hill, Marshall, Shaw,[10] 1962	65	29	5	11.2
Baker et al,[11] 1962	60	26	31	19.5
Howell, Talow, Feldman,[12] 1964	92	30		10.0
Enger and Boysen,[13] 1965	49	16	38	4.8
McDowell and McDevitt,[14] 1965	99	22	32	7.9
Robinson, Demirel, LeBeau,[15] 1968	535	42		21.0
Baker, Schwartz, Ranseyer,[16] 1968	430	26		7.0
Acheson and Hutchinson,[17] 1970	349	53	35	12.9
Whisnant, Fitzgibbons, Kurland, et al,[18] 1971	302	26	53	

higher subsequent mortality, attempts at prevention of stroke recurrence are justified if the surgical procedures improve upon the natural history of this disease.

SURGICAL THERAPY FOR ACUTE STABLE STROKE

Carotid reconstruction was originally performed on symptomatic patients to reverse completed strokes in the presence of carotid occlusion. In 1957, Rob[19] described several patients in whom a major deficit disappeared after emergency carotid reconstruction. This led to the postulate that cellular viability was preserved for some time after the clinical onset of ischemia, and urgent revascularization would be of benefit. Several centers subsequently published reports about operations for acute stroke and severe neurologic deficit. Rob reported his own series of patients with acute completed or progressing stroke.[19] In patients with completed stroke, only 7% were improved by the time of discharge after early operation. The perioperative mortality of 21% was commonly due to cerebral hemorrhage. Wylie and co-workers[20] reported that five of nine patients operated on for acute stroke died of intracranial hemorrhage. The Joint Study of Extracranial Arterial Occlusion reported on 50 patients who underwent carotid endarterectomy within 2 weeks of an acute stroke.[8] Although 34% of patients were improved, the operative mortality was 42%. Bruetman's 1963 report has previously been noted. These disappointing results led to a reappraisal of urgent carotid endarterectomy after acute stroke. Although some patients improved dramatically, there was and still is no reliable way to predict which group would have a favorable outcome. Therefore, during the 1960s and 1970s, carotid endarterectomy for acute stroke or any acute neurologic deficit was rarely performed.

After the initial unfavorable reports on early operations for acute stroke, individuals began investigating the period of time required to wait before proceeding with carotid endarterectomy after an acute stroke. Radionuclide brain scans reveal some instability in the cerebral vascular bed (i.e., blood-brain barrier) after acute ischemic infarction lasting for approximately 6 weeks.[21] On the basis of this information it was proposed that surgery for acute strokes be delayed beyond this 6-week interval to allow for stabilization of the vascular bed, which would decrease the risk of hemorrhagic infarction. These data and other factors led to an almost universally accepted arbitrary delay of 4 to 6 weeks before carotid endarterectomy should be performed after an acute stroke. With use of this arbitrary 4- to 6-week delay, an operative mortality of 1.9% to 11% and a perioperative stroke risk of 2% to 15%, with a mean of approximately 5%,[22–30] have been reported (Table 2). Morbidity and mortality rates after carotid artery endarterectomy for acute stroke are higher than those reported for elective operations, yet they compare favorably with the natural history of patients not surgically treated.

Concern was then raised about the incidence of new stroke during the 4- to 6-week delay from the acute stroke to carotid artery endarterectomy. Dosick and colleagues[30] retrospectively reviewed patients who were followed after an acute stroke and who were going to undergo carotid endarterectomy after the 4- to 6-week delay, and they found that 21% had a second stroke during this time period. A subsequent prospective study[31] of

TABLE 2.
Morbidity and Mortality of CAE After Stroke (>4-Week Delay)

Author	No. of Patients	% Perioperative Stroke	% Perioperative Death
Cornell,[22] 1978	35	6.0	11.0
Duke, Slaymaker, Lamberth, et al,[23] 1979	51	4.0	1.9
Kremer and Ahlquist,[24] 1979	13	15.0	0
White, Sirinek, Root, et al,[25] 1981	31	10.0	10.0
Lees and Hertzer,[26] 1981	50	10.0	
Bardin, Bernstein, Humber, et al,[27] 1982	107	3.9	3.1
Takolander, Bergentz, Ericsson,[28] 1983	60	8.3	5.9
Baker, Littooy, Hayes, et al,[29] 1984	161	2.5	0.6
Dosick, Whalen, Gale, et al[30] 1986	51	2.0	2.0

CAE = carotid artery endarterectomy

74 patients who had an acute onset of neurologic symptoms that persisted for longer than 24 hours and had CT scan–verified cortical infarcts showed that after a 4- to 6-week wait, 9.5% of patients had a second neurologic episode of either transient cerebral ischemia or infarction. Although there were only a few publications regarding this issue, several individuals began to challenge this arbitrary 4- to 6-week delay before performing carotid endarterectomy after acute stroke. Whittemore and associates[32] reported a series of 28 patients operated on less than 4 weeks after an acute stroke who had an operative mortality of 3.7% and no new perioperative strokes. The requirement for the intraoperative use of a shunt based on EEG criteria, however, was noted to be substantially higher (40%) in this acute group than in their elective patients (18%). Rosenthal and co-workers[33] performed carotid endarterectomy on 104 patients after an acute stroke: 29 patients were operated on within 3 weeks of the acute stroke and 75 patients had their operations after a delay of more than 3 weeks. There was no difference in operative morbidity or mortality between the two groups. Piotrowski and associates[31] reported a retrospective analysis comparing the operative complication rate of carotid endarterectomy at various times after the occurrence of an acute stroke. They compared patients operated on at 1 to 2 weeks, 3 to 4 weeks, and 5 to 6 weeks after an acute stroke and found that there was no significant differ-

ence in morbidity and mortality between any of these subgroups. The overall postoperative complication rate was 11.6%, with strokes accounting for only 2.3% of the morbidity; these rates are comparable to those reported for elective carotid artery endarterectomy. They concluded that there was no evidence to support an arbitrary delay of 6 weeks after stroke before performing carotid endarterectomy and that there may be some increased risk of a second stroke during this waiting period.

AN APPROACH TO THE PATIENT WITH AN ACUTE STROKE

The patient with an acute stroke does not undergo immediate surgical intervention until the improvement in neurologic condition reaches a pla-

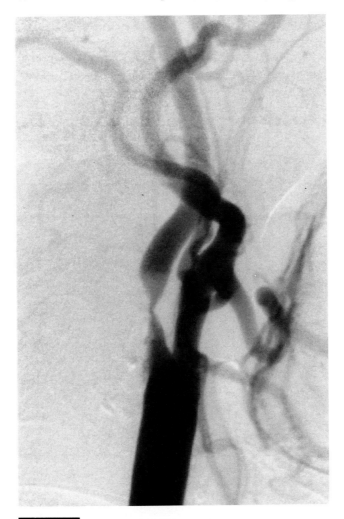

FIGURE 1.

Carotid arteriogram showing a high-grade lesion at the proximal right internal carotid artery in a 67-year-old man who had a right hemispheric stroke 3 weeks previously that manifested as left hemiparesis. His neurologic condition has improved and stabilized with persistent left arm weakness. He underwent a right carotid artery endarterectomy during the fourth week after his stroke and has done well with the persistent neurologic deficit of left arm weakness.

teau. During this interval, the patient's investigation should include a CT scan or MRI of the head to look for intracerebral pathology, and a Duplex scan of the carotid arteries to identify a potential surgically correctable lesion as the cause of the event. After a plateau of neurologic recovery, the patient undergoes cerebral angiography if there is any question as to the nature of extracranial arterial occlusive disease by noninvasive evaluation (Fig 1). Simultaneously, the patient's medical condition is optimized and all causes for increased operative morbidity and mortality are corrected. Operative therapy is then instituted based on preoperative angiography or Duplex findings and current recommendations for surgical repair of carotid artery occlusive disease. The timing of operation is based not on an arbitrary waiting period but rather on a plateau in the patient's neurologic condition (Fig 2). The time required to reach this plateau has been highly variable, ranging from a few days to a few weeks. Contraindications to surgical treatment in this setting are total occlusion of the internal carotid artery in question, severe uncontrolled hypertension, and a fixed neurologic deficit large enough that no meaningful additional impairment would ensue from a subsequent infarction.

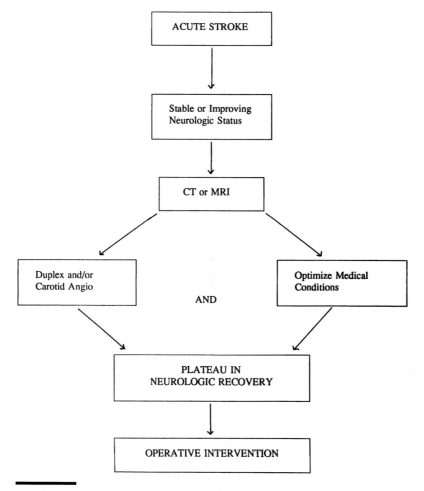

FIGURE 2.
Algorithm for management of a patient with an acute stroke.

PROGRESSING STROKE

Progressing stroke, also known as a deteriorating stroke, stroke in evolution, incomplete stroke, or stroke in progression, describes a variety of cerebral vascular events with a neurologic deficit of varying etiologies. Unfortunately, the definition and clinical syndrome are ill-defined. A mild neurologic deficit may, over the course of a few hours or days, progress to a severe stroke. The initial neurologic deficit may show some recovery, although incomplete, only to reappear later as a more severe pattern with waxing and waning symptoms that occur over hours to days. Some have arbitrarily attempted to define a 24-hour time limit beyond which an evolving stroke would be classified as a completed stroke, but this has been shown not to be true, and the progression may occur much later (Fig 3). Crescendo transient ischemic attacks (TIAs) should be included in the category of progressing stroke. These are cerebral ischemic events that usually last a few minutes to hours, leaving no residual signs or symptoms between the attacks. The usual pattern is that of a series of attacks that increase abruptly in frequency or severity (Fig 4).

A review of the literature suggests that progressing stroke is probably a more frequent clinical entity than generally appreciated. Progressing stroke was more common than sudden onset stroke in reports of the Harvard Stroke Registry. In a report of acute strokes by Jones and colleagues,[34]

PROGRESSING STROKE

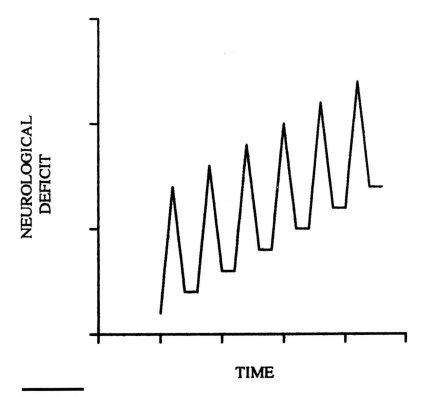

FIGURE 3.

Graphic representation of a progressing stroke.

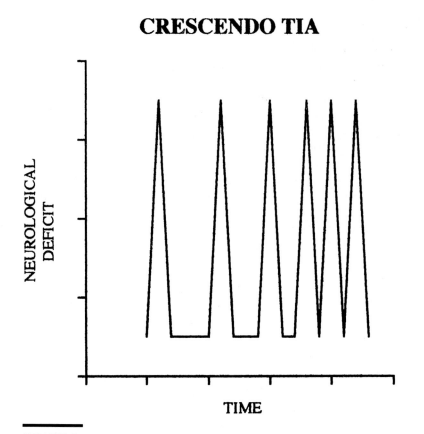

FIGURE 4.
Graphic representation of crescendo TIAs.

it was the pattern of onset in 29% of the patients. Interestingly, in this series it was found more commonly in the vertebrobasilar than in the carotid system.

It was initially postulated that progressing stroke was the clinical expression of progressive thrombosis of the involved artery. However, recent investigations have shown this not to be the case. Progressing stroke can result from a variety of mechanisms, including extension of thrombus with obliteration of collaterals, recurrent embolization, or increasing brain edema and deterioration of the general condition of the patient. Regardless of etiology, the diagnosis of progressing stroke should be made promptly so that immediate action may be taken to favorably alter the dismal natural history of this condition.

NATURAL HISTORY OF PROGRESSING STROKE

Few reports are available on the natural history of progressing stroke. Millikan[35] reported on the natural history of 204 patients diagnosed with progressing stroke. After 2 weeks, 12% of patients had no new neurologic deficit, 14% died, 69% were hemiparetic, and 5% were monoparetic. The administration of heparin has not been associated with significant improvement in outcomes. A study by Mentzen and colleagues[36] suggests that the natural history of crescendo TIA is in most instances progression to a moderate or severe neurologic deficit. Several clinical reviews by leading neurologists have supported these findings.

SURGICAL THERAPY OF PROGRESSING STROKE

Because of the dismal results of nonoperative management of progressing stroke, some individuals began to reconsider early operative intervention. Goldstone and Moore[37] reported a series of 12 patients treated at the VA Medical Center in San Francisco for an unstable neurologic condition, either crescendo TIA or a stroke in evolution. All 12 patients underwent preoperative angiography, and those patients subjected to surgical therapy had a critical or unstable arterial lesion (defined as preocclusive stenosis with or without identifiable mural or intraluminal thrombus) appropriate to the side of the cerebral symptoms. Operative details included selective use of a shunt in the four patients with crescendo TIAs based on low stump pressures, but use of a shunt in all seven patients operated on for stroke in evolution because of concern for the presence of cerebral infarction. Eleven of the 12 patients in this study had patent internal carotid arteries. The one patient with total carotid occlusion received no operation and died of a cerebral infarction. Of the 11 operated patients, 10 had a complete recovery, and there was no operative mortality. On the basis of this experience, Goldstone and Moore[37] recommended that an aggressive diagnostic approach be taken in patients with a rapidly changing or atypical neurologic condition. They did not advocate angiography or operation for patients with severe fixed neurologic deficits, especially with depressed levels of consciousness. Greenhalgh and associates[38] reported on 22 patients who underwent an urgent carotid operation for unstable neurologic conditions. Fifteen patients in their series had progressing stroke, and progression of stroke was arrested in all by operation. Six patients had complete recovery, and eight had improvement in their neurologic deficit after operation. Overall, 14 out of the 15 (93%) benefited from operation. The other patient initially had an arrest of neurologic progression but then suffered an ipsilateral recurrent stroke 7 days later. Of the seven patients operated on for crescendo TIAs, five had no deficit after surgery. One patient, who had no further TIAs, was found to have a small neurologic deficit by CT scan. Six out of seven (87%) patients with crescendo TIAs benefited greatly from surgery, although one had a fatal stroke; the operative mortality was 13%. In this series, CT scans were performed on 13 of the 15 patients, and urgent arch angiography was performed on all patients. All patients in this series were fully conscious and well oriented. Shunts were selectively used in patients who had stump pressures of less than 50 mm Hg. The authors concluded that good results can be achieved for emergency carotid endarterectomy for either crescendo TIAs or progressing strokes. In another publication, Lenzi and associates[39] reported on 22 patients with crescendo TIAs or progressing stroke who underwent emergency carotid operations. There were no postoperative neurologic complications and 1 death due to a myocardial infarction. Gertler and co-workers[40] reported their experience with carotid endarterectomy for unstable neurologic conditions at the

Massachusetts General Hospital. Three of the groups in this study included:

1. Stroke in evolution with a tight carotid stenosis
2. Crescendo TIAs continuing with heparin therapy
3. Crescendo TIAs ceasing with heparin therapy

The overall results of emergency carotid endarterectomy in these groups were that 97.3% of the patients improved or stabilized after operation with an operative mortality of 2.9%. Five of the patients treated had acute carotid artery occlusion. One had mild preoperative symptoms and had a good neurologic result. The remaining four patients had profound neurologic deficits and underwent operation within 3 hours of the onset of symptoms. Symptoms in three of the four patients improved; however, only one patient's outcome could be considered satisfactory. Gertler[40] concluded that carotid endarterectomy can be performed on properly selected patients with unstable neurologic symptoms with low operative morbidity and mortality rates. A literature review[41-43] shows a satisfactory outcome in 61% of patients operated on before 1970 with a 31% mortality, whereas patients operated on after 1970 have a satisfactory outcome 84% of the time with only a 5% operative mortality.

AN APPROACH TO PROGRESSING STROKE

The primary treatment objective for patients with progressing stroke is to prevent cerebral infarction or progression of cerebral infarction if it has already begun. There is currently no known method for reversal of cerebral infarction. However, evidence does suggest that there is a limited time period during which treatment can be effective in preventing further cerebral infarction.[44] Diagnostic evaluation should proceed on an urgent basis in patients with an acute unstable neurologic deficit.

A rapid but thorough history and physical examination is one of the best diagnostic tools in these clinical situations. When a mild to moderate neurologic deficit is present with no depression in the level of consciousness, a CT scan or MRI should be performed to evaluate the brain. Although the limitations of CT are well known, and infarctions may be difficult to diagnose in the first 24 to 36 hours after ischemic injury, this is an important study that may identify other pathologic causes for the symptom complex seen clinically, such as intracerebral hematoma, arteriovenous malformation, or brain tumor. Hemorrhagic infarctions may also be detected on CT scanning. These various pathologic causes would have an important impact on further decision making for patients with a clinically progressing stroke. Magnetic resonance imaging, although a relatively new diagnostic modality, has achieved widespread use. Its main advantage is the ability to discriminate tissue differences (including ischemic tissue injury) in the period immediately after cerebral infarction in a much more sensitive manner than with conventional CT scanning. In addition, it may allow for earlier confirmation of an ischemic process.

The patient is immediately anticoagulated if the results of the CT or MRI scan are normal or do not reveal other pathology thought to be the cause of symptoms. There are few contemporary studies on the use of anticoagulation in progressing strokes. Baker and colleagues[45] reported a significant reduction in the progression of infarction in an anticoagulated group when compared with controls. Although this finding has not been substantiated by others, it has been shown that heparin can be safely administered in the situation of a progressing stroke without increasing the risk of cerebral hemorrhage. Given these facts, it would seem that the potential advantages far outweigh any disadvantages of the use of heparin therapy for progressing stroke, especially when the types of carotid lesions that are usually found are considered.

After CT or MRI, arteriography should be the next diagnostic procedure to consider. Many clinicians are reluctant to have a patient with a progressing stroke undergo angiography because of the fear of exacerbating the neurologic symptoms, but these fears are unfounded. In the Joint Study of Extracranial Arterial Occlusion,[46] the stroke rate from angiogra-

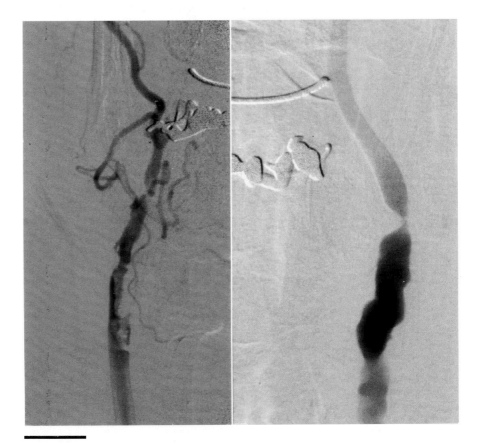

FIGURE 5.
Bilateral carotid arteriograms showing an occluded right internal carotid artery and a high-grade lesion of the left internal carotid artery in a 72-year-old man who was experiencing episodes of right hemiparesis increasing in frequency from one every 3 days to three episodes per day. His neurologic status returned to normal between episodes. Urgent arteriography was performed, and the patient underwent an emergency left carotid artery endarterectomy. Postoperatively, the patient noted complete symptom relief.

phy was only 0.5% among the nearly 4,800 patients subjected to four-vessel cerebral angiography, and in patients with severe progressing neurologic deficits the stroke rate was only 1%. Angiography is now usually performed via the retrograde transfemoral approach with use of digital subtraction, small catheters, and small amounts of contrast medium. It is usually important to limit the studies in these neurologically unstable patients; therefore, aortic arch and vertebral artery views are not routinely requested. When a critical carotid lesion is identified that is appropriate to the patient's symptoms, the examination is usually terminated. It is important to obtain adequate visualization of the carotid bifurcation to ensure that the internal carotid artery is not occluded (Fig 5). Heparin therapy is usually not discontinued unless the transaxillary route is required for angiography. Patients with progressing stroke are frequently found to have critical arterial lesions; these, as described earlier, produce a 95% or greater reduction in diameter of the internal carotid artery and/or associated thrombus seen on arteriogram, which seems to be freely floating within the vessel or attached to the vessel wall. These preocclusive

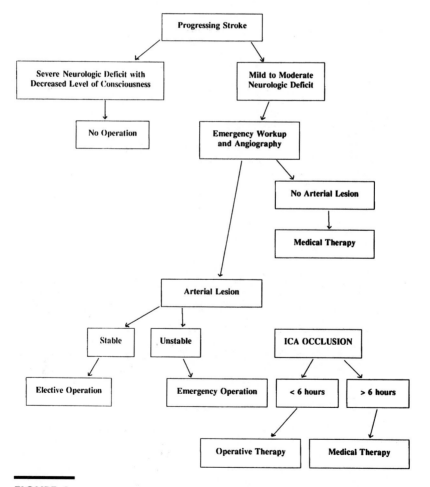

FIGURE 6.

Algorithm for management of a patient with a progressing stroke.

and thrombotic lesions are unstable because of their propensity to totally thrombose or embolize. Ulcerated, nonstenotic atherosclerotic lesions are not usually classified as critical in this sense. They may release multiple emboli into the bloodstream, and in the clinical setting of progressing stroke they have the same surgical significance as a critical lesion. They tend to occur more frequently in patients with crescendo TIA. Other diagnostic tests, such as EEGs, static brain scans, routine blood tests, and cerebrospinal fluid analysis, will not usually add clinically significant or useful information that aids decision making. B-mode imaging and Duplex scans of the carotid bifurcation, although able to identify the types of unstable or critical arterial lesions generally responsible for ischemic strokes, do not visualize some portions of the extracranial carotid system and do not preclude angiography, although more and more teams are omitting catheter angiography in the routine evaluation of patients with carotid-territory lesions and symptoms. Patients with progressing strokes and unstable arterial lesions should undergo carotid artery endarterectomy as soon as possible after limited medical preparation. This approach provides the best opportunity for reversing or preventing progression of the neurologic deficit. If a patient has a noncritical arterial lesion and the neurologic symptoms stabilize with heparin therapy, carotid endarterectomy can be delayed until further workup is completed and medical conditions optimized.

Operations should not be performed on patients with progressing stroke or severe neurologic deficits when the patient has a depressed level of consciousness. In addition, operations to establish flow in a totally occluded internal carotid artery are not recommended unless patency and flow can be restored within 4 to 6 hours of the onset of occlusion. For practical purposes, this limits this approach to patients who are already hospitalized when the process becomes clinically detected or who gain access to hospital facilities very soon after the onset of neurologic symptoms (Fig 6).

REFERENCES

1. Thompson JE: The development of carotid artery surgery. *Arch Surg* 107:643, 1973.
2. NASCET Collaborators: Beneficial effect of carotid endarterectomy in symptomatic patients with high grade carotid stenosis. *N Engl J Med* 325:445–453, 1991.
3. The Asymptomatic Carotid Atherosclerosis Study Group: Study design for randomized prospective trial of carotid endarterectomy for asymptomatic atherosclerosis. *Stroke* 20:844–849, 1989.
4. Bruetman ME, Fields WS, Crawford ES, et al: Cerebral hemorrhage in carotid artery surgery. *Arch Neurol* 9:458, 1963.
5. Garcia JH, Lowry SL, Briggs L, et al: Brain capillaries expand and rupture in areas of ischemia and reperfusion, in Reivich M, Hurtig HL (eds): *Cerebrovascular diseases.* New York, 1983, Ravel Press, p 169.
6. Meyer JS: Importance of ischemic damage to small vessels in experimental cerebral infarction. *J Neuropathol Exp Neurol* 17:571, 1958.
7. Gonzales LL, Lewis CM: Cerebral hemorrhage following successful endarterectomy of the internal carotid artery. *Surg Gynecol Obstet* 123:773, 1966.

8. Blaisdell WF, Claus RH, Galbraith JG, et al: Joint study of extracranial arterial occlusion. IV. A review of surgical considerations. *JAMA* 209:1889–1895, 1969.

9. Matsumoto N, Whisnant JP, Kurland LT, et al: Natural history of stroke in Rochester, Minnesota, 1955 through 1969: An extension of a previous study, 1945 through 1954. *Stroke* 4:20–29, 1973.

10. Hill AB, Marshall J, Shaw DA: Cerebrovascular disease: Trial of longterm anticoagulant therapy. *Br Med J* 2:1003–1006, 1962.

11. Baker RN, Broward JA, Fang HC, et al: Anticoagulant therapy in cerebral infarction. *Neurology* 12:823–835, 1962.

12. Howell DA, Talow SFT, Feldman G: Observations of anticoagulant therapy in thromboembolic disease of the brain. *Can Med Assoc J* 90:611–614, 1964.

13. Enger E, Boysen S: Long term anticoagulant therapy in patients with cerebral infarction. A controlled clinical study. *Acta Med Scand* 178(suppl 438):1–61, 1965.

14. McDowell F, McDevitt E: Treatment of the completed stroke with long-term anticoagulant: Six and one-half years' experience, in Siekert RG, Whismant JB (eds): *Cerebral vascular diseases: Transactions of the Fourth Princeton Conference.* New York, 1965, Grune & Stratton, pp 185–199.

15. Robinson RW, Demirel M, LeBeau RJ: Natural history of cerebral thrombosis: Nine to 19 year follow-up. *J Chronic Dis* 21:221–229, 1968.

16. Baker RN, Schwartz WS, Ranseyer JC: Prognosis among survivors of ischemic stroke. *Neurology* 18:933–941, 1968.

17. Acheson J, Hutchinson EC: The natural history of 'focal cerebral vascular disease.' *Q J Med* 40:15–23, 1970.

18. Whisnant JP, Fitzgibbons JP, Kurland LT, et al: Natural history of stroke in Rochester, Minnesota, 1945 through 1954. *Stroke* 2:11–21, 1971.

19. Rob GC: Operation for completed stroke due to thrombosis of the internal carotid artery. *Surgery* 65:862–865, 1969.

20. Wylie EJ, Hein MF, Adams JE: Intracranial hemorrhage following surgical revascularization for treatment of acute strokes. *Neurosurgery* 21:212, 1964.

21. Sandmann W, Kniemeyer HW, Jaeschock R, et al: Indication for carotid reconstruction in patients with established stroke, in Greenlaugh RM (ed): *Indications in vascular surgery.* Philadelphia, 1988, WB Saunders, pp 25–32.

22. Cornell WP: Carotid endarterectomy: Results in 100 patients. *Ann Thorac Surg* 25:122–126, 1978.

23. Duke LJ, Slaymaker EE, Lamberth WC Jr, et al: Carotid arterial reconstruction: Ten-year experience. *Am Surg* 45:281–288, 1979.

24. Kremer RM, Ahlquist RE Jr: The prophylactic carotid thromboendarterectomy. *Am Surg* 45:703–708, 1979.

25. White JS, Sirinek KR, Root D, et al: Morbidity and mortality of carotid endarterectomy: Rates of occurrence in asymptomatic and symptomatic patients. *Arch Surg* 116:409–412, 1981.

26. Lees CD, Hertzer NR: Postoperative stroke and late neurologic complications after carotid endarterectomy. *Arch Surg* 116:1561–1568, 1981.

27. Bardin JA, Bernstein EF, Humber PB, et al: Is carotid endarterectomy beneficial in prevention of recurrent stroke? *Arch Surg* 117:1401–1407, 1982.

28. Takolander RJ, Bergentz SE, Ericsson BR: Carotid artery surgery in patients with minor stroke. *Br J Surg* 70:13–16, 1983.

29. Baker WH, Littooy FN, Hayes AC, et al: Carotid endarterectomy without a shunt: The control series. *J Vasc Surg* 1:50–56, 1984.

30. Dosick SM, Whalen RC, Gale SS, et al: Carotid endarterectomy in the stroke patient: Computerized axial tomography to determine timing. *J Vasc Surg* 2:214–219, 1986.

31. Piotrowski JJ, Bernhard VM, Rubin JR, et al: Timing of carotid endarterectomy after acute stroke. *J Vasc Surg* 11:45–52, 1990.
32. Whittemore AD, Ruby ST, Couch NP, et al: Early carotid endarterectomy in patients with small fixed neurologic deficit. *J Vasc Surg* 1:795–799, 1984.
33. Rosenthal D, Borrero E, Clark MD, et al: Carotid endarterectomy after reversible ischemic neurologic deficit or stroke: Is it of value? *J Vasc Surg* 8:527–534, 1988.
34. Jones HR, Millikan CH: Temporal profile (clinical course) of acute carotid system cerebral infarction. *Stroke* 7:64, 1976.
35. Millikan CH: Clinical management of cerebral ischemia, in McDowell FH, Brennan RW (eds): *Cerebral vascular disease. Eighth Princeton Conference.* New York, 1973, Grune & Stratton, p 209.
36. Mentzer RM, Finkelmeir BA, Crosby IK, et al: Emergency carotid endarterectomy for fluctuating neurologic deficits. *Surgery* 89:60, 1981.
37. Goldstone J, Moore WS: Emergency carotid artery surgery in neurologically unstable patients. *Arch Surg* 111:1284, 1976.
38. Greenhalgh RM, Cuming R, Perkin GD, et al: Urgent carotid surgery for high risk patients. *Eur J Vasc Surg* 7:25–32, 1993.
39. Lenzi GL, Rasura M, Ventura M, et al: Surgical treatment of unstable and acute cerebral ischaemia: Indications and results in the light of pathophysiological data, in Courgier R (ed): *Basis for a classification of cerebral arterial diseases,* vol 1. Amsterdam, 1985, Excerpta Medica, p 189.
40. Gertler JP, Blankensteijn JD, Brewster DC, et al: Carotid endarterectomy for unstable and compelling neurologic conditions: Do results justify an aggressive approach? *J Vasc Surg* 19:32–42, 1994.
41. DeBakey ME, Crawford ES, Cooley DA, et al: Cerebral arterial insufficiency: One to 11-year results following arterial reconstructive operation. *Ann Surg* 161:921–945, 1963.
42. Ojemann RG, Crowell RM, Roberson GH, et al: Surgical treatment of extracranial carotid occlusive disease. *Clin Neurosurg* 22:215–263, 1975.
43. Bourke BM, McCollum CN, Greenhalgh RM: Carotid endarterectomy in patients with actively changing neurological deficits—Correlations with CT brain scans. *Aust N Z J Surg* 55:335–340, 1985.
44. Carter LP, Yamagata S, Erspamer R: Time limits of reversible cortical ischemia. *Neurosurg* 12:620–668, 1983.
45. Baker RW, Broward JA, Fang HC, et al: Anticoagulant therapy in cerebral infarction: Report on cooperative study. *Neurology* 12:823, 1962.
46. Hass WK, Fields WS, North RR, et al: Joint Study of Extracranial Arterial Occlusion. *JAMA* 203:961–968, 1968.

Management of Acute Postendarterectomy Neurologic Deficits

Joseph Patrick Archie, Jr., M.D., Ph.D.
Clinical Professor of Surgery, University of North Carolina at Chapel Hill School of Medicine, Chapel Hill, North Carolina; Adjunct Professor of Mechanical and Aerospace Engineering, North Carolina State University, Raleigh, North Carolina

The development of a new central neurologic deficit after carotid endarterectomy can be a devastating event for both patient and surgeon. It demands immediate analysis of the probable cause and, in appropriate cases, intervention. Many neurologic deficits are surgeon related, yet we have only recently begun to critically analyze our own contribution to morbidity and mortality. Most critical analyses of vascular surgical procedures have been directed at either systemic patient-related risk factors, such as cardiac, pulmonary, and renal dysfunction, or local procedure options, such as the choice of conduit and location for lower extremity bypass and the use of both shunt and patch for carotid endarterectomy. The role of intraoperative decisions, technique, and experience on the outcome of vascular surgical procedures has been infrequently addressed. Many operations are performed with incomplete or suboptimal preoperative information. The operative evaluation of arteries often yields new and sometimes critical information necessary for optimizing vascular reconstructions. Operative decisions and technique are often the primary determinant of outcome, particularly with respect to carotid endarterectomy. The brain is an extremely sensitive end-point detector of technical errors and suboptimal decisions. Nowhere else in vascular surgery does there exist such a well-documented wide spectrum of outcome results. Analysis of the cause, management, and prevention of neurologic complications of carotid endarterectomy is of vital importance.

A new neurologic deficit after carotid endarterectomy is sometimes difficult for the surgeon to accept, and some degree of denial as to the true cause may be anticipated. Failure of surgeons to review in detail the course of their operations and learn from adverse results is a greater tragedy than the isolated event itself. Fortunately, many perioperative neurologic deficits are minor at onset and produce minimal or no permanent deficits. For every symptomatic early postoperative internal carotid artery occlusion there are several asymptomatic ones, and similarly, for every symptomatic perioperative embolus there are probably multiple subclinical events. Clinically evident neurologic events are only the tip of

Advances in Vascular Surgery®, vol. 3
© 1995, Mosby–Year Book, Inc.

the iceberg. A surgeon with a neurologic morbidity and mortality for carotid endarterectomy greater than 3% or 4% is likely to be making frequent judgment and/or technical errors. The key to management of these events is prevention, and prevention begins with analysis of the causes.

Most early postoperative central neurologic deficits are due to either internal carotid artery thrombosis or perioperative embolization, whereas delayed postoperative events may result from the hyperperfusion syndrome. The incidence of post–carotid endarterectomy neurologic deficits in general, and severe disabling or fatal strokes in particular, has decreased significantly over the past four decades. The current accepted standard of excellence of 3% or less stroke and mortality for carotid endarterectomy is the result of a number of factors, including patient selection, timing of surgery, optimal decision making, refined technique, and experience. Some surgeons who are on the learning curve or perform this operation infrequently do not meet this gold standard. However, both highly experienced and inexperienced surgeons will occasionally be faced with the unhappy situation of a new postoperative central neurologic deficit. There are no controlled or randomized studies that identify the best management protocol for this problem. Retrospective analysis of our own experience and that of others is all that is available. The fundamental question concerns the specific cause of the neurologic deficit. Is it the result of intraoperative embolization or hypoperfusion ischemia, postoperative embolization of atheromatous debris or platelet aggregates, or internal carotid artery occlusion, cerebral hyperperfusion, or cerebral hemorrhage? Although protocols and algorithms for management of post-endarterectomy neurologic deficits have been proposed,[1-3] management decisions are often difficult because the etiology of the deficit is not clear. The operating surgeon has the most information about both the patient and the course of the operation and is therefore the optimal person to make the management decisions. At first glance, it may appear that these decisions are straightforward: reoperate to restore blood flow if the internal carotid artery is suspected or confirmed to be occluded, or give anticoagulants or antiplatelet or rheologic agents if the internal carotid artery is open and there is no hemorrhagic cerebral infarction. However, reoperation is not without risk, and rapid confirmation that the internal carotid artery is patent short of reoperation can sometimes be difficult, and an artery proved by duplex scanning to be patent may harbor a residual intimal flap or significant platelet aggregate. This chapter addresses these critical issues and reviews the causes, diagnosis, management, and prevention of these events. Management of ischemic strokes per se should follow well-established guidelines.[4]

CAUSES AND MANAGEMENT OPTIONS OF POSTOPERATIVE NEUROLOGIC DEFICITS

The high incidence of postendarterectomy internal carotid artery occlusion reported in some series is a disturbing statistic. Although Hertzer and colleagues[5] found a 2% incidence of early internal carotid artery occlusion after carotid endarterectomy when primary closure reconstruction was used, Van Alphen and Polman[6] reported that 16 of 96 (18.5%) primarily closed carotid endarterectomies had an internal carotid artery occlusion identified 4 months after operation. However, only 3 of the 16 (18%) patients with an occlusion were symptomatic. Most postendarterectomy internal carotid artery occlusions are asymptomatic and go undetected unless discovered by duplex scan or arteriography. In a large series, Rosenthal and associates reported a less than 2% incidence of postoperative internal carotid artery occlusion after carotid endarterectomy using both primary closure and patch reconstruction. In a recent report, Riles and co-workers[8] found that almost all of the 15 patients who had a stroke secondary to a postendarterectomy internal carotid artery occlusion tolerated carotid clamping under local or cervical block anesthesia. This suggests that distal embolization may be a component of symptomatic postoperative internal carotid artery thrombosis. However, the duration of occlusion is also important. Both Boysen's[9] and Sundt's[10] measurements of cerebral blood flow during and after carotid clamping indicate that the carotid occlusion time in patients with marginal collateral blood flow is a major factor in determining neurologic dysfunction and reversible and irreversible neurologic cell ischemia. Clinical evidence supports this observation; therefore, urgent reoperation is advised when an internal carotid artery occlusion is suspected or confirmed early after endarterectomy.

Reoperation for symptomatic early postoperative internal carotid artery occlusion is the only therapeutic intervention that may produce an immediate benefit. However, less than half of the patients with an occlusion will be improved by the restoration of blood flow.[1, 2, 8, 11] Even in large series, the number of patients with immediate clear-cut improvement in neurologic status after reoperation is small. Even so, reoperation is the one chance to reverse the deficit, and the decision to do so must be made promptly. In general, if a patient awakes from anesthesia with, or subsequently develops, a dense ipsilateral stroke, it must be assumed that the internal carotid artery has occluded, and the patient should be immediately returned to the operating room. There are situations when the surgeon is highly suspicious that interoperative embolization has occurred. When this is the case, or when a mild deficit or a transient ischemic attack (TIA) occurs, immediate evaluation with a duplex scan or an angiogram is indicated to determine if the internal carotid artery is occluded, contains thrombus, or has a major defect. Transcranial Doppler may also be useful to evaluate the presence or absence of flow in the proximal middle cerebral artery. None of these modalities, however, may detect a small but significant platelet thrombus/aggregate as the source of emboli. Reoperation, however, has an associated risk and should be avoided if possible. Patients with a patent internal carotid artery and a new neurologic event after endarterectomy should ultimately undergo a computed axial tomography (CAT) or magnetic resonance imaging (MRI) scan to make sure there is no intracerebral hemorrhage prior to initiation of anticoagulation, antiplatelet, or rheologic therapy.

The development of neurologic deficits after carotid endarterectomy has a biphasic temporal course. The early peak is the first 24 hours after operation. These deficits are usually caused by internal carotid occlusion or emboli and are most likely surgeon related. The second peak occurs 5 to 12 days after carotid endarterectomy, usually after the patient has been discharged from the hospital, and is caused by the hyperperfusion syndrome. This syndrome occurs in 0.5% to 2% of patients undergoing carotid endarterectomy.[11–16] It is most common in patients with evidence of poor collateral perfusion prior to reconstruction of a high-grade carotid stenosis. Patients with these risk factors have a much higher postendarterectomy cerebral blood flow than normal.[10, 13] Chronic cerebral ischemia can produce a loss of autoregulation that results in hyperperfusion and cerebral edema when normal blood flow and pressure are restored. This may produce ipsilateral headache, with progression to seizure activity, cerebral infarction, or hemorrhage, and in some cases death. When the hyperperfusion syndrome is suspected, pharmacologic control of blood pressure to prevent hypertension is clearly advisable. If lateralizing epileptiform discharges are noted on electroencephalogram, anticonvulsant therapy should be initiated. A CAT or MRI scan may be normal or show edema, infarction, or hemorrhage. Patients should remain hospitalized until the symptoms abate.

Various causes of stroke associated with carotid endarterectomy have been identified over several decades.[1, 2, 8, 11, 17–20] Perdue[1] reported 31 post–carotid endarterectomy neurologic deficits after 1,023 operations (3.1%). Seventeen (1.7%) patients had a focal or minor deficit, nine of which occurred after a lucid period after general anesthesia. Of the 14 (1.4%) patients who sustained a severe stroke, 7 died, and 5 had a permanent deficit. Four strokes were inappropriate to the side of operation. Six of the 31 patients (19%) had an internal carotid artery occlusion and underwent reoperation, but only two (6%) had a complete recovery. Rosenthal and colleagues[2] reviewed 818 patients undergoing carotid endarterectomy and found that 37 (4.5%) had a new neurologic deficit. Of these, 22 (2.7%) patients had a minor transient deficit and returned to normal. Fifteen (1.8%) patients had a profound deficit. Seven were caused by internal carotid artery thrombosis, three were thought to be caused by emboli, and five were caused by an unknown etiology. Roughly one third of their patients were operated on with a shunt and general anesthesia, one third without a shunt and general anesthesia, and one third awake with a local or regional block and selective shunting. There was no statistically significant difference between the incidence of TIAs and permanent neurologic deficits in these three groups. Krul and associates[19] reviewed the distribution of 42 ischemic strokes after 658 carotid endarterectomies (4.8%). Of these, 34 had diagnostic studies that allowed analysis. Seven had a hemodynamically induced or watershed stroke presumed to be caused by inadequate cerebral infusion during the procedure. Several of these were bilateral. Twenty-seven were thought to be embolic in nature, 20 of which were in the middle cerebral artery territory. Unfortunately, the status of the internal carotid artery after surgery and the events of the operations were not clarified, so the underlying causes could not be identified. The ratio of thromboembolic to hemodynamic or watershed-induced strokes was approximately 3:1.

From a series of almost 2,000 operations, Sundt[11] reported 15 post-endarterectomy internal carotid artery occlusions that were immediately reoperated on with return of blood flow. Seven of these patients had no subsequent deficit, five had a major stroke, and three had a minor stroke. The hyperperfusion syndrome occurred in 2% of this series, 1% of which had a transient ischemic attack; the other 1% had a disabling stroke or died. Riles and co-workers[8] reviewed a 26-year experience with 3,062 carotid endarterectomies. Twenty mechanisms of perioperative stroke were identified in 66 operations. Of these, 63 had the mechanism of stroke defined. These were placed into five categories. Ten strokes were produced by ischemia during carotid clamping, 25 were caused by postoperative thrombosis and/or embolization, 8 were caused by other mechanisms associated with the operation, 12 were caused by an intracerebral hemorrhage with or without a hyperperfusion syndrome, and 8 were unrelated to the reconstructed carotid artery. Over almost three decades they found that the incidence of ischemia due to clamping and the incidence of hemorrhagic stroke decreased significantly with improved patient selection and operative management. The majority of the intracerebral hemorrhages in this series occurred early and were in patients who had a preoperative stroke. The hyperperfusion syndrome was identified in only one patient in their series. Sixty-five percent of the perioperative strokes were identified as being secondary to a surgeon-related technical defect.

PERSONAL SERIES

The cause, management, and outcome of neurologic deficits that occurred during or immediately after 1,202 consecutive primary and redo carotid endarterectomies performed by me between 1982 and 1994 were reviewed. The indications for operation were transient ischemic attack in 483 (40.2%), reversible ischemic neurologic deficit in 34 (2.8%), completed stroke in 182 (15.1%), global nonlateralizing ischemia in 121 (10.1%), and asymptomatic stenosis (75% or greater diameter) in 382 (31.8%). Of these, 67 (5.6%) carotid endarterectomies were performed concomitant with a cardiac operation, and 9 (0.7%) with a peripheral vascular or general surgical procedure. Reconstruction was by primary closure in 125 (10.4%), synthetic patch in 137 (11.4%), greater saphenous vein patch in 927 (77.1%), and interposition vein bypass in 12 (1.0%). There were 42 (3.5%) redo operations, only 6 of which came from the same patient population. The collateral cerebral perfusion pressure modification of the carotid stump back-pressure method was used to determine the necessity for a shunt.[20–22] After 1986, all stump back-pressure measurements were confirmed for accuracy by use of previously described methods.[23] The 123 (10.2%) patients with a perfusion pressure less than 18 mm Hg were shunted. The occlusion time for endarterectomy without a shunt was 27 ± 6.6 minutes (mean ± 1 SD). When a shunt was used, the occlusion time for placement was 1.6 ± 0.7 minutes, and for removal 1.9 ± 1.3 minutes. The shunt time was 30 ± 8.0 minutes. All but 2 (0.2%) operations were performed under general anesthesia. Intraoperative confirmation of an adequate reconstruction with continuous-wave Doppler was used in all 1,202 operations. All major defects identified were repaired.

Twenty-nine (2.4%) new central neurologic deficits were identified within the first 10 days of operation. The causes and time of occurrence of these events are given in Table 1. The distribution of these events was evenly spaced among the indications for operations. It is interesting that four patients had TIAs that were identical in presentation to the preoperative symptoms and resolved. This is most likely due to a single preoperative embolic event that produced a focal ischemic zone that triggered identical TIA symptoms for several days or weeks independent of carotid endarterectomy. There were 16 (1.3%) strokes, 8 of which were severe and 8 mild. The outcome of these 16 strokes is given in Table 2. One patient who died had an internal carotid artery occlusion, one an intracerebral hemorrhage with the hyperperfusion syndrome, and the third a malignant cardiac arrhythmia, hypotension, and a metabolic-induced stroke. Of the remaining five patients with an initially dense stroke, two improved significantly. Six of the 10 patients with a mild stroke completely recovered in 6 months. Three of the eight patients who awoke with a new deficit underwent reoperation. Of these, two had an internal carotid occlusion that was successfully reopened. However, one died from the stroke and the other was not improved and had a severe permanent deficit. Both had primary closure reconstruction. The third patient had no operative event that could explain the neurologic deficit and underwent immediate reoperation without waiting for a duplex scan. The carotid artery was patent and no abnormality was found. This patient im-

TABLE 1.

Causes and Time of Occurrence of 29 Postendarterectomy Neurologic Defects*

	Time of Occurrence			
	Awoke With	**1–24 Hrs**	**1–10 Days**	**Total**
Internal carotid occlusion	2 (2)		1	3 (2)
Emboli from common carotid	1 (1)	1	1	3 (1)
Emboli from external carotid	1 (1)			1 (1)
Emboli from shunt	1 (1)			1 (1)
Emboli of unknown etiology	2	1 (1)	1 (1)	4 (2)
Metabolic-cardiac			1 (1)	1 (1)
Unrelated to carotid endarterectomy	1 (1)		3 (3)	4 (4)
Hyperperfusion syndrome			8 (4)	8 (4)
TIA identical to preoperative TIA		1	3	4
Total	8 (6)	3 (1)	18 (9)	29 (16)

*The number of events that resulted in strokes is given in parentheses. TIA = transient ischemic attack.

TABLE 2.

Six-Month Outcome of 16 Strokes

	Awoke With	1–24 Hrs	1–10 Days With HPS*	1–10 Days No HPS	Total
Died	1	0	1	1	3
Severe deficit	1	1	1	1	4
Mild deficit	1	0	1	1	3
No deficit	3	0	1	2	6
Total	6	1	4	5	16

*HPS = hyperperfusion syndrome.

proved with only a mild permanent deficit. The stroke was presumed to be caused by an embolus that occurred during or immediately after carotid endarterectomy. The remaining five patients who awoke with a new neurologic deficit had either a mild focal deficit or a clear explanation for the event (see Table 1). All five had immediate duplex scanning that confirmed both patency and normality of the reconstructed carotid arteries. The management algorithm I tended to follow is given in Figure 1. The major unanswered question in this algorithm is reoperation when there is a major but nonocclusive defect in the artery.

Several observations of this analysis and management of post–carotid

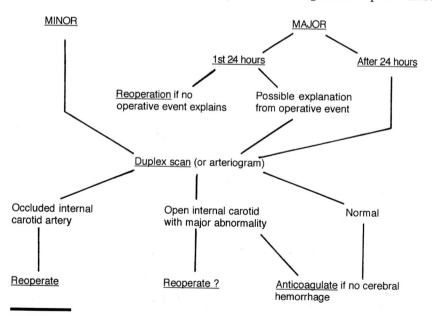

FIGURE 1.

Algorithm used by the author for management of postendarterectomy neurologic deficits.

endarterectomy neurologic deficits are worthy of mention. First, 7 of the 16 strokes were surgeon related and therefore potentially preventable. Second, reoperation was performed only three times. In each case there was a profound neurologic deficit, yet no intraoperative technical problem that could have produced emboli was identified. Reoperation was not helpful in these three cases. Third, duplex scanning is invaluable in confirming patency and normality of the internal carotid artery in patients with a deficit suspected to have been produced by a perioperative embolus, or in patients with a minor focal deficit. All of the patients in this category had patent internal carotid arteries, and many of the minor deficits resolved. Reoperation was not performed in this group, and I do not believe it was indicated. Fourth, the most frequent cause of neurologic deficits in this series was the hyperperfusion syndrome. Of the eight (0.7%) patients who had this syndrome, four had strokes from which two died and two survived with permanent deficits. Finally, on a preventative note, the collateral cerebral perfusion pressure modification of the carotid stump back-pressure technique for determining selective shunting is reliable. Only two patients awoke with a new deficit of unknown etiology, and both were minor and resolved.

Review of this data, as well as that of others,[1, 2, 8, 11] may suggest that analysis and management decisions are clear-cut and easily made. I have not found this to be the case. Each event must be assessed individually by the operating surgeon. Reoperation is not without hazard. One of the minor strokes in this series was caused by an embolus produced while manipulating the carotid artery in a patient who was reoperated on for excessive hemorrhage. The policy of immediate reoperation for patients who awake with a new major unexplained neurologic deficit is based on the assumption that the internal carotid artery has occluded or has a major defect. If a duplex scan can be obtained immediately, reoperation can be prevented in patients who clearly have a patent and normal reconstruction. Such patients bear careful watching, however; if the deficit increases, reoperation for evolving occlusion may prove necessary. I have no experience with performing angiography in this setting, but it is an excellent alternative technique. In patients with a patent internal carotid artery, a CAT scan should be obtained to rule out intracerebral hemorrhage, thus making the decision for anticoagulation, antiplatelet, or rheologic therapy possible.

SELECTED CASE MANAGEMENT

The nine cases briefly presented below are drawn from my personal knowledge of operations performed by other surgeons when the facts were clearly established, and from my own experience. They illustrate the importance of selective management of individual situations as opposed to strict adherence to a predetermined algorithm.

CASE REPORTS

Case 1. Man, 63, was seen with crescendo left body motor TIAs. He was admitted to the hospital. A CAT scan was negative, and an arteriogram demonstrated an 85% right internal carotid artery stenosis. Because of five TIAs in a 24-hour period, semiurgent surgical intervention was advised. In preoperative holding before surgery, the patient had another event and was thought to have a mild left-sided motor weakness before induction of anesthesia. The patient underwent a standard carotid endarterectomy with primary closure that was described by the operating surgeon as uneventful. On awakening from general anesthesia, the patient was lucid but had a dense left hemiplegia. The surgeon assumed that the stroke had occurred "just prior to surgery." No assessment of the internal carotid artery was made. The patient was begun on heparin, and a subsequent CAT scan showed a right cerebral ischemic infarction and no evidence of hemorrhage. A duplex scan 21 weeks later showed the right internal carotid artery to be occluded. The patient had a significant permanent neurologic deficit.

Comment. This is an example of a missed opportunity to reoperate for what was most likely an occluded internal carotid artery. The patient should have been returned immediately to the operating room if there was any question regarding whether or not the artery was patent. If it was believed that reintervention would be too dangerous because the patient was unstable, a duplex scan or an arteriogram should have been obtained to confirm patency. Heparin should not have been given prior to confirmation by CAT or MRI scan that there was no intracerebral hemorrhage. This is perhaps an example of "surgeon denial."

Case 2. Man, 72, underwent a right carotid endarterectomy for an asymptomatic 80% stenosis. He awoke from general anesthesia and had a lucid period of approximately 2 hours, and then developed left arm and leg paralysis. The operation was performed late in the afternoon and the surgeon was not available when the deficit occurred. Vascular surgical consultation was obtained by the on-call surgeon. A duplex scan indicated that the internal carotid artery was occluded. The patient was returned to the operating room within 30 minutes of the onset of the neurologic deficit. At reoperation it was discovered that the internal carotid artery had been externally wrapped with polytetrafluoroethylene (PTFE). The internal carotid artery distal to this had a normal continuous-wave Doppler velocity, as did the common and external carotid arteries. The ultrasound would not penetrate the PTFE wrap. The artery was not opened. The patient was anticoagulated after a CAT scan confirmed no intracerebral hemorrhage. The operating surgeon subsequently noted that the original operation had been difficult, the endarterectomy primarily closed, and a PTFE wrap placed around the reconstructed internal carotid. The patient gradually improved but had a moderate permanent deficit. On follow-up duplex scan there was a residual 75% internal carotid artery stenosis, subsequently confirmed to be at the distal end of the endarterectomy (Fig 2).

Comment. If the operating surgeon had been available or there had been an adequate description of the procedure in the chart, the reoperating surgeon would have known that the operation was difficult and that a PTFE wrap had been placed. PTFE has multiple tiny air pockets that can persist for several hours, and through which ultrasound will not penetrate. This can give a false-positive Doppler ultra

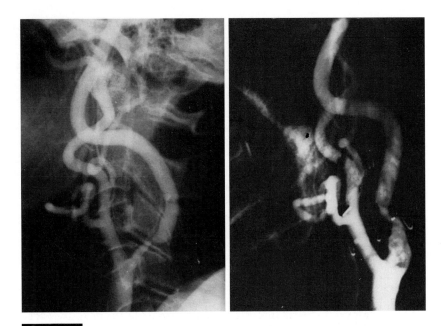

FIGURE 2.

Carotid arteriograms showing stenosis before carotid endarterectomy (*left*) and residual stenosis caused by an endarterectomy end-point technical error and a major postoperative stroke (*right*).

sound diagnosis of internal carotid artery occlusion. I have had similar difficulty interrogating PTFE-patched arteries in the operating room and early after operation. The PTFE wrap also precluded intraoperative Doppler ultrasound interrogation of the endarterectomized segment. An operative arteriogram would have demonstrated the defect, which was most likely an intimal flap or residual stenosis at the distal internal carotid end point that produced an embolus. Repair at the time of reoperation would not have improved the neurologic status but would have prevented the subsequent reoperation necessary 6 months later.

Case 3. Man, 68, with TIAs underwent an uneventful left carotid endarterectomy with Dacron patch reconstruction and was dismissed from the hospital on the second postoperative day. He was brought to the emergency room on the fifth postoperative day with a moderate right hemiparesis. A duplex scan showed a 5-mm-thick thrombus on the endarterectomized and patched segment of the internal and common carotid bulb but no significant obstruction of the lumen. The patient was anticoagulated with heparin and converted to Coumadin, which was continued for 6 weeks. He had no further neurologic deficits, and the stroke subsequently cleared. A repeat duplex scan at 3 months showed only minor wall thickening.

Comment. The management of patients with fresh partial or nonocclusive thrombus on the endarterectomized segment that produces embolic symptoms is controversial. Whether this patient should have been reoperated on and the artery reconstructed is not clear. Management with anticoagulation in this case was satisfactory in that no further clinically evident embolization occurred. However, the decision to reoperate with thrombectomy and re-repair or interposition vein by-pass grafting also would have been a satisfactory choice.

Case 4. Man, 57, underwent an uneventful left carotid endarterectomy for a mild stroke that had resolved. He was discharged on the second postoperative day in satisfactory condition on aspirin. On the sixth postoperative day he had an episode of expressive dysphasia and mild right arm weakness that lasted 5 minutes. A duplex scan showed a sharp 3-mm common carotid artery step at the proximal endarterectomy end point (Fig 3) but no thrombus, residual stenosis, flap, or other abnormality. He was continued on aspirin, and the following day had a similar event. He was hospitalized, placed on heparin, and converted to Coumadin for 6 weeks. A repeat duplex scan was unchanged. He had no further transient ischemic attacks.

Comment. This is an example of a symptomatic technical defect at the proximal end of the endarterectomy in an atherosclerotic common carotid artery.

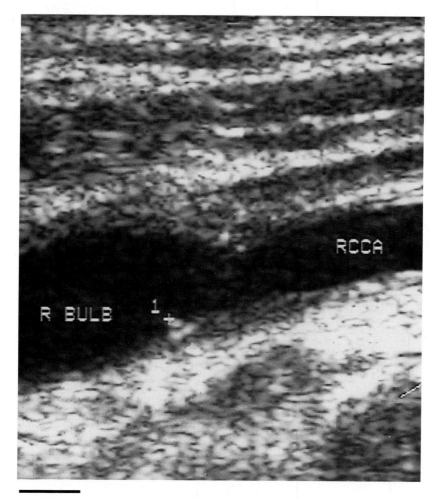

FIGURE 3.
Early postoperative duplex scan showing a common carotid step defect at the proximal end of an endarterectomy that produced two TIAs.

Case 5. Woman, 76, with an asymptomatic 90+% right internal carotid artery stenosis underwent carotid endarterectomy. She had a carotid stump back-pressure of 15 mm Hg and a collateral cerebral perfusion pressure of 9 mm Hg. Upon placement of the proximal end of a Javid shunt into the common carotid artery and flushing, a large amount of atheroma was noted in the shunt to the degree that it completely plugged it up. The shunt was removed, the common carotid artery flushed, and a second shunt placed. This was flushed, no further embolic material was noted, and the operation proceeded in an eventful manner. When the patient awoke from general anesthesia, her level of consciousness was diminished and she had a moderate left hemiparesis. A duplex scan demonstrated a normal patch reconstruction and normal flow velocity in the internal carotid artery. Anticoagulation was begun after a CAT scan showed no evidence of hemorrhage. Over the next 6 weeks she cleared and had no permanent neurologic deficit. Approximately 6 months after carotid endarterectomy, she developed atheroembolization to her lower extremities, kidneys, and mesentery and subsequently died of the complications of multiple emboli from a shaggy aortic arch and descending thoracic aorta.

Comment. This patient had shaggy atheroma in most of her aortic arch and branch vessels and was noted to have atheroemboli in the shunt; therefore, the presence of a neurologic deficit after manipulation of the common carotid artery was not surprising. However, confirmation that the internal carotid artery was opened by duplex scanning was clearly indicated with reoperation only if the artery was occluded.

Case 6. Man, 63, with an ulcerated and 80% stenotic internal carotid artery and a high bifurcation had a left carotid endarterectomy after two episodes of amaurosis fugax. During the procedure it was noted that the external carotid artery was severely diseased and branched early. Eversion endarterectomy of the external carotid was not successful. The remainder of the endarterectomy was uncomplicated. After restoration of blood flow, continuous-wave Doppler interrogation demonstrated very low flow in the external carotid artery. An isolated external carotid repair was performed by use of vessel loop occlusion on the branches and a small metal vascular clamp on the origin of the external carotid. On opening the artery, atheroma was observed in the proximal clamp. The clamp was briefly removed and the atheroma cleared from the lumen. An external carotid endarterectomy was completed, and repeat Doppler exam was normal. On awakening from general anesthesia, no neurologic deficit was noted; however, when the patient was ambulated the next day, he had a mild weakness in his left leg and foot. A duplex scan was normal. He gradually improved over the next 3 months.

Comment. This patient in all likelihood had embolization from the loose incompletely removed atheroma in the proximal external carotid when the clamp was placed. Because inadequate repair of the external carotid artery can be a source of postendarterectomy emboli, this vessel must be managed with the same care given the internal and common carotid arteries.

Case 7. Woman, 49, was seen with a moderately stenosed and severely ulcerated left internal carotid artery. She had frequent identical right arm and hand TIAs the week before carotid endarterectomy. She awoke neurologically intact from an uneventful left carotid endarterectomy, but approximately 2 hours later developed a TIA identical to the preoperative TIAs. A duplex scan was normal. The patient had another identical TIA on the second postoperative day and a third after being discharged from the hospital. She was maintained on aspirin.

Comment. I have had four patients with postoperative TIAs identical to the preoperative TIAs. These may continue for several weeks after surgery. I presume that there is a small ischemic zone that produces the symptoms for a short time. Carotid endarterectomy probably plays no role in this except to prevent further embolization.

Case 8. After a mild sensory TIA, a man, 72, had a duplex scan that demonstrated greater than 80% internal carotid artery stenosis with a flaplike mobile intraluminal thrombus attached to the distal end of the stenosis. When the arteriotomy was completed distal to the plaque, the thrombus was not present. The patient awoke from an otherwise uneventful carotid endarterectomy with a mild neurologic deficit. A duplex scan was normal.

Comment. This patient most likely had embolization of the thrombus during manipulation of the artery before clamp placement. Immediate reoperation was not advisable because the operating surgeon was relatively confident about the cause of the problem. It was appropriate to obtain a duplex scan to confirm that the internal carotid artery was patent and normal.

Case 9. Man, 69, was seen with asymptomatic bilateral 90% internal carotid artery stenosis. Two weeks after an uneventful right carotid endarterectomy, the left side was done. At the first operation, the carotid stump back-pressure was 23 mm Hg, and at the second it was 27 mm Hg. The patient was discharged on the second postoperative day and returned 2 days later with seizures and a 24-hour history of severe headache ipsilateral to the second carotid endarterectomy. He was admitted to the hospital and begun on antihypertensive and anticonvulsive therapy. A CAT scan showed ipsilateral cerebral edema but no infarction. A duplex scan was normal bilaterally. He had recurrent severe seizures and developed an ipsilateral ischemic stroke and a severe permanent neurologic deficit.

Comment. This is an example of the severe form of the hyperperfusion syndrome in a patient with major risk factors bilaterally, namely, poor collateral hemodynamics and high-grade stenosis.

REOPERATIVE TECHNIQUE AND MANAGEMENT

Reoperation for internal carotid artery occlusion and restoration of blood flow is the one intervention for a postoperative neurologic deficit that may dramatically improve the patient's condition. Most authors report that only 10% to 20% of patients with a new neurologic deficit are reoperated on for this problem and have, at best, a 50% probability of immediate improvement. The two major goals of reoperation are to directly evaluate the carotid arteries for occlusion, thrombosis, or major defect, and, if present, to restore patency and correct any underlying technical defect. After reopening the incision, the carotid arteries should be interrogated to determine patency and assess the presence of major abnormalities produced by technical error, dissection, or thrombus. Although palpation of the internal carotid artery distal to the reconstruction provides information about patency, a standard method of evaluation should be used. This is when in-depth experience with a routine method of confirmation of the adequacy of a carotid artery reconstruction is invaluable. The operating surgeon should have completed such an interrogation a few minutes or hours previously and thus can reassess the artery with knowledge of the prior postendarterectomy operative findings. Continuous-wave Doppler is an inexpensive and readily available technique not only for determining patency but also for establishing that the velocity waveform is normal, and for qualitatively interrogating the entire endarterectomized and reconstruction segments. Four possibilities exist: the internal carotid artery is occluded, the internal carotid artery is patent but there is an abnormal flow pattern and a qualitative velocity abnormality, the internal carotid is patent and the interrogation is normal, or the arteries are patent but normality of the endarterectomized and reconstructed segment cannot be adequately confirmed. If a duplex scan is available in the operating room, a more quantitative analysis can be obtained. As mentioned before, I have no experience with operative angiography, but this is an excellent method for investigating a patent but possibly abnormal arterial reconstruction without opening the artery.

The patient should be reheparinized before opening the artery. A shunt and a 3F or 4F balloon embolectomy catheter should be available. If a saphenous vein patch was not used at the first reconstruction, it is wise to prep the thigh for a possible vein harvest should the need arise for a patch or an interposition graft. I prefer elastic vessel loops for occlusion of the common and external carotid arteries, and these are carefully placed. If the internal carotid artery is thrombosed, an occlusion device should not be placed until the artery has been cleared because of the possibility of producing distal embolization. The arteriotomy is opened, the clot gently extracted from the internal carotid artery, and back bleeding observed briefly. Inspection of the distal tail of the thrombus is helpful in determining if there is retained partially occluding thrombus distally. A smooth, tapered thrombus and back bleeding consistent with that observed at the primary operation are indications of an open and clear internal carotid artery. Measurement of stump back-pressure is not helpful in determining if there is partially occluding thrombus. If there is confirmed or suspected retained thrombus in the internal carotid artery, a balloon catheter is advanced and withdrawn with very gentle balloon pressure lest vessel rupture or a cavernous sinus arterial venous malformation be produced. If the internal carotid artery cannot be opened or just a trickle of blood returns, it should be ligated and the external carotid artery reconstructed. After the artery is opened and the thrombus is removed, a shunt should be placed even if one was not used at the initial operation. If the patient was initially operated on with use of local or regional anesthesia without a shunt, the surgeon must assume that distal embolization from the occluded internal carotid artery occurred, and the new ischemic zone should be protected as soon as possible with a shunt. If the patient was operated on under general anesthesia without a shunt and awoke with a deficit, either low-flow or emboli-induced ischemia occurred, and a shunt may be beneficial.

After the internal carotid artery is cleared of thrombus and a shunt is placed, attention is turned to reconstruction. If there is an internal carotid artery end-point flap or defect, a technical problem with primary closure, or a kink, the new reconstruction must be tailored to correct the problem and prevent a recurrent thrombosis.[16] If no obvious defect is found, one must assume that some combination of a thrombogenic endarterectomized surface and a hypercoagulable state exists. Sundt[11] reported heparin-induced thrombocytopenia to be the cause of internal carotid artery thrombosis in 4 of 15 patients with early postendarterectomy internal carotid artery occlusions. This is worthy of consideration if the patient was on heparin preoperatively. If heparin cannot be given postoperatively, low-molecular-weight dextran is advisable. If the artery was initially primarily closed, patch reconstruction, preferably with greater saphenous vein, should be used. If there is redundancy of the endarterectomized internal carotid artery segment, it should be shortened to prevent kinking by transverse eversion plication. Perhaps the best revascularization technique in the setting of a thrombosed internal carotid artery with no identifiable defect is interposition bypass grafting with greater saphenous vein.

NONOPERATIVE MANAGEMENT

Depending on the etiology of the deficit, anticoagulation, antiplatelet, or rheologic therapy should be considered once it has been established that the artery is patent and a CAT or MRI scan confirms that there is no intracerebral hemorrhage. Most patients in whom a neurologic deficit is known or considered to be of embolic origin should be given heparin, particularly when it is unclear when the embolus occurred or what its origin was. When heparin cannot be used, low-molecular-weight dextran (30–50 mL per hour) should be considered. Patients with an abnormality demonstrated on duplex scan but not reoperated on should be anticoagulated with heparin. Therapeutic or low-dose Coumadin is normally given for 6 to 12 weeks, particularly if there is an unrepaired defect in the carotid artery. Consideration should be given to the use of ticlopidine, which has been demonstrated to minimize shear-induced platelet aggregation in patients with cerebral ischemia, whereas aspirin does not.[24] Hopefully, this drug will prove to be useful perioperatively. My experience with nonoperative management of minor neurologic deficits produced by emboli is that no further events are likely to occur.

PREVENTION

The best management of post–carotid endarterectomy neurologic deficits is prevention. Although it is generally agreed that the probability of perioperative stroke is highest in patients who had a preoperative stroke and lowest in patients with minimal or no symptoms,[1, 2, 17, 18] surgeon-related factors play a major role in perioperative stroke. Riles and colleagues[8] found that two thirds of their strokes were surgeon related and therefore potentially preventable. Similarly, one third of my patients with a perioperative stroke had an associated intraoperative event. Like Sundt,[11] I had a significant proportion of postoperative neurologic events that were caused by the hyperperfusion syndrome. Prevention of stroke in this latter group remains a clinical challenge and requires prompt recognition of patients at risk, blood pressure control, close observation, and evaluation with electroencephalogram (EEG) and CAT or MRI scans.

The operative prevention of stroke is founded on attention to multiple details of carotid endarterectomy. These include meticulous dissection with minimal manipulation of the carotid bulb, selective or obligatory use of a shunt (although only 1%–2% of patients may actually need it[25]), good completion end points of all three carotid arteries, optimal hemodynamic reconstruction that includes eversion plication shortening and patching or interposition grafting when indicated, and confirmation of an adequate reconstruction. Reconstruction should be customized to the operative findings and the condition of the endarterectomized artery to provide a hemodynamically optimal geometry.[26] Disturbed flow fields, particularly over a thrombogenic surface, are harbingers of thrombosis.[27–29] Turbulence in the carotid bulb after carotid endarterectomy has been shown to be associated with both residual stenosis and restenosis.[30] Complete endarterectomy and optimal reconstruction based on operative findings[16] should minimize the probability of internal carotid thrombosis and postoperative embolization. Our goal should be to eliminate these two preventable causes of neurologic deficits after carotid endarterectomy.

REFERENCES

1. Perdue GD: Management of postendarterectomy neurologic deficits. *Arch Surg* 117:1079–1081, 1982.
2. Rosenthal D, Zeichner WD, Lamis PA, et al: Neurologic deficit after carotid endarterectomy: Pathogenesis and management. *Surgery* 94:776–780, 1983.
3. Moore WS, Quinones-Baldrich WJ: Extracranial cerebrovascular disease. In Moore WS, editor: *Vascular surgery*. Philadelphia, 1991, WB Saunders, pp 459–461.
4. Adams HP, Brett TJ, Crowell RM, et al: Guidelines for the management of patients with acute ischemic stroke. *Stroke* 25:1901–1914, 1994.
5. Hertzer NR, Beven EG, Modic MT, et al: Early patency of the carotid artery after endarterectomy: Digital subtraction angiography after two hundred sixty-two operations. *Surgery* 92:1049–1053, 1982.
6. Van Alphen HAM, Polman CH: Carotid endarterectomy: How does it work? A clinical and angiographic evaluation. *Stroke* 17:1251–1253, 1986.
7. Rosenthal D, Archie JP, Garcia-Rinaldi R, et al: Carotid patch angioplasty: Immediate and long-term results. *J Vasc Surg* 12:326–333, 1990.
8. Riles TS, Imparato AM, Jacobowitz GR, et al: The cause of perioperative stroke after carotid endarterectomy. *J Vasc Surg* 19:206–216, 1994.
9. Boysen G: Cerebral blood flow measurement as a safeguard during carotid endarterectomy. *Stroke* 2:1–10, 1971.
10. Sundt TM: The ischemic tolerance of neural tissue and the need for monitor-

ing and selective shunting during carotid endarterectomy. *Stroke* 14:93–98, 1983.

11. Sundt TM: *Occlusive cerebrovascular disease: Diagnosis and surgical management.* Philadelphia, 1987, WB Saunders, pp 229, 252–258.

12. Lord RSA: *Surgery of occlusive cerebrovascular disease.* St. Louis, 1986, Mosby, pp 227–280.

13. Reigel MM, Hollier LH, Sundt TM, et al: Cerebral hyperperfusion syndrome: A cause of neurologic dysfunction after carotid endarterectomy. *J Vasc Surg* 5:628–634, 1987.

14. Pomposelli FB, Lamparello PL, Riles TS, et al: Intracranial hemorrhage after carotid endarterectomy. *J Vasc Surg* 7:248–255, 1988.

15. Harrison PB, Wong MJ, Belzberg A, et al: Hyperperfusion syndrome after carotid endarterectomy. *Neuroradiology* 33:106–110, 1991.

16. Archie JP: Carotid endarterectomy with reconstruction techniques tailored to operative findings. *J Vasc Surg* 17:141–151, 1993.

17. Collins GJ, Rich NM, Anderson CA, et al: Stroke associated with carotid endarterectomy. *Am J Surg* 83:306–312, 1978.

18. Steed DL, Peitzman AB, Grundy BI, et al: Causes of stroke in carotid endarterectomy. *Surgery* 92:634–641, 1982.

19. Krul JMJ, VanGijn J, Acherstaft RGA, et al: Site and pathogenesis of infarcts associated with carotid endarterectomy. *Stroke* 20:324–328, 1989.

20. Archie JP: Hemodynamics of carotid back pressure and cerebral flow during endarterectomy. *J Surg Res* 23:223–232, 1977.

21. Archie JP, Feldtman RW: Determinants of cerebral perfusion pressure during carotid endarterectomy. *Arch Surg* 117:319–322, 1982.

22. Archie JP, Feldtman RW: Linear response of collateral cerebral perfusion pressure during carotid clamping. *J Surg Res* 46:253–255, 1989.

23. Archie JP: Technique and clinical results of carotid stump back-pressure to determine selective shunting during carotid endarterectomy. *J Vasc Surg* 13:319–327, 1991.

24. Uchiyama S, Yamazaki M, Maruyama S, et al: Shear-induced platelet aggregation in cerebral ischemia. *Stroke* 25:1547–1551, 1994.

25. Baker WH, Littooy FN, Haynes AC, et al: Carotid endarterectomy without a shunt: The control series. *J Vasc Surg* 1:50–56, 1984.

26. Kleinstreuer C, Nazemi M, Archie JP: Hemodynamics analysis of a stenosed carotid bifurcation and its plaque-mitigating design. *ASME J Biomech Eng* 113:330–335, 1991.

27. Stain PD, Sabbah HN: Measured turbulence and its effect on thrombus formation. *Circ Res* 35:608–614, 1974.

28. Goldsmith HL, Turitto VT: Rheological aspects of thrombosis and haemostasis: Basic principles and applications. *Thromb Haemost* 55:415–435, 1986.

29. Gregory K, Basmadjian D: An analysis of the contact phase of blood coagulation: Effects of shear rate and surface are intertwined. *Ann Biomed Eng* 22:184–193, 1994.

30. Bandyk DF, Kaebnick HW, Adams MB, et al: Turbulence occurring after carotid endarterectomy: A harbinger of residual and recurrent stenosis. *J Vasc Surg* 7:261–274, 1988.

Intraoperative, Postendarterectomy Duplex Evaluation

William H. Baker, M.D.

Professor and Chief, Section of Peripheral Vascular Surgery, Loyola University of Chicago Stritch School of Medicine, Maywood, Illinois

Carotid endarterectomy has been established as the treatment of choice for patients who clinically have transient ischemic attacks or mild strokes and an appropriate, severe carotid artery stenosis.[1, 2] Patients who have the above symptoms and only a moderate stenosis may be treated with either operation or medical therapy. These patients are currently being randomly allocated to each treatment arm in the ongoing North American Symptomatic Carotid Endarterectomy Trial (NASCET). Those patients with neurologic symptoms that are associated with mild carotid stenosis are usually treated with the best medical therapy, except under unusual and special circumstances. Finally, those patients who are asymptomatic but who harbor a severe carotid stenosis are best protected from stroke by prophylactic carotid endarterectomy.[3, 4]

All of the aforementioned clinical decisions assume that operation can be safely performed. Past studies have underscored that the stroke and death rate associated with carotid endarterectomy is highly variable. Whereas numerous studies have reported a combined stroke and death rate of approximately 2%, others have suggested that it is 10% overall in the United States.[5, 6] Furthermore, Hsia and colleagues[7] have pointed out that death rates after operation in the community hospital are in general higher than those in university hospitals, casting doubt as to the widespread applicability of carotid endarterectomy if indeed the indications for operation are based on university-established stroke and death rates. The recently announced Asymptomatic Carotid Atherosclerosis Study (ACAS) had a stroke and death rate of 2.3%.[3] This figure includes five strokes (1.2%) suffered at the time of carotid angiography. This low stroke and death rate associated with operation was achieved in 39 different centers, many of which would be classified as community hospitals. This stroke and death rate demonstrates that a low morbidity and mortality can be achieved and thus should be the goal of all surgeons caring for patients with atherosclerosis.

Although there are many causes of stroke associated with operation, most surgeons agree that the sine qua non of a successful operation is technical perfection. The most common cause of operation-related stroke is either intraoperative embolization, postoperative embolization, or postoperative occlusion. Intraoperative embolization may be minimized by gentle operative techniques. Postoperative embolization and occlusion usually arise from technical imperfections. Thus, postclosure intraoperative assessment is desirable to detect such imperfections.

Surgeons have attempted to assess their operations in a variety of ways. The ideal method is time efficient, not costly, and risk free, and it identifies abnormalities that, if corrected, improve patient care. Intraoperative arteriography has been used for many years.[8, 9] The common carotid artery is punctured with a needle, and potentially dangerous contrast material is injected. From a practical point of view, it is rare to have complications associated with this procedure. Approximately 10 mL of contrast material is injected and a film obtained. The carotid artery is usually visualized in one plane only. The aggravation associated with operative arteriography, be it with positioning of the patient, timing of the films, or delay due to technician or machine unavailability, has made this a cumbersome surveillance technique. The older cited series had revision rates of 26% and 8%. However, many of these revisions were in the external carotid artery only, a procedure that may or may not have lessened the risk of postoperative stroke in these patients.

Intraoperative endoscopy has been used for years to visualize the external and distal internal carotid artery.[10] The old rigid endoscopes were too bulky for vascular use; thus, one third of the arteries could not be visualized. The magnification obtained by endoscopy makes relatively small defects appear larger than they are. It is very difficult to visualize the common carotid shelf in a meaningful fashion because the flow of irrigation fluid runs countercurrent to the usual flow of blood. The arterioscope can inspect some of the distal closure but obviously cannot inspect the entire closure because the scope is inserted through the arteriotomy. Use of the intraoperative endoscope may add as much as 5 minutes of time to a patient's ischemia. In some patients who require a temporary indwelling shunt, this may become critical.

Intraoperative auscultation with a hand-held Doppler allows the surgeon to listen to the Doppler-derived signal. Clearly, gross abnormalities and turbulent flow will be discovered by use of this technique. Abnormalities that do not disturb flow will be missed. There have been no studies to date to determine whether or not all significant abnormalities can be detected by this technique.

At Loyola University Chicago, we prefer to interrogate the operated carotid with duplex ultrasonography. This allows us to both assess the systolic and diastolic flow patterns and visualize the operated artery in two planes. Large and small abnormalities of the operated carotid artery can be visualized with this technique.[11]

METHOD OF THE EXAMINATION

After the carotid arteriotomy has been closed and hemostasis obtained, the duplex scanner (Advanced Technology Laboratories, Bothel, Washington) that is used in our peripheral vascular laboratory is rolled into the operating room. A 10-MHz probe is encased in a sterile plastic covering into which coupling gel has been inserted. The probe and sheath are placed into the wound, and ultrasonic coupling between the sheath and the artery is achieved by flooding the wound with saline. The large size of the 10-MHz probe makes some examinations more difficult. However, with practice, this becomes a relatively easy exercise.

Interrogation is begun proximal to the endarterectomized segment in the common carotid artery and continued distally. The proximal common carotid end point is visualized and the thickness of the proximal common carotid intima is noted. The carotid bulb is next interrogated, and an experienced ultrasonographer can easily differentiate the external from the internal carotid arteries. In some patients, rather tortuous vessels are more difficult to examine. These examinations are sometimes best completed with some traction on the carotid artery, either to rotate the artery into view or to straighten a difficult-to-examine tortuous carotid. The distal end point may be difficult to visualize if this end point has extended much beyond the angle of the mandible. After a normal examination has been completed, the wound is closed in the usual fashion.

In our review, we observed all small defects less than 2 to 3 mm in size, unless the surgeon believed that the defect represented thrombus. Larger abnormalities were usually corrected. Separate arteriotomies on the large common carotid artery were sometimes performed to avoid re-opening the entire original arteriotomy. If the arteriotomy was reopened, the secondary closure usually involved patch angioplasty.

RESULTS OF INTRAOPERATIVE DUPLEX SCANNING

We recently published our results of 316 intraoperative duplex scans performed in 283 patients.[11] One hundred and four patients were women and 212 were men. The mean age was 66 years, with a range of 42 to 82 years. A scan was not performed on all carotid endarterectomies because either the scanner or technologist was not available on 42 occasions.

The intraoperative duplex examination was unequivocally normal in 254 (80.4%) of our patients. That is, these scans demonstrated perfectly normal frequencies and no turbulent flow, and no small fronds were seen in any aspect of the artery. A thickened proximal common carotid shelf was not seen.

A defect was seen in 62 (19.6%) of the carotid arteries examined. Fifty-three of these 62 defects (85.5%) were not explored, whereas nine (14.5%) were (Fig 1).

The minor defects that were not re-explored were mostly thickened proximal end points of the common carotid artery (N = 35). If a thickened common carotid shelf adherent to the carotid wall was seen, and this shelf appeared to be a 10% stenosis or less, it was not re-explored. Five patients had small (<2–3 mm in size) fronds or other defects in the internal carotid artery. Two patients had like defects in the external carotid artery. Two patients had a small frond that was seen in the bulb only (Fig 2). Interestingly, two patients had a thickened wall of a vein patch. Seven patients had a kink of the internal carotid artery distal to the endarterectomy site, and two of these were associated with minimal retained atheroma.

The decision to explore or not re-explore is sometimes difficult. Some

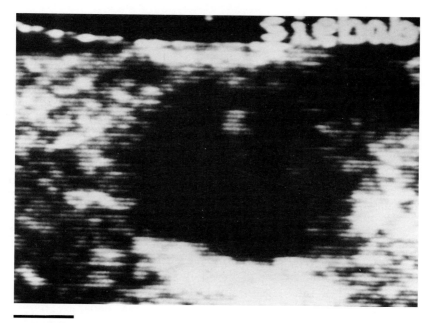

FIGURE 1.
This defect was hanging from the suture line. At exploration, a 3–4-mm thrombus was removed.

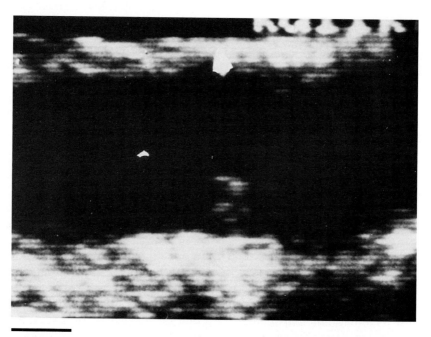

FIGURE 2.
A 3-mm frond was seen waving during systole and diastole. This was not explored. The patient did well.

authors believe that small defects that occur after endarterectomy are of no consequence.[12] Animal studies seem to verify this opinion.[13] Later on in this chapter, our late results will be presented. These late results suggest that all defects should be explored.

EARLY RESULTS

The early (0–30 days) stroke rate for these 316 operations was 1.6%. The presence or absence of minor ultrasound abnormalities did not appear to influence the clinical result. Of the patients with a normal intraoperative duplex examination, four (1.3%) had a stroke. Three of these four patients had a stroke due to an early internal carotid artery occlusion. One of these patients died.

There was one stroke (1.9%) among the 53 patients who had unrepaired, minor defects that were not re-explored. This one stroke was due to an early internal carotid artery occlusion. No occlusions or new strokes occurred in the nine patients who underwent re-exploration for offending duplex abnormalities. Thus, the incidence of early stroke was equal in all groups. Residual, minor defects were not associated with early postoperative stroke.

Regardless, intraoperative duplex scanning did influence the performance of our operation. Almost immediately we began to extend the common carotid arteriotomy proximally to ensure that the offending shelf of the proximal common carotid atheroma was more completely removed. Others would suggest that this is not necessary. Courbier and associates[14] reported that 17 of 21 proximal common carotid shelfs resolved in their patients. Only four of their patients progressed, and all of these progressed to a <50% stenosis. Gonzalez and co-workers[15] suggested that this shelf is benign and later blends to become less distinct. Nonetheless, we were offended by its visual presence. One of our patients early in our experience had a nonadherent, flapping, retained thickened atheroma at this area, which undoubtedly influenced our opinion in this regard (Figs 3 and 4).

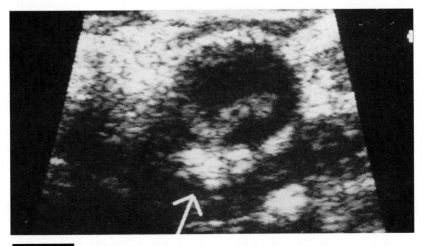

FIGURE 3.
A cross-sectional view of the waving proximal common carotid end point.

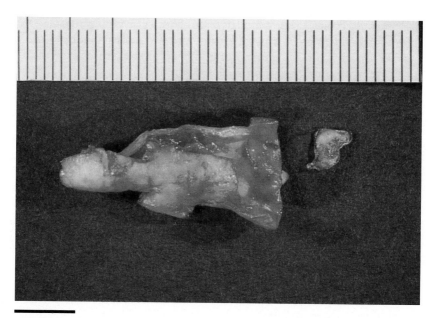

FIGURE 4.

At exploration, this impressive atheroma was removed from the patient imaged in Figure 3.

INFLUENCE OF SCANNING OVER THE YEARS

Intraoperative duplex scanning was initiated in 1986. Four of our re-explorations based on duplex scanning occurred in the first year of the study. After a year in which no re-explorations were performed, two were performed in 1988. In the next 3 years, no re-explorations were performed. However, three patients in 1992 required re-exploration, underscoring the continued importance of intraoperative surveillance. We believe that this intraoperative surveillance has been instrumental in helping us to improve and maintain our operative technique over time.

LATE RESULTS

Follow-up examination was performed on all of our 283 patients a mean of 21.6 months after operation. Of the surviving patients with 251 patent carotid arteries whose initial intraoperative duplex examination was normal, four were found to be stenotic (PSF > 8000 Hz) on postoperative day 1, and four additional patients returned with a significant (>75% area) stenosis at 6, 7, 19, and 90 months. Three of these later stenoses were in the internal carotid artery, and all were within the endarterectomized segment. Two may have been within the endarterectomized segment but were quite proximal and could also have been related to a proximal end point. None of the patients who returned with stenoses had hemispheric symptoms.

There were 53 patients who had minimal defects but were not re-explored. Of the 52 patent carotid arteries that were available for re-examination, nine arteries in eight patients (17.3%) had a <75% area stenosis. Six were noted on postoperative day 1, and the remainder were noted at 27, 32, and 80 months. One artery that was stenotic on postoperative day 1 was occluded on postoperative day 30. Interestingly, all of these stenoses were within the endarterectomized segment of the bulb and internal carotid artery. No patient returned with hemispheric symptoms. Chi-square analysis comparing the recurrence rate between the patients who had a normal intraoperative duplex scan and the patients who had a minimal defect was highly significant ($P = 0.002$).

There were nine patients who had their carotid endarterectomy site revised. Whereas eight of these patients were normal, one patient returned with a significant stenosis in the endarterectomized segment at 6 months (11.1%).

It is of interest that our patients were fairly evenly divided between those who had primary closure (N = 162) and those who had patch angioplasty (N = 153). There were five strokes in total. Three of these strokes occurred in patients closed with use of patch angioplasty, and two occurred after primary closure. Four operation-related occlusions were discovered. None of these occlusions occurred in patients with patch angioplasty closure.

The late follow-up of these patients was likewise interesting. Four restenoses occurred in the patch angioplasty patients, whereas 11 restenoses (plus the four immediate occlusions) occurred in the primarily closed vessels (chi-square $P = 0.025$).

In the entire series, there have been no late strokes in follow-up. One of our patients who had bilateral carotid endarterectomies has a progressive hemiparesis related to the second endarterectomy. Despite his clinical condition, he has normal computed tomography and magnetic resonance scan. Three additional patients have returned with transient ischemic attacks. None of these patients had a demonstrated stenosis.

COMMENT

The incidence of neurologic symptoms after carotid endarterectomy is known to be low. The results in our most recent series are excellent. The late clinical results in both the NASCET and the ACAS studies are also excellent and underscore the value of carotid endarterectomy in stroke prevention. If, indeed, stroke prevention is linked to a widely patent internal carotid artery, then it is important that our patients have an operation that results in long-term patency.

The incidence of severe, late internal carotid artery restenosis after operation has been reported to be as low as 3%[16] and as high as 23%.[17] Some years ago we published a restenosis rate of 10% in a series of 133 serially tested carotid arteries.[18] It will be interesting to note the incidence of restenosis in the ACAS patients. This is the only study that has standardized the criteria for significant stenosis among its participating diagnostic laboratories. If the incidence of restenosis late after operation in this series is low, this will further support the use of operation in asymptomatic patients.

The causes of recurrent carotid stenosis are clearly multifactorial. Patients who are hypercholesterolemic and continue to smoke tend to have an increased incidence of restenosis. Interestingly, hypertension does not appear to be related to recurrent carotid stenosis, despite its importance as a risk factor for atherosclerosis. Recurrent internal carotid artery stenosis is said to be more common in women. It has been hypothesized that this recurrence in women may be because of the smaller arterial diameter noted in women. However, accelerated atherosclerosis in these females cannot be ruled out. Furthermore, the finding that recurrent stenosis is more common in women is not universal.

The importance of intraoperative monitoring cannot be overemphasized. Originally, we believed that this technology would improve our immediate operative results; particularly, we hoped it would help eliminate postoperative occlusions. Interestingly, although our incidence of postoperative occlusion is low, this problem has not been eliminated. Furthermore, three of the four strokes in our patients who had a normal intraoperative scan were due to internal carotid artery occlusion. Clearly, the presence of a normal intraoperative scan does not rule out the possibility that postoperative occlusion can occur. The operating surgeon cannot deny prompt reoperation to a patient who has a stroke in the recovery room on the basis of a previously normal intraoperative scan.

The finding that even small abnormalities on intraoperative scanning could lead to an increased incidence of late postoperative restenosis was somewhat surprising. Other authors, however, have had identical experiences. Dr. Barnes[19] in 1986 used intraoperative monitoring with Doppler spectrum analysis. He detected 10 internal carotid artery stenoses after 125 carotid endarterectomies (8.0%). He suggested that late recurrent carotid artery stenosis may actually be residual carotid artery stenosis. That is, spectral abnormalities were present from the beginning. Sanders and colleagues[20] used both ultrasound duplex scanning and intravenous digital subtraction angiography to study 109 patients with internal carotid endarterectomies. Their rate of restenosis at 3, 6, 12, and 24 months was 6%, 12%, 6%, and 8%, respectively. Like Barnes, they noted that approximately one half of their significant restenoses seen at 1 year had already been demonstrated at 1 week. Bandyk and associates[21] from Milwaukee studied 250 carotid endarterectomies with pulse-wave Doppler spectral analysis as well as arteriography. He found 68 arteries with residual flow disturbances. These arteries had a restenosis/occlusion rate of 21% at 2 years' follow-up. This was compared with his patients with a normal examination, who had a recurrent stenosis rate of 9%. Salvian and co-workers[22] from UCLA reported that gross technical problems were seen in the operative reports in 75% of their patients in whom restenosis developed. Our data agree with this opinion. Thirteen of the 21 restenoses identified in this study were present on postoperative day 1. All of the above-cited papers, as well as our series, strongly suggest that late recurrence of stenosis is directly related to operative imperfection.

One can only speculate about the exact pathogenesis of these restenoses. Perhaps minor defects lead to local flow disturbances. These flow disturbances may favor platelet deposition and enhance a hyperplastic healing response. Until the exact mechanism of this process is understood, surgeons can only hope to modify the process by performing a technically superior operation. Does patch angioplasty modify this response regardless of the intraoperative duplex scan? The relatively small number of recurrences in our series makes such an analysis statistically invalid. However, it is interesting to note that the number of recurrences in our patients closed with a patch angioplasty technique was indeed lower ($P = 0.025$) when compared with the number of recurrences in patients who had a primary closure. It may well be that enlargement of the carotid bulb minimizes the significance of small defects seen on intraoperative scanning.

CONCLUSION

Early and late post—carotid endarterectomy stenosis/occlusion appears to be directly related to the technical performance of the operation. Intraoperative duplex ultrasonography accurately assesses the postendarterectomy carotid artery and is recommended as a valuable tool to ensure the best possible result.

REFERENCES

1. North American Symptomatic Carotid Endarterectomy Trial Collaborators: Beneficial effect of carotid endarterectomy in symptomatic patients with high-grade carotid stenosis. *N Engl J Med* 325:445–453, 1991.
2. European Carotid Surgery Trialists' Collaborative Group: MRC European Carotid Surgery Trial: Interim results for symptomatic patients with severe (70–99%) or with mild (0–29%) carotid stenosis. *Lancet* 337:1235–1257, 1991.
3. Executive Committee for the Asymptomatic Carotid Atherosclerosis Study: Endarterectomy for Asymptomatic Carotid Artery Stenosis. *JAMA* 273:1421–1428, 1995.
4. Hobson RW, Weiss DG, Fields WS, et al: Efficacy of carotid endarterectomy for asymptomatic carotid stenosis. *N Engl J Med* 328:221–227, 1993.
5. Baker WH, Littooy FN, Hayes AC, et al: Carotid endarterectomy without a shunt: The control series. *J Vasc Surg* 1:50–56, 1984.
6. Winslow CM, Solomon DH, Chassin MR, et al: The appropriateness of carotid endarterectomy. *N Engl J Med* 318:721–727, 1988.
7. Hsia DC, Krushat WM, Moscoe LM: Epidemiology of carotid endarterectomies among Medicare beneficiaries. *J Vasc Surg* 16:201–208, 1992.
8. Blaisdell FW, Lim R Jr, Hall AD: Technical results of carotid endarterectomy: Arteriographic assessment. *Am J Surg* 114:239, 1967.
9. Rosental JJ, Gaspar MR, Movius HJ: Intraoperative arteriography in carotid thromboendarterectomy. *Arch Surg* 106:806, 1973.
10. Towne JB, Bernhard VM: Vascular endoscopy: Usable tool or interesting toy. *Surgery* 82:415, 1977.
11. Baker WH, Koustas G, Burke K, et al: Intraoperative duplex scanning and late carotid artery stenosis. *J Vasc Surg* 19:829–833, 1994.
12. Flanigan DP, Douglas DJ, Machi J: Intraoperative ultrasonic imaging of the carotid artery during carotid endarterectomy. *Surgery* 5:893–898, 1986.
13. Coelho JCU, Sigel B, Flanigan DP, et al: Detection of arterial defects by real-time ultrasound scanning during vascular surgery: An experimental study. *J Surg Res* 30:535–543, 1981.
14. Courbier R, Ferdani M: Criteria for immediate reoperation following carotid surgery. In Bergan JJ, Yao JST, editors: *Reoperative arterial surgery.* Orlando, 1986, Grune & Stratton, pp 495–507.
15. Gonzalez LL, Partusch L, Wirth P: Noninvasive carotid artery evaluation following endarterectomy. *J Vasc Surg* 1:403–408, 1984.

16. Sundt TM, Whisnant JP, Houser OW, et al: Prospective study of the effectiveness and durability of carotid endarterectomy. *Mayo Clin Proc* 65:625–635, 1990.
17. Zbornikova V, Elfstrom J, Lassvik C, et al: Restenosis and occlusion after carotid surgery assessed by duplex scanning and digital subtraction angiography. *Stroke* 17:1137–1142, 1986.
18. Baker WH, Hayes AC, Mahler D, et al: Durability of carotid endarterectomy. *Surgery* 94:112–115, 1983.
19. Barnes RW, Nix ML, Nichols BT, et al: Recurrent versus residual carotid stenosis. *Ann Surg* 203:652–660, 1986.
20. Sanders EACM, Hoeneveld H, Eikelboom BC, et al: Residual lesions and early recurrent stenosis after carotid endarterectomy. *J Vasc Surg* 5:731–737, 1987.
21. Bandyk DF, Kaebnick HW, Adams MB, et al: Turbulence occurring after carotid bifurcation endarterectomy: A harbinger of residual and recurrent carotid stenosis. *J Vasc Surg* 7:261–274, 1988.
22. Salvian A, Baker JD, Machleder HI, et al: Cause and noninvasive detection of restenosis after carotid endarterectomy. *Am J Surg* 146:29–34, 1983.

PART III

Aorta

Ruptured Abdominal Aortic Aneurysm: From Diagnosis to Discharge*

Thomas F. Lindsay, M.D., F.R.C.S.(C.)

Division of Vascular Surgery, The Toronto Hospital, Toronto, Ontario, Canada;
Assistant Professor of Surgery, University of Toronto, Toronto, Ontario, Canada

K. Wayne Johnston, M.D., F.R.C.S.(C.)

Division of Vascular Surgery, The Toronto Hospital, Toronto, Ontario, Canada;
Professor of Surgery and Chairman, Division of Vascular Surgery, University of
Toronto, Toronto, Ontario, Canada

Rupture of an abdominal aortic aneurysm (AAA) remains a lethal condition. Although reports of the in-hospital mortality rates are between 40% and 70%,[1-6] the overall mortality, including patients who die before admission to hospital, is 90%.[1] No decline in the mortality rate for ruptured AAA has been observed despite advances in all phases of the care of these patients, but there has been a decline in mortality rates for patients having elective AAA repair.[7] Improved results for elective AAA have not created an improved rate of survival for patients with ruptured AAA. In this chapter, the key features related to diagnosis, resuscitation, operative approaches, results, and complications will be reviewed.

DEFINITION

A ruptured AAA can be defined as disruption of the dilated aortic wall that leads to extravasation of blood outside the aorta. A further subclassification differentiates retroperitoneal rupture from free rupture. With a retroperitoneal rupture, bleeding is contained in the retroperitoneal space, whereas with a free rupture, either the direction of the rupture or expansion of the retroperitoneal hematoma leads to uncontained bleeding into the peritoneal cavity. The prognosis of a free rupture is significantly worse.[8]

Patients with symptomatic aneurysms who present with severe back and abdominal pain may have pain that is indistinguishable from that experienced by ruptured patients; however, at laparotomy, blood has not leaked beyond the wall of the aorta, and consequently they are not considered to have ruptured AAA. In this case, the etiology of the pain may

*Supported by the Physicians of Ontario through the Physician Services Incorporated Foundation.

Advances in Vascular Surgery®, vol. 3
© 1995, Mosby-Year Book, Inc.

be related to acute expansion of the wall, intramural hemorrhage, bleeding into the mural thrombus, or degeneration of the wall; however, these patients must be considered separately from ruptured AAA patients and are excluded from reports of ruptured AAA.

INCIDENCE

The incidence of aortic aneurysms varies with the age and gender of the population. An increase in incidence has been noted in two Mayo Clinic studies that reported an increase from 12.2 per 100,000 to 36.2 per 100,000 over a period of 30 years from 1951 to 1980.[9, 10] Two studies from Sweden have reported the incidence of ruptured aortic aneurysm in stable populations. The strength of these studies is that the autopsy rate is between 85% and 100%; thus, the cause of death was confirmed in most cases. The first study from Malmö noted that the rate of ruptured AAA did not increase between 1971 and 1986 when results were age and sex standardized.[11] These authors noted that the incidence of ruptured AAA increased with age, peaking between 80 and 89 years for men, with an incidence of 112.7 per 100,000, and above 90 years for women, with an incidence of 67.6 per 100,000. A second Swedish study from Göteborg noted a dramatic increase in the incidence of ruptured AAA cases between 1952 and 1988.[2] This study was standardized for age and noted a 2.4% per year increase in the incidence of ruptured AAA. During the same period of time, the rate of ruptured thoracic aneurysm did not increase. Over the most recent period (1980–1988), the proportion of ruptured abdominal aortic aneurysms operated upon increased to 37%; between 1952 and 1959, only 3.6% of patients underwent operative intervention, with a 100% mortality rate. The 30-day survival of operated cases increased to 50%. The study confirmed that many patients died outside the hospital. Taking these cases into account, the overall mortality was 85%.

The incidence of abdominal aortic aneurysm is estimated to be 5% in patients over the age of 65. The ratio of men to women with aneurysms is 4 to 1.

The incidence of ruptured AAA in North America has not been well documented; however, in 1988, 14,982 deaths resulted from AAA in people older than 55 years of age.[1] Ruptured aneurysm is the tenth leading cause of death in the United States of men over the age of 55. Studies from Great Britain have also suggested an increase in the incidence of ruptured aneurysms. If the incidence in North America is similar to that being observed in Sweden and Britain, then it is expected that the burden of suffering and the associated dollar costs, which are already substantial, are going to increase with aging of the population.

RISK OF ANEURYSM RUPTURE AND PREDISPOSING FACTORS

Every patient requires individual attention with respect to their risk of rupture and benefit of repair; however, it is helpful to understand which factors have been demonstrated to be associated with an increase in the risk of rupture. The risk of aneurysm rupture varies with the size of the aneurysm and other factors. The risk of rupture of a 5-cm aneurysm is 14.4 events per 100 patient years of observation.[12] An autopsy study from Rome examined 297 pathologic cases of intact and ruptured AAA to identify risk factors associated with rupture.[13] Rupture was independently predicted in a multivariate analysis by size of the AAA, arterial hypertension, and the presence of bronchiectasis. Univariate analysis noted that saccular aneurysms were more likely to rupture than fusiform ones. These factors enable the clinician to include individual patient characteristics when a decision is made with regard to the risks and benefits of repair.

DIAGNOSIS

CLINICAL FEATURES

A good clinical history and appropriate physical findings on examination are sufficient diagnostic information to mandate immediate surgical referral for operative intervention. The sudden onset of severe abdominal and/or back pain and syncope form a clinical history that should alert medical personnel to entertain the diagnosis of ruptured AAA.[14] Other historical features may include a known history of AAA and vomiting. Pertinent factors on physical examination include hypotension, tachycardia, the presence of an abdominal mass, and abdominal tenderness, frequently in the area of rupture. A pulsatile mass may be absent or difficult to palpate in patients with large abdominal girth. Several case reports have noted that the presenting diagnosis can be incarceration of an inguinal hernia secondary to the increased intra-abdominal pressure, and in these cases the attendant abdominal pain has been ascribed to traction on the mesentery or bowel obstruction.[15] A patient with an aortocaval fistula may demonstrate distended neck veins, congestive heart failure, a murmur in the abdomen, and hematuria, which can be macro- and/or microscopic, but this situation is uncommon. Other communications between aortic aneurysms and major veins include rupture into the iliac veins or into the left renal vein. The latter has also been observed as an acute left varicocele or hematuria.[16]

DIFFERENTIAL DIAGNOSIS

The differential diagnosis includes renal colic, diverticulitis, and, less frequently, appendicitis, pancreatitis, gastrointestinal hemorrhage, inferior myocardial infarction, and perforated ulcer. Clinical presentations of ruptured AAA vary dramatically from clear-cut cases to subtle cases, where significant delays often occur. Frequently, an increase in the intensity of the pain or the onset of hypotension suggests the diagnosis in cases in which the presentation was subtle initially. Marston and colleagues[14] noted a misdiagnosis rate of 30% in their series, where the most common diagnoses were renal colic, diverticulitis, and gastrointestinal hemorrhage. In patients who were initially misdiagnosed, a high incidence of shock, abdominal pain, and back pain was noted; however, a pulsatile mass was noted in only 26%, compared with 76% for the properly diagnosed group. The classic triad of abdominal and back pain, shock, and a pulsatile mass was found in only 9% of those patients who were initially misdiagnosed, compared with 34% in the correctly diagnosed group. This was frequently due to the lack of a palpable mass that was noted later on examination by a surgical consultant. The presence of a palpable mass on initial examination was associated with a misdiagnosis rate of 14%, whereas the lack of one was associated with a misdiagnosis rate of 53%. Thus, the inability to detect a pulsatile mass frequently confused the diagnosis of ruptured AAA. Paradoxically, those in whom the initial diagnosis was incorrect had a mortality rate of 44%, compared with 58% for the correctly diagnosed patients. This negative correlation between delay of diagnosis and death was attributed to selection bias, because patients who were able to survive a prolonged delay had less severe rupture. The authors stress that the diagnosis of a ruptured AAA should be considered in all elderly men with abdominal or back pain and with any episode of hypotension. Careful examination for a palpable mass should be performed by an experienced examiner in any suspected case. A reduction in the number of patients who are incorrectly diagnosed should result in an increased survival rate for ruptured AAA.

PLAIN RADIOGRAPHS

In patients who show subtle findings but have a suspected ruptured AAA, several diagnostic modalities may be used, including plain radiographs of the abdomen. Loughran[17] reviewed 31 cases of ruptured AAA retrospectively and noted evidence of the diagnosis on 90% of the plain films. Calcification within the aortic wall well beyond the limits of the normal aorta was noted in 65%, loss of one or both psoas shadows was present in 75%, and obliteration of one or both renal outlines was found in 78%. These findings suggest that in a stable patient, plain radiographs may be useful when reviewed with an expert radiologist.

ABDOMINAL ULTRASOUND

The diagnostic role of abdominal ultrasound examination in the emergency department has been evaluated in 60 consecutive patients at Harborview Medical Center.[18] The majority of patients were initially evaluated by paramedics, and the sonographer was called to the emergency department before the patient actually arrived at the hospital. A rapid study (1 minute) was performed to evaluate the aorta and adjacent areas while intravenous access, assessment of vital signs, and phlebotomy were being performed. An aneurysm was correctly identified in 31 of 32 patients who proved to have an AAA at surgery or on subsequent computed tomography (CT) scan. At surgery, 24 patients were found to have a ruptured AAA, but ultrasound documented extramural blood in only one patient. Thus, rapid ultrasound in the emergency department can accurately diagnose AAA; however, it is not sensitive for detecting extraluminal blood.

COMPUTED TOMOGRAPHIC SCAN

Several studies have retrospectively examined the accuracy of computed tomography (CT scan) in cases of suspected ruptured AAA. When the presence of retroperitoneal blood was used as the gold standard, one study[19] found that the sensitivity of CT in the detection of AAA rupture was 77%, the specificity 100%, the false-negative rate 23%, and the false-positive rate 0%. The overall accuracy was 92%, with a positive predictive value of 100% and a negative predictive value of 89%. In a second study, 65 hemodynamically stable patients with suspected ruptured AAA were scanned and 18 were diagnosed as having a rupture by CT scan; 17 of these ruptures were proved at surgery.[20] Three patients had no AAA, whereas 44 were found to have an AAA but no leak on CT scan. Only one of these patients with a negative CT scan had a ruptured AAA, which was repaired the next day. Thirteen had other causes of pain identified, and 24 underwent elective surgical repair for intact AAAs. The authors concluded that CT scanning is useful in hemodynamically stable patients for detecting AAA and evaluating the possibility of rupture, and that this approach does not adversely affect the outcome. Siegel and Cohan[20] suggest that CT is the technique of choice when the diagnosis of ruptured AAA is being considered. Fortunately, false-negative studies (i.e., no leak on CT but a ruptured AAA at surgery) are rare, because this could lead to delayed surgery or death. Thus, even in those patients with an apparently unruptured AAA on CT scan, operative management should be performed expeditiously if the clinical history includes any hypotension and/or if the patient continues to have pain. Otherwise, observation in hospital and semielective repair are recommended.

RESUSCITATION AND TRANSFER

Patients who show the symptoms and signs of ruptured AAA should have rapid intravenous access established and blood drawn for crossmatch, and they should be transferred immediately to the operating room. In this setting, with the help of trained nursing and technical personnel, the establishment of large-bore venous access, resuscitation, and preparation for operative intervention can then proceed simultaneously. In the operating room, any deterioration in the patient's condition will necessitate rapid operative intervention and the securing of proximal aortic control.

Those patients who arrive at hospitals without the facilities or manpower to repair ruptured AAAs require resuscitation followed by rapid transfer to a hospital with the required resources. Controversy exists regarding the degree of resuscitation that should be conducted during this preoperative transfer. Crawford[21] suggested that blood pressure should be maintained at 50 to 70 mm Hg with small volumes of whole blood or crystalloid until the aorta is clamped. He believed that blood volume expansion would raise the blood pressure and dislodge the clot, with a resumption of or increase in bleeding. The major argument against minimal resuscitation is that the initial blood pressure is closely linked to survival and that the duration of shock is associated with the incidence of multisystem organ failure.[6, 22] Although Crawford makes his point with some vigor, many would argue that a blood pressure of 50 to 70 mm Hg is too low for prolonged periods of time. Our policy has been to advise fluid resuscitation during transport from the referring hospital to maintain the blood pressure between 80 and 100 mm Hg. If blood is available at the time of transfer, it is sent with the patient and may be given en route if the patient begins to deteriorate. Transfer from the referring hospital should not be delayed pending a full crossmatch of blood.

A recent randomized trial in patients with penetrating trauma demonstrated improved survival in those patients who received minimal fluid resuscitation until they arrived at the operating room.[23] It is important to note, however, that the incidence of multiple organ failure and death (30% to 38%) was lower than that observed in patients with ruptured AAA (50% to 75%). These results may not be directly applicable to patients with ruptured AAA, because those in this trauma series were younger (mean age, 31) males who did not have underlying coronary artery disease, chronic obstructive pulmonary disease, or diminished renal function. Although the mortality rate was high (30% to 38%), the incidence of adult respiratory distress syndrome, sepsis syndrome, and acute renal failure was low. Despite these differences, perhaps minimal resuscitation to keep the blood pressure between 80 and 100 mm Hg may be a better choice. A definitive trial in ruptured AAA is required to answer this question.

The use of a MAST (Military Antishock Trousers) garment during transport of unstable patients with ruptured AAA has been advocated by Gustafson and associates.[3] They reported their use in eight consecutive patients and compared them with historical controls. Patients who had application of the garment had lower systolic blood pressure yet had only a 25% mortality rate at 30 days, compared with 100% in controls. In addition, they noted that the volume of blood transfused was reduced in the MAST group, as was the incidence of respiratory and multiple organ failure. This initial report supporting the use of MAST in ruptured AAA appears to stand alone in the literature.[3] A prospective randomized trial of MAST in trauma victims demonstrated that those who had them applied had an increase in overall mortality despite the ability of MAST to increase blood pressure.[24] In the subgroup with abdominal vascular injuries, the application of MAST did *not* increase survival, and logistic regression demonstrated that MAST applications significantly contributed to the likelihood of death. Thus, we do not recommend MAST garments for patients with ruptured AAA.

OPERATIVE STRATEGY AND TECHNICAL DETAILS

INITIAL ANESTHETIC MANAGEMENT

Once the patient is transferred to the operating room table, the initial goal is to establish sufficient large-bore intravenous access to allow rapid administration of fluid and blood products. Next, arterial access will allow accurate blood pressure measurements and sampling of hematocrit and blood gases. These procedures are performed with the patient awake while the surgical instruments are prepared and the team is gowning. The patient is prepared and draped awake and rapidly inducted and intubated; this is followed by rapid aortic control. Anesthesia can be induced with ketamine or fentanyl plus a muscle relaxant. The placement of central venous access and a Swan-Ganz catheter can be completed after induction during the initial phases of the operation.

INCISION AND PROXIMAL CONTROL

The key element in the initial phase of operative treatment is achieving safe and rapid proximal control of the aorta. Our preferred approach to obtain proximal control is to dissect the aorta at the infrarenal level. Critics of this approach note the potential for venous injuries to the inferior mesenteric vein and left renal vein. However, this is the approach that most surgeons are familiar with if they perform elective aortic surgery. Traction on the aneurysm in a caudal direction by the first assistant will increase exposure of the neck of the aneurysm. Clamping at the infrarenal level will increase afterload but will not cause direct ischemia to the liver, intestine, or kidneys. Occasionally, clamping above the renal arteries and below the superior mesenteric artery will be required, and this can also be achieved by use of this approach.

Several large centers advocate that proximal control be achieved at the diaphragmatic hiatus where the aorta enters the abdomen.[5, 21] Once this is achieved, the AAA can be entered and the proximal anastomosis performed from within the AAA at the infrarenal level. This approach offers several advantages: it raises the blood pressure to a greater degree secondary to increased afterload caused by clamping above the visceral arteries, and it allows the anesthetist time for resuscitation before the clamp is moved to the infrarenal level. More important, it reduces the likelihood of venous injury during dissection in a large pararenal hematoma. Disadvantages consist primarily of ischemia to those organs supplied by the celiac and superior mesenteric arteries. Further ischemic injury to the liver and gut in addition to that induced by hemorrhagic shock may contribute to multisystem organ failure, as discussed below.

An alternative approach to proximal control is to clamp the lower thoracic aorta through a separate thoracic incision or a thoracoabdominal incision. In patients with many previous abdominal procedures that suggest a hostile abdomen, a thoracic incision will allow rapid control of the aorta. A thoracoabdominal incision should be considered in patients suspected of proximal extension of the aneurysm above the renal arteries (i.e., no space between the aneurysm and the costal margin) by examination or radiologic investigations. If a thoracic incision is considered, elevation of the chest with a sandbag will help with exposure, whereas for a thoracoabdominal approach, the chest may be rotated 45 to 60 degrees.

Another approach to repair of the ruptured AAA has been use of the retroperitoneal incision, which begins in the tenth interspace at the posterior axillary line and extends to the lateral border of the rectus muscle. In a nonrandomized series, the transperitoneal and retroperitoneal approaches have been compared by a group from Albany, New York.[25] This retrospective series excluded 13 ruptures with unusual features but compared 38 transperitoneal and 25 retroperitoneal approaches. There were few significant differences in pre- and intraoperative parameters, although the operative time was longer in the retroperitoneal approach and there was more intraoperative hypotension in the transperitoneal group. Although not significant, the number of hypotensive patients in the transperitoneal group was greater and the degree of hypotension was not recorded in the study. The transperitoneal group had a longer length of stay and a greater delay in the initiation of alimentation. The mortality was lower in the retroperitoneal group (12% vs. 35%). This series serves to document that for those performing this approach routinely, ruptured aneurysms can also be repaired through a retroperitoneal incision; however, for those not familiar with it, the transperitoneal approach is probably safer.

Some authors advocate using devices to obtain proximal aortic control.[26] These include a brachial cutdown with insertion of a large Fogarty catheter into the distal thoracic aorta and then occlusion by balloon inflation. A similar approach with use of the femoral artery and percutaneous insertion has also been reported. A commercially available aortic balloon catheter can be inserted once the abdomen is opened. It can be inserted directly through the opened aorta or through a small incision in the anterior wall of the aorta, fed proximally, and inflated. An aortic compressor is available, which is designed to compress the aorta at the hiatus onto the lumbar vertebral bodies. All of these balloon techniques and the aortic compressor are blind and are prone to migration of the balloon and/or dislodgment. For these reasons, we are most satisfied with a direct approach to aortic control.

DISTAL CONTROL

Distal control can usually be obtained by clamping the common iliac arteries. However, the use of balloon occlusion catheters placed from inside the AAA, once it has been opened, provides rapid distal control.

ANESTHETIC MANAGEMENT

After the aorta has been controlled, it is imperative that the anesthetist be allowed sufficient time to "catch up" before the AAA is opened, because blood loss can be anticipated. During the procedure, the results of arterial blood gas measurements will direct the administration of bicarbonate, and the hematocrit will guide blood replacement. One unit of fresh frozen plasma is given for every five to six units of blood, whereas six units of platelets are given after eight to ten units of blood. Coordination with anesthesia prior to unclamping is critical to the success of the procedure. Providing the anesthetist with 3 to 5 minutes of advance notice of unclamping will allow the reduction of inhalational agents (which cause myocardial depression) and the increase of cardiac preload with blood or fluid administration. Gradual release of the clamp over several minutes avoids dramatic reductions in the blood pressure.

AAA OPENING

The AAA is opened longitudinally and the proximal and distal ends explored. Back bleeding from lumbar vessels and the inferior mesenteric artery can then be controlled with interrupted sutures. Rapid and uncontrolled bleeding that is not due to inadequate proximal or distal control may be secondary to an aortocaval fistula. Although these are rare, immediate digital compression over the area is frequently required to control the bleeding and prevent air embolism. The use of two sponge sticks to apply pressure on either side of the fistula is recommended to control the bleeding and permit primary suture closure. Compression must avoid dislodging thrombus or other aortic debris into the venous circulation. No attempt should be made to gain formal control of the vena cava. Direct suture of the area, incorporating the aortic wall and adherent inferior vena cava, will ensure secure and rapid closure. If bleeding cannot be controlled with direct local pressure, control may be possible by passing two large Fogarty catheters up from the saphenous vein or femoral vein into the vena cava and positioning the balloons on either side of the fistula.

GRAFT TYPE

A low-porosity graft of appropriate size is selected for aortic replacement. A tube graft is preferred because less dissection is necessary and a more expeditious operation can be performed. Exceptions are made if the distal aorta at the bifurcation is significantly dilated, the iliac arteries are aneurysmal, or the iliac vessel is responsible for the rupture. If an aortobiiliac or aortobifemoral graft is required, flow should be maintained to at least one internal iliac artery to minimize the incidence of ischemic colitis.

HEPARINIZATION

In our experience, systemic heparin is usually *not* given, although local heparin can be administered down the iliac vessels by use of the irrigation port of the occlusion catheters. A brief back-flush of the iliac arteries with pressure on the groins will dislodge any soft red thrombus that may have formed. Because many of these patients develop a coagulopathy secondary to massive transfusion and shock, avoiding the use of heparin may reduce the incidence of subsequent bleeding, and in our experience this does not potentiate thrombotic complications.

CELL SAVER

The use of a cell-saver device to allow autotransfusion in a ruptured AAA is recommended but is not always available. The returned blood usually contains small amounts of free heparin and heparin bound to the red cells, which may require reversal to prevent potentiation of a coagulopathy. Coagulation factors are removed and must be replaced as noted above.

ANATOMIC ANOMALIES

Anatomic abnormalities and variants can dramatically increase the complexity of surgical management in patients with a ruptured AAA. The incidence of injuries to normal arterial and venous anatomy at the time of ruptured AAA repair is higher than in elective cases and contributes to the increased mortality rate. The discovery of venous, renal, or arterial anomalies further increases the complexity of the surgical repair.

Venous abnormalities include retroaortic left renal vein, circumaortic renal venous collar, and persistent left-sided vena cava and aortocaval fistula (already discussed). The retroaortic left renal vein can be injured by the jaws of the aortic clamp as it is applied, releasing a torrent of venous bleeding. Repair is accomplished by direct suture or division of the vein, but access to this vein is difficult and is best achieved by moving the aortic clamp to a more proximal site, retracting the aorta, or dividing the aorta. With division of the aorta, the proximal cuff can be elevated to expose the injury. A persistent left-sided vena cava frequently crosses the aorta at or near the level of the renal vessels. It has an oblique course over the aorta and can impede access to the neck of the aortic aneurysm. Elevation and mobilization are required to gain access to the aorta, or the inferior vena cava may have to be divided to permit aortic repair.

The discovery of a horseshoe kidney at laparotomy for ruptured AAA can present a difficult technical challenge because it lies anterior to the distal aorta and its bifurcation, and anomalies of the renal arteries, veins, and ureters are common. These kidneys are of variable size, location, and degree of attachment. The two problems that need immediate attention are the blood supply of the kidney and the access to the aorta. In 80% of cases, the arterial supply is from multiple renal vessels that can come from the distal aorta or iliac arteries.[27] With a ruptured AAA, proximal control must be achieved as quickly as possible. However, this may be at the expense of ischemia to the horseshoe kidney if there are multiple distal renal arteries. The location of the kidney can impede access to gain control of the distal aorta. Rarely, the kidneys are tethered together by just a fibrous cord that can be divided. More commonly, the isthmus is solid and consists of renal tissue and blood supply, and can also be the site of ureteric drainage. In this case, the inferior aspect of the isthmus must be dissected to permit access to the iliac arteries and control of the vessels at this site. To permit further exposure of the aortic bifurcation, the isthmus must be elevated. Every effort is made to avoid division of the isthmus. With mobilization and retraction of the isthmus, the aorta can be opened and a careful search made for large anomalous renal artery origins that will have to be reimplanted with buttons of aortic wall used as a Carrel patch; alternatively, several arteries can be incorporated into a patch for reattachment to the body of the aortic graft. Renal arteries that arise from the iliac arteries will be reperfused when the aorta is unclamped. Care must be taken to avoid injury to the ureters because they may also travel in aberrant directions. Recognition of the horseshoe kidney preoperatively would permit a retroperitoneal approach, which would avoid many of the exposure problems inherent in the anterior approach.

Discovery of an inflammatory aneurysm with the desmoplastic reaction extending up to and involving the duodenum will frequently require placement of the aortic clamp at the suprarenal level. As in elective cases, minimal mobilization of the duodenum is performed to prevent injury. After proximal control is achieved, balloon occlusion of the iliac vessels will reduce the dissection required.

RESULTS

The immediate and late survival rates after repair of a ruptured AAA remain low in spite of improvements in surgical care. The following sections review the results of treatment of ruptured AAA and include the data from the Canadian Aneurysm Study, the details of which have been published previously.[6] In this prospective study, follow-up of a cohort of 147 patients with ruptured AAA operated on during a 9-month period in 1986 by 51 surgeons provides the database to identify the preoperative, intraoperative, and postoperative variables that were associated with survival. Regular follow-up was maintained at 6- to 9-month intervals to determine the patient's status, cause of death, complications, and intercurrent diseases. The Kaplan-Meier method was used to calculate the cumulative percent survival rate versus time of follow-up,[28, 29] and the Cox proportional hazards model was used for multivariate analysis of the factors associated with late survival.[30]

OPERATIVE FINDINGS AND PATHOLOGY FROM THE CANADIAN ANEURYSM STUDY

Of the 147 patients studied in the Canadian Aneurysm Study, a ruptured AAA was present in 145 patients and a ruptured iliac aneurysm was present in 2 patients. The average age was 72 years, and 86% were male. In addition to a ruptured aneurysm, other vascular pathologic findings included aortocaval fistula (4), inflammatory aneurysm (1), mycotic aneurysm (1), horseshoe kidney (1), accessory renal artery (2), and bilateral femoral aneurysms requiring repair (2). Associated intra-abdominal procedures included cholecystectomy (2), division of isthmus of horseshoe kidney (1), and placement of a peritoneal dialysis catheter (1). Heparin was administered in 47.6% of patients.

EARLY SURVIVAL RATE

In the Canadian Aneurysm Study, the in-hospital survival rate was 50% and at 1 month was 49%. These data are comparable to the 46% survival rate for 278 ruptured AAAs repaired by 190 surgeons in New York State[31] and the 53% survival rate reported by Callam and colleagues[32] from collected series.

Individual Predictors of Early Survival

The individual variables that were found to be associated with early survival included preinduction systolic blood pressure (≤70 mm Hg 36% early survival; 71–119 mm Hg 38%; ≥120 mm Hg 75%), creatinine (≤1.3 mg/dL 77%; >1.3 mg/dL 47%), total intraoperative urine output (0 mL 4%; 1–199 mL 55%; ≥200 mL 70%), total volume of blood administered (≤1800 mL 68%; 1801–3499 mL 53%; ≥3500 mL 35%), site of aortic cross clamp (infrarenal 56%; suprarenal 29%), and aortic cross clamp time (<60 minutes 67%; ≥60 minutes 43%). The development of the following postoperative complications was associated with a significantly lower survival rate: bleeding (31%), distal arterial thrombosis (31%), paraplegia (0%), cerebrovascular event (0%), postoperative myocardial infarction

(19%), cardiac arrhythmia (46%), congestive heart failure (41%), respiratory failure (47%), renal damage manifested by a creatinine rise (53%), renal failure requiring dialysis (33%), and coagulopathy (23%).

Multiple Predictors of Early Survival

The following variables were independently predictive of a poor early survival: preoperative variables—elevated serum creatinine and low induction blood pressure; intraoperative variables—aortic clamp site above the renal arteries, large volume of blood administered, and low total urine output; preoperative and intraoperative variables—elevated preoperative creatinine, low intraoperative urine output, and aortic clamp site above the renal arteries; postoperative variables—occurrence of a myocardial infarction, respiratory failure, renal damage, and/or coagulopathy; all preoperative, intraoperative, and postoperative variables—aortic cross clamping above renal arteries and occurrence of a myocardial infarction, respiratory failure, renal damage, and coagulopathy.

Data from Other Studies

Other studies have generally been retrospective and have frequently used univariate analysis. A summary of the results of many trials is given in Table 1. Gloviczki and associates[8] used multivariate analysis and found that the following were associated with higher mortality: poor APACHE II score, hypotension, low hematocrit, and chronic obstructive lung disease. Johansen and colleagues,[5] in an urban center with a paramedic resuscitation team, noted an overall 30-day survival rate of only 30% and found that the following were associated with a better survival ($P < .05$): no preoperative cardiac arrest, female gender, blood pressure stabilized, requirement for transfusion of <15 units. For 73 patients who survived to reach the operating room, AbuRahma and associates[34] noted that the following factors were associated with a higher mortality ($P < .05$): syncope, low systolic blood pressure, symptoms for less than 1 day, time from emergency department to induction of anesthesia >2 hours, and intraperitoneal rupture. Ouriel and colleagues[35] noted a better prognosis if the patient was hemodynamically stable, and did not have chronic obstructive lung disease or renal insufficiency. Murphy and co-workers[36] used multiple variables to develop a discriminant function model that was correct in predicting survival in 87% of cases, but they believed that it was not precise enough for clinical application. Amundsen and colleagues,[37] using logistic regression analysis in 114 cases for the Norwegian Aneurysm Trial, noted that systolic blood pressure >92 and age <72 were jointly associated with better survival. Vohra and associates[38] examined the relationship between 12 variables and survival in 103 patients, 61% of whom survived, and they found that improved survival was related only to volume of blood transfused ($P < .05$). Donaldson and co-workers[39] used discriminant function analysis and concluded that many of the significant factors were beyond the surgeon's control (age >76, gender, medical comorbidity, low admission blood pressure, EKG abnormality, rupture site) but that others could potentially be modified (prompt diagnosis, time to operation, hemodynamic status, and technical complications). Fielding and colleagues[40] noted that only the amount of blood transfused was of prognostic value and concluded that no *single* risk factor contra-

TABLE 1.
Literature Review of Variables Associated With High Early Mortality Rates*

Author	Variables Associated With High In-Hospital Mortality Rates
Johnston[6] Prospective; logistic regression analysis	Creatinine >1.3; intraoperative urine output <200 mL; suprarenal aortic clamp
Gloviczki et al.[8] Logistic regression analysis	High APACHE II score; hypotension; low hematocrit; chronic lung disease
Harris et al.[4] Logistic regression analysis	Renal failure
Johansen et al.[5]	Preoperative cardiac arrest; male sex; unstable BP; transfusion >15 units
AbuRahma et al.[34]	Syncope; low systolic BP; symptoms <1 day; >2 hours from emergency to OR; intraperitoneal rupture
Ouriel et al.[35]	Hemodynamically unstable; chronic lung disease; renal insufficiency
Amundsen et al.[37] Logistic regression analysis	Systolic BP <92; age >72 years
Vohra et al.[42]	Large volume of blood transfused
Donaldson et al.[39]	Age >76 years; hematocrit <30%; acute electrocardiographic abnormality; persistent low BP; technical complications; organ failure
Fielding et al.[40]	Volume blood transfused
Wakefield et al.[41]	Hypotension; abnormal BUN; abnormal creatinine level; duration hypotension; volume blood transfused; volume fluid administered

*Abstracted from Johnston KW: *J Vasc Surg* 19:898, 1994. Used by permission.
BP = blood pressure; OR = operating room; BUN = blood urea nitrogen

indicated surgery. Wakefield and associates,[41] in a retrospective, univariate analysis of 116 cases from 1964 to 1980, found that the significant preoperative variables that predicted outcome were blood pressure, BUN, and creatinine, and that the significant intraoperative variables were the duration of hypotension, blood transfusion, and volume of fluids administered.

Application of Information
Although operation is the only hope for survival in a patient with ruptured AAA, some patients have such a low chance of in-hospital survival that it is reasonable to question if all patients with a ruptured AAA should have surgery. Because no combination of preoperative variables predicted a near-zero percent chance of early or late survival, we believe that all patients should be offered surgery unless major comorbid conditions are identified. Note that this opinion is contrary to the view of Johansen and colleagues,[5] who believed that certain clinical features helped predict ex-

tremely high early mortality and that these patients should not have surgery. However, the data from the Canadian Aneurysm Study show that useful prognostic information can be obtained when intraoperative and postoperative data are considered together. The chances of early and late survival are very poor when multiple negative prognostic variables are recorded intra- or postoperatively. We concluded the following:

> After surgery (when information on intra-operative and pre-operative variables is available) and in the intensive care unit (when additional information on post-operative variables is available), the results of this study provide justification for the surgeon to use these prognostic variables to assist his/her clinical judgment and guide discussions on prognosis with the family and identify those patients who have such a low chance of early and late survival that further aggressive treatment may be futile.[6]

LATE SURVIVAL RATE AFTER RUPTURED AAA

Canadian Aneurysm Study Data

The survival, calculated by the Kaplan-Meier method, at 1 month was 49%, at 1 year 43%, at 2 years 37%, at 3 years 35%, at 4 years 29%, and at 5 years 26%.

The common causes of late deaths were coronary artery disease in 29%, cancer in 16%, pulmonary in 16%, gastrointestinal bleeding (not aortoenteric fistula) in 10%, and renal failure in 7%.

For those patients who survived the operation and the first month, the survival rate was 53% at 5 years. This is significantly less than the 71% 5-year survival rates for patients who survived operation for nonruptured AAA. This observation is in contrast to that in other reports[40, 42] and may be explained by the fact that the Canadian Aneurysm Study was a contemporary study, and the data were not obtained from retrospective analysis.

Review of Other Literature

The long-term survival rates obtained in the Canadian Aneurysm Study are in the middle of the range observed in other studies. All other reports were retrospective, and in some studies patient entry spanned more than a decade and the follow-up was incomplete or not current. Olsen and colleagues[43] studied 218 patients between 1979 and 1988. The immediate survival rate was 63% and the cumulative 5-year survival rate was 48%. It is not clear if the follow-up was complete and current for the 137 patients who were potentially available for follow-up. Vohra and co-workers[38] studied 92 patients who were to have operations, but 11 died before surgery could be undertaken. The 30-day survival was 71%, and approximately 66% of those patients who survived hospitalization lived for 4 years; hence, the estimated 4-year survival was 47%. For 65 patients with ruptured AAA between 1977 and 1987, Rohrer and associates[44] found that the hospital mortality rate was 36.9%, and for the 41 who survived hospitalization, the actuarial 5-year survival rate was 51%. Nachbur and colleagues[45] studied 112 patients operated on between 1978 and 1984. The initial mortality rate was 46.6%, and the 5-year survival rate from their Kaplan-Meier plot was 29%. Soreide and associates[46] noted

Moving?

I'd like to receive my *Advances in Vascular Surgery* without interruption.
Please note the following change of address, effective:

Name: _____

New Address: _____

_____

City: _____ State: _____ Zip: _____

Old Address: _____

_____

City: _____ State: _____ Zip: _____

Reservation Card

Yes, I would like my own copy of *Advances in Vascular Surgery*. Please begin my subscription with the current edition according to the terms described below.* I understand that I will have 30 days to examine each annual edition. If satisfied, I will pay just $72.95 plus sales tax, postage and handling (price subject to change without notice).

Name: _____

Address: _____

City: _____ State: _____ Zip: _____

Method of Payment
○ Visa   ○ Mastercard   ○ AmEx   ○ Bill me   ○ Check (in US dollars, payable to Mosby, Inc.)

Card number: _____ Exp date: _____

Signature: _____

LS-0909

*Your *Advances* Service Guarantee:

When you subscribe to *Advances*, we'll send you an advance notice of future volumes about two months before they publish. This automatic notice system is designed to take up as little of your time as possible. If you do not want *Advances*, the advance notice makes it quick and easy for you to let us know your decision, and you will always have at least 20 days to decide. If we don't hear from you, we'll send you the new volume as soon as it's available. And, of course, *Advances* is yours to examine free of charge for 30 days (postage, handling and applicable sales tax are added to each shipment.).

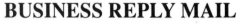

BUSINESS REPLY MAIL

FIRST CLASS MAIL   PERMIT No. 762   CHICAGO, IL

POSTAGE WILL BE PAID BY ADDRESSEE

Chris Hughes
Mosby-Year Book, Inc.
200 N. LaSalle Street
Suite 2600
Chicago, IL 60601-9981

BUSINESS REPLY MAIL

FIRST CLASS MAIL   PERMIT No. 762   CHICAGO, IL

POSTAGE WILL BE PAID BY ADDRESSEE

Chris Hughes
Mosby-Year Book, Inc.
200 N. LaSalle Street
Suite 2600
Chicago, IL 60601-9981

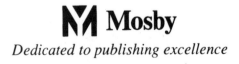

M Mosby

Dedicated to publishing excellence

that for 125 patients operated on for ruptured AAA between 1967 and 1979, the initial survival rate was 41.6% and the 5-year survival rate was 30.5%. In the series reported by Fielding and co-workers[47] from 1960 to 1979, of the 100/174 patients who survived hospitalization, 65 could be followed, and they had a 57.1% actuarial survival rate. Appleberg and colleagues[48] noted that late survival of 65 patients who were discharged from the hospital between 1961 and 1978 was the same as for the average matched Australian population. Unfortunately, the cumulative survival curves were not calculated by standard life table methods, and the raw data do not allow recalculation.

Predictors of Late Survival
Other studies in the literature do not address the predictors of late survival in detail. In the Canadian Aneurysm Study, of the preoperative variables, preinduction systolic blood pressure and creatinine were significant in relation to long-term survival. The only intraoperative variable that was significant was the total urine output. Considering the preoperative and intraoperative variables together, the patient's age and total urine output during the procedure predicted survival. For the postoperative variables, the significant predictors were renal damage, respiratory failure, and myocardial infarction.

When all significant variables were considered together, the chances of long-term survival were predicted by intraoperative urine output, respiratory failure, and myocardial infarction. When urine output was zero or low and complications occurred postoperatively, late prognosis was poor.

Implications of Observations
Preoperative variables do not clearly identify patients with ruptured AAA who may obtain long-term survival; hence, when seen in the emergency situation, most should have the benefit of surgical repair. The results of the Canadian Aneurysm Study show that after surgery and in the intensive care unit when additional information becomes available, useful prognostic information can be obtained when both intraoperative and postoperative information are considered. It is possible to identify those patients who have such a low chance of early and late survival that further aggressive treatment may be futile. When information identifies that the chances of early and late survival are very poor, the surgeon can use these prognostic variables to assist his/her clinical judgment in decision making and to guide discussions on prognosis with the family.[6]

COMPLICATIONS AND CAUSES OF DEATH

As described above, many potential complications may develop after ruptured AAA repair, and they can be broadly classified as vascular (both local and generalized) or systemic complications. The complications are closely linked to the causes of death.

LOCAL VASCULAR COMPLICATIONS
Local vascular complications include bleeding requiring repeat laparotomy, which is frequently confounded by the development of a coagu-

lopathy. The incidence of coagulopathy and postoperative bleeding was noted to be 12% and 14.4%, respectively.[6] Distal thrombosis (requiring embolectomy) or "trash" foot secondary to the embolization of intra-aortic debris is also infrequent (11.7%); however, it is much higher than would be expected in elective patients. Paraplegia or paraparesis may develop secondary to the reduced perfusion pressure in combination with interruption of lumbar and pelvic collaterals. This complication is rare (2.8%– 5.1%); however, it has been associated with a 50% mortality rate.[6, 8] Colon ischemia has a multifactorial etiology, which includes the duration and degree of hypotension, the patency of the inferior mesenteric artery prior to rupture, and the degree of collateral supply from the superior mesenteric artery and pelvic circulation. Colonic injury can range in severity from partial mucosal necrosis to full-thickness bowel necrosis that may result in perforation. The incidence has been reported to be between 3% and 13%; however, it is associated with a mortality rate that ranges from 73% to 100%.[8, 39–41]

SYSTEMIC COMPLICATIONS

Systemic complications occur frequently in these patients and with a much higher incidence than in multiple trauma patients who are younger and frequently suffer similar degrees of hypotension but do not have atherosclerotic occlusive disease.[6, 23] The most frequently cited general postoperative complications include respiratory failure, renal failure, myocardial infarction, arrhythmia, congestive heart failure, hyperbilirubinemia, sepsis, and multiple organ failure. Other complications, including stroke, wound dehiscence, hyperamylasemia, deep venous thrombosis, and pulmonary embolus, are variably reported.[33] The following sections discuss the etiology and prevention of some of the complications that are common in patients with ruptured AAA.

Respiratory Failure

The development of respiratory insufficiency and its relationship to mortality have been noted frequently in clinical series.[5, 6, 8, 39] The incidence has been reported to vary from 26% to 47% with mortality rates between 34% and 68%. The exact nature and etiology of the respiratory failure have not been specifically investigated; however, increases in lung permeability and a decrease in compliance similar to those in the adult respiratory distress syndrome are noted. Predisposing factors include large volumes of infused crystalloid, blood, and blood products. Predictors of postoperative pulmonary dysfunction include the presence of preoperative pulmonary disease and the duration of the aortic cross clamp.[49] The latter suggests that the relative lower torso ischemia produced during ruptured AAA repair may release mediators that are responsible for the induction of pulmonary dysfunction.

Renal Failure

Olsen and colleagues[43] have reviewed the incidence and consequences of renal failure after elective and ruptured AAA repair. They noted that the incidence of renal failure was related to the urgency of repair: ruptured AAA 26%, elective repair 4%, and acute repair of nonruptured AAA

9%. In patients with ruptured AAA, 90% had preoperative, in-hospital hypotension with a duration greater than 5 minutes, 82% were anuric preoperatively, and only 25% developed renal failure. The amount of perioperative bleeding was related to the incidence of renal failure. After ruptured AAA, the 30-day mortality rate of patients with renal failure was 59% compared with 31% for those without renal failure. In the Canadian Aneurysm Study, the in-hospital mortality rate was 19% for patients without renal damage, 47% for those who had a rise in serum creatinine, and 89% for those who required dialysis.[6] Bauer et al.[49] noted that the suprarenal position and duration of the aortic cross clamp, as well as preexisting renal disease, shock, and age, were predictors of postoperative renal failure. Thus, the surgeon can influence the development of renal failure by placing the clamp in the infrarenal position when possible or minimizing the duration of suprarenal clamping.

The etiology of renal failure after ruptured AAA is related to the preoperative renal status, severity and duration of hypotension, and intraoperative renal ischemia, whereas the intraoperative urine output reflects all of these variables. Although the etiology of renal failure after ruptured AAA repair is multifactorial, those patients who develop it frequently have sustained injury to other organs, such as liver and lungs, indicating that a greater systemic insult has taken place.

Myocardial Infarction

Cardiac events, which include infarction, arrhythmia, arrest, and congestive heart failure, occur with a frequency of 20% to 42%, which is associated with a 47% early survival, compared with 87% for those without a cardiac event.[6] The etiologic factors responsible for this dramatic increase in cardiac complications, compared with those in elective patients, are likely secondary to the sudden alterations in cardiac perfusion pressure (blood pressure) in the face of rapidly changing requirements. The predictive factors for the development of myocardial insufficiency include preexisting coronary artery disease, intraoperative fluid volume given, the position of the clamp, and the presence of preoperative shock.[49] Thus, infrarenal clamp placement for the shortest possible time is the only factor that can be modified by the surgeon. Prompt recognition of a myocardial infarction postoperatively allows for consideration of therapeutic interventions that may prevent further complications.

Irreversible Shock

Johansen and associates[5] noted that 14% of their deaths occurred in the operating room and were attributed to cardiogenic shock and/or circulatory collapse. Patients in this group are frequently those who, despite the application of the aortic clamp and appropriate fluid resuscitation, fail to have a positive response in their blood pressure. These individuals remain unresponsive to further pharmacologic interventions and frequently die in the operating room with cardiac arrest as the final event. Few authors specifically comment upon irreversible shock as a cause of death, and the etiologic factors responsible are poorly defined.

Hepatic Failure

Early descriptions[50] of patients who developed sequential system failure after ruptured AAA reported that the lung failure was an early phenomenon but that liver failure occurred later at about postoperative day 5, with central nervous system, heart, and gastrointestinal failure occurring in the days that followed. Hermreck and associates[51] described severe jaundice in a group of patients after ruptured AAA repair. In addition to hepatic dysfunction, they noted that all had acute renal failure, and the majority had significant respiratory failure. Liver morphology did not demonstrate recent or resolving hepatic necrosis but did demonstrate cholestasis with both canalicular and ductal bile thrombi. The causes of the hepatic failure were suggested to be an increase in the load of bile pigment (secondary to hematoma and transfusion) and hepatocyte dysfunction secondary to the hypoxic injury associated with shock. These patients with severe jaundice had an overall mortality of 83%. The insult required to produce jaundice in this group of patients with ruptured AAA was severe enough to produce multiple organ failure as well. It took several days for the jaundice to develop in these patients, suggesting that acute organ failure after ruptured AAA is a dynamic process that evolves over time. No major predictive factors have been identified.

Multiple Organ Failure

In the preceding paragraphs we have discussed failure of individual organs including the lung, kidney, and liver. The dysfunction of these organs rarely occurs in isolation. An early monograph on postoperative respiratory failure described clinical cases that initiated this event and a case of ruptured AAA was among those described.[52] Tilney and colleagues,[50] in a 1973 review of renal failure in patients after ruptured AAA, noted progressive failure of other organs and systems that ultimately led to a mortality of over 90%. Multiorgan failure was noted to be responsible for 21% of deaths in a study of ruptured AAA in Norway.[46] Johansen and co-workers[5] noted that multiple organ failure was the most common cause of death in the intensive care unit. Thus, patients who have suffered from a ruptured AAA develop sequelae similar to those of many general surgical and trauma patients who frequently develop multiple organ failure. In the latter group of patients, an acute inflammatory event, such as pancreatitis or a perforated viscus, is frequently suspected to be the initiator of multiple organ failure. The development of multiple organ failure is a similar end point in ruptured AAA patients. However, the initiator of the syndrome in this group of patients is less obvious. The pathophysiologic mechanisms that result in organ injury and failure and are initiated by rupture and surgical repair of an abdominal aortic aneurysm have yet to be elucidated.

Repair of an aortic aneurysm requires a brief period of lower torso ischemia, and several authors suggest that the preferred method of control is achieved in the supraceliac level. The suprarenal position (vs. infrarenal) and the duration of aortic cross clamping have also been related to early postoperative death.[49] Suprarenal or supraceliac cross clamping induces further ischemic injury to these organs during repair.

One hypothesis that would account for the high incidence of death and multiple organ failure after ruptured AAA might be stated as follows. Ruptured AAA is a combination of two events: ischemia and reperfusion. The pathophysiologic mechanisms initiated by the first ischemic event, hemorrhagic shock,[53] may be compounded and augmented by the second ischemic event, relative lower torso ischemia. Reperfusion occurs during resuscitation and after the release of the aortic clamp reperfusing the lower torso (and all the abdominal organs if a supraceliac clamp placement is used). The combination of these events, which occur sequentially, may result in a synergistic effect that initiates pathophysiologic mechanisms that result in organ failure, which contributes to the development of complications and mortality. Should this hypothesis be proven there would be implications for potential new therapeutic interventions designed to interrupt the pathophysiologic mechanisms of ischemia/reperfusion injury.

QUALITY OF LIFE AFTER RUPTURED AAA

Several studies have addressed the quality of a patient's life after elective or ruptured aneurysm surgery. Rohrer and colleagues[44] adapted a Life Function Scale questionnaire, a tool used previously in geriatric populations, and administered it to survivors of 65 ruptured and 100 elective aneurysms. Responses were obtained from 26 of 29 ruptured AAA patients still alive at the time of the study and from 76 of the 94 elective AAA patients. In the overall score, there was no difference between the elective and the ruptured groups. When individual questions were analyzed, the elective group reported a higher sense of general well-being compared with the ruptured AAA group. The physical independence of the patients with ruptured AAA and nonruptured AAA was similar. No difference in overall score was noted in the ruptured AAA group when stratified by age above 70 years. By contrast, the elective AAA patients older than 70 years had significantly lower scores than those younger than 70 years. This study indicates that those who survive ruptured AAA can be returned to an acceptable quality of life.

Magee and colleagues[54] used a Rosser index questionnaire, administered postoperatively, to determine the level of disability and distress before and after elective and after ruptured AAA repair. A total of 86 elective and 45 ruptured AAA patients were administered the questionnaire at a personal interview. The elective patients did not demonstrate any significant reduction in the quality of life. However, the group that had a ruptured AAA did suffer a reduction. The authors stress that in the ruptured AAA group, this represents a significant deterioration in the level of functional capacity. Taken together, these two studies suggest that individuals with ruptured AAA may suffer a greater degree of disability compared with the elective patients, and they reinforce the fact that elective repair is clearly a better alternative. Nonetheless, after ruptured AAA repair, patients are able to return to an acceptable level of function.

CONCLUSIONS AND FUTURE DIRECTIONS

Rupture of AAA continues to be a lethal event in 90% of patients. Several strategies can be developed to reduce the mortality. Ultrasound screening programs could increase the frequency of elective repair, but this has not proved to be cost-effective, particularly because the average national mortality rate is about 5% for elective repair. Improved education of primary care physicians, stressing the importance of examining carefully for an enlarged aorta in patients over the age of 60 years and referring patients for elective repair, may be helpful. Improved awareness by emergency physicians may result in prompt recognition of a ruptured AAA and early referral for surgical treatment. Despite all efforts at education, screening, and increases in the safety of elective repair, a percentage of patients with AAA will continue to have their first clinical presentation as aortic rupture. Thus, to improve mortality rates, it is necessary to investigate the pathophysiologic mechanisms that result in the development of multiple organ failure. Improvements in understanding these mechanisms may allow the development of strategies and interventions to decrease the incidence of organ failure that accounts for a large percentage of the mortality from this condition.

ACKNOWLEDGMENTS

The authors gratefully thank Pam Purdy and Anna Schulze for their assistance in preparation of the manuscript, and Dr. Paul M. Walker for helpful discussions.

REFERENCES

1. Ernst CB: Abdominal aortic aneurysm. *N Engl J Med* 328:1167–1172, 1993.
2. Drott C, Arfvidsson B, ¨Ortenwall P, et al: Age-standardized incidence of ruptured aortic aneurysm in a defined Swedish population between 1952 and 1988: Mortality rate and operative results. *Br J Surg* 79:175–179, 1992.
3. Gustafson RA, McDowell DE, Savrin RA: The use of the MAST suit in ruptured abdominal aortic aneurysms. *Am Surg* 49:454–459, 1983.
4. Harris LM, Faggioli GL, Fiedler R, et al: Ruptured abdominal aortic aneurysms: Factors affecting mortality rates. *J Vasc Surg* 14:812–820, 1991.
5. Johansen K, Kohler TR, Nicholls SC, et al: Ruptured abdominal aortic aneurysm: The Harborview experience. *J Vasc Surg* 13:240–247, 1991.
6. Johnston KW: Ruptured abdominal aortic aneurysm: Six-year follow-up results of a multicenter prospective study. *J Vasc Surg* 19:888–900, 1994.
7. Katz DJ, Stanley JC, Zelenock GB: Operative mortality rates for intact and ruptured abdominal aortic aneurysms in Michigan: An eleven-year statewide experience. *J Vasc Surg* 12:28–33, 1990.
8. Gloviczki P, Pairolero PC, Mucha P, et al: Ruptured abdominal aortic aneurysms: Repair should not be denied. *J Vasc Surg* 15:851–859, 1992.
9. Melton LJ III, Bickerstaff LK, Hollier LH, et al: Changing incidence of abdominal aortic aneurysm: A population based study. *Am J Epidemiol* 120:379–386, 1984.
10. Bickerstaff LK, Hollier LH, Van Peenen HJ, et al: Abdominal aortic aneurysms: The changing natural history. *J Vasc Surg* 1:6–12, 1984.
11. Bengtson H, Bergqvist D: Ruptured abdominal aortic aneurysm: A population-based study. *J Vasc Surg* 18:74–80, 1993.
12. Katz DA, Littenberg B, Cronenwett JL: Management of small abdominal aortic aneurysms. *JAMA* 268:2678–2686, 1992.
13. Sterpetti AV, Cavallaro A, Cavallari N, et al: Factors influencing the rupture of abdominal aortic aneurysms. *Surg Gynecol Obstet* 173:175–178, 1991.
14. Marston WA, Ahlquist R, Johnson G, et al: Misdiagnosis of ruptured abdominal aortic aneurysms. *J Vasc Surg* 16:17–22, 1992.

15. Khan H, Sottiurai VS, Craighead CC, et al: Ruptured abdominal aortic aneurysm presenting as symptomatic inguinal mass: Report of six cases. *J Vasc Surg* 4:384–389, 1986.
16. Linsell JC, Rowe PH, Owen WS: Rupture of an aortic aneurysm into the renal vein presenting as a left sided varicocele. Case report. *Acta Chir Scand* 153:477–478, 1987.
17. Loughran CF: A review of the plain abdominal radiograph in acute ruptured abdominal aortic aneurysms. *Clin Radiol* 37:383–387, 1986.
18. Shuman WP, Hastrup W, Kohler TR, et al: Suspected leaking abdominal aortic aneurysm: Use of sonography in the emergency room. *Radiology* 168:117–119, 1988.
19. Weinbaum FI, Dubner S, Turner JW, et al: The accuracy of computed tomography in the diagnosis of retroperitoneal blood in the presence of abdominal aortic aneurysm. *J Vasc Surg* 6:11–16, 1987.
20. Siegel CL, Cohan RH: CT of abdominal aortic aneurysms. *AJR* 163:17–29, 1994.
21. Crawford ES: Ruptured abdominal aortic aneurysm: An editorial. *J Vasc Surg* 13:348–350, 1991.
22. Brimacombe J, Berry A: A review of anaesthesia for ruptured abdominal aortic aneurysm with special emphasis on preclamping fluid resuscitation. *Anaesth Intensive Care* 21:311–323, 1993.
23. Bickell WH, Wall MJ Jr, Pepe PE, et al: Immediate versus delayed fluid resuscitation for hypotensive patients with penetrating torso injuries. *N Engl J Med* 331:1105–1109, 1994.
24. Mattox KL, Bickell W, Pepe PE, et al: Prospective MAST study in 911 patients. *J Trauma* 29:1104–1112, 1989.
25. Chang BB, Shah DM, Paty PSK, et al: Can the retroperitoneal approach be used for ruptured abdominal aortic aneurysms? *J Vasc Surg* 11:326–330, 1990.
26. Wolf RK, Williams EL II, Kisler PC: Transbrachial balloon catheter tamponade of ruptured abdominal aortic aneurysms without fluoroscopic control. *Surg Gyn & Obstet* 164:463–465, 1987.
27. McCarthy WJ, Schneider JR, Shah P, et al: Management of aortic aneurysm and associated urologic problems. In Yao JST, Pearce WH eds: *Aneurysms— New Findings and Treatments.* Norwalk, Conn, 1994, Appleton and Lange, 6(23):275–286.
28. Coldman AJ, Elwood JM: Examining survival data. *Can Med Assoc J* 121:1065–1071, 1979.
29. Steinberg D, Colla P: *Survival: A Supplementary Module for SYSTAT.* Evanston, IL, 1988, SYSTAT.
30. Hopkins A: *Survival Analysis With Covariates: Cox Models,* 1983. BMDP Statistical Software, pp 576–594.
31. Hannan EL, Kilburn H Jr, O'Donnell JF, et al: A longitudinal analysis of the relationship between in-hospital mortality in New York State and the volume of abdominal aortic aneurysm surgeries performed. *Health Serv* 27, 1992, pp 517–542.
32. Callam MJ, Haiart D, Murie JA, et al: Ruptured aortic aneurysm. A proposed classification. *Br J Surg* 178:1126–1129, 1991.
33. Crawford ES, Saleh SA, Babb JW III, et al: Infrarenal abdominal aortic aneurysm. Factors influencing survival after operation performed over a 25-year period. *Ann Surg* 193:699–709, 1981.
34. AbuRahma AF, Woodruff BA, Lucente FC, et al: Factors affecting survival of patients with ruptured abdominal aortic aneurysms in a West Virginia community. *Surgery* 172:377–382, 1991.

35. Ouriel K, Geary K, Green RM, et al: Factors determining survival after ruptured aortic aneurysm: The hospital, the surgeon, and the patient. *J Vasc Surg* 11:493–496, 1990.

36. Murphy JL, Barber GG, McPhail NV, et al: Factors affecting survival after rupture of abdominal aortic aneurysm: Effect of size on management and outcome. *Can J Surg* 33:201–205, 1990.

37. Amundsen S, Skjaerven R, Trippestad A, et al: Abdominal aortic aneurysms—A study of factors influencing postoperative mortality. *Eur J Vasc Surg* 3:405–409, 1989.

38. Vohra R, Reid D, Groome J, et al: Long-term survival in patients undergoing resection of abdominal aortic aneurysm. *Ann Vasc Surg* 4:460–465, 1990.

39. Donaldson MC, Rosenberg JM, Bucknam CA: Factors affecting survival after ruptured abdominal aortic aneurysm. *J Vasc Surg* 2:564–570, 1985.

40. Fielding JWL, Black J, Ashton F, et al: Ruptured aortic aneurysms: Postoperative complications and their aetiology. *Br J Surg* 71:487–491, 1984.

41. Wakefield TW, Whitehouse WM Jr, Wu S-C, et al: Abdominal aortic aneurysm rupture: Statistical analysis of factors affecting outcome of surgical treatment. *Surgery* 91:586–596, 1982.

42. Vohra R, Abdool-Carrim ATO, Groome J, et al: Evaluation of factors influencing survival in ruptured aortic aneurysms. *Ann Vasc Surg* 2:340–344, 1988.

43. Olsen PS, Schroeder T, Agerskov K, et al: Surgery for abdominal aortic aneurysms: A survey of 656 patients. *J Cardiovasc Surg* 32:636–642, 1991.

44. Rohrer MJ, Cutler BS, Wheeler HB: Long-term survival and quality of life following ruptured abdominal aortic aneurysm. *Arch Surg* 123:1213–1217, 1988.

45. Nachbur R, Gut A, Sigrist S: Prognostic factors in the surgical treatment of aorto-iliac aneurysmal disease. *J Cardiovasc Surgery* 28:469–478, 1987.

46. Soreide O, Grimsgaard C, Myhre HO, et al: Time and cause of death for 301 patients operated on for abdominal aortic aneurysms. *Age Ageing* 11:256–260, 1982.

47. Fielding JWL, Black J, Ashton F, et al: Diagnosis and management of 528 abdominal aortic aneurysms. *Br Med J* 283:355–359, 1981.

48. Appleberg M, Coupland GAE, Reeves TS: Ruptured abdominal aortic aneurysm: Long-term survival after operation. *Aust N Z J Surg* 50:28–32, 1980.

49. Bauer EP, Redaelli C, von Segesser LK, et al: Ruptured abdominal aortic aneurysms: Predictors for early complications and death. *Surgery* 114:31–35, 1993.

50. Tilney NL, Bailey G, Morgan AP: Sequential system failure after rupture of abdominal aortic aneurysms: An unsolved problem in post-operative care. *Ann Surg* 178:117–122, 1973.

51. Hermreck AS, Proberts KS, Thomas JH: Severe jaundice after rupture of abdominal aortic aneurysm. *Am J Surg* 134:745–748, 1977.

52. Moore FD, Lyons JH Jr, Pierce EC Jr, et al: *Post-Traumatic Pulmonary Insufficiency*. Toronto, 1969, WB Saunders, pp 42–78.

53. Vedder NB, Winn RK, Rice CL, et al: A monoclonal antibody to the adherence-promoting leukocyte glycoprotein, CD18, reduces organ injury and improves survival from haemorrhagic shock and resuscitation in rabbits. *J Clin Invest* 81:939–944, 1988.

54. Magee TR, Scott DJ, Dunkley A, et al: Quality of life following surgery for abdominal aortic aneurysm. *Br J Surg* 79:1014–1016, 1992.

PART IV

Infrainguinal Reconstruction

The Impact of Endoluminal Pathology on Vein Grafts: The Role of Routine Angioscopy for Vein Preparation

Arnold Miller, M.B., Ch.B., F.R.C.S., F.R.C.S.(C.), F.A.C.S.
Assistant Clinical Professor of Surgery, Harvard Medical School, Boston
Massachusetts; Attending Surgeon, MetroWest Medical Center, Framingham,
Massachusetts, and New England Deaconess Hospital, Boston, Massachusetts

Juha P. Salenius, M.D., Ph.D.
Vascular Research Fellow, Harvard Medical School, MetroWest Medical Center,
Framingham and New England Deaconess Hospital, Boston, Massachusetts;
Assistant Professor of Vascular Surgery, Tampere University, Tampere, Finland;
Attending Vascular Surgeon, University Hospital, Tampere, Finland

S ince the introduction of femoropopliteal bypass grafting with saphenous vein by Kunlin[1] in 1949, autogenous vein has remained the conduit of choice for infrainguinal bypass grafting. Despite intense efforts in research and development over the last half century, the durability and long-term patency of autogenous vein remain superior to those of all currently available synthetic or biologic grafts. However, the incidence of graft failure is not insignificant. The 5-year primary patency rates of recent series of mixed groups of femoropopliteal and femorodistal bypass grafts range between 59% and 80%, with secondary patency rates between 76% and 85%.[2–5] Although some factors, if recognized, can be avoided or even corrected, others, particularly those associated with graft biology, remain unresponsive to known therapeutic interventions.

Angioscopy, introduced into clinical surgery over the last two decades, is the only method currently available that allows the surgeon to visualize directly the interior of the graft conduit, anastomoses, and native vessels before, during, and after bypass grafting. Since our first successful clinical angioscopic examination in 1987, we have attempted to evaluate the efficacy of angioscopy and delineate its role in vascular surgery. We have used angioscopy routinely to prepare vein conduit and monitor the technical results of primary, redo, and revision bypass surgery. To date, we have performed angioscopy during more than 1,250 infrainguinal bypass procedures. In addition, we have used angioscopy rou-

Advances in Vascular Surgery®, vol. 3
© 1995, Mosby–Year Book, Inc.

tinely in graft or arterial thrombectomy and embolectomy, carotid endarterectomy, and vascular access surgery.

In this chapter we will briefly review the factors contributing to vein graft failure as currently understood, describe the endoluminal pathology detected by routine angioscopy, and discuss the impact of these findings in the preparation of the optimal vein graft conduit.

REVIEW OF FACTORS CONTRIBUTING TO VEIN GRAFT FAILURE

The causes of primary autogenous vein graft failure, in addition to the influence of the anatomy of the bypass graft, source of the vein, and configuration of the final vein conduit, may be divided into those factors intrinsic or extrinsic to the vein (Table 1). The intrinsic factors account for almost two thirds of the causes of graft failure and include problems associated with surgical technique and proficiency, and the quality and biology of the vein and native vessels. Extrinsic factors account for the remaining one third of causes of graft failure.[6] Of these, the most common problem encountered is a compromised arterial inflow or runoff situation, usually resulting from misinterpretation of the preoperative angiogram, clinical presentation, or perioperative findings. More unusual are problems associated with hypercoagulability, low cardiac output, and graft infection.

TABLE 1.
Factors Contributing to Vein Graft Failure

Intrinsic factors
   Technical factors
      Valvulotome injury
      Retained competent valve leaflets
      Graft entrapment/kinks/torsion
      Arteriovenous fistula
      Clamp injury
      Intimal dissection/intimal flaps
      Anastomotic technical deficits
      Incorrect siting of anastomosis
   Stenosis
      Perianastomotic/midgraft/diffuse (intimal hyperplasia, fibrosis,
        sclerosis, thrombus, recanalization)
   Aneurysmal degeneration
      Perianastomotic/vein conduit
Extrinsic factors
   Progression of atherosclerotic disease in native vessels and vein graft
     conduit
   Thromboembolism
   Hypercoagulable states
   Low cardiac output states
   Graft infection

The occurrence of graft failure after bypass surgery and the underlying etiology are well recognized. The predominant causes of failure in the first postoperative month are technical or judgmental errors, such as valvulotome or clamp injury, retained competent valve leaflets in the in situ and nonreversed vein, intimal flaps, anastomotic narrowing, and twisting or kinking of the graft.[6-10] Most of these will manifest within the first 72 hours. Embolization or thrombus formation with or without associated coagulation disorders, such as AT III, protein S, and protein C deficiencies; immune-mediated heparin-induced thrombocytopenia; and lupus anticoagulant,[8, 11, 12] are responsible for an occasional and unexpected early graft failure. Modern surgical techniques and intraoperative monitoring have reduced the incidence of early graft occlusion to as low as 3% to 5%.[13-17]

Graft stenosis, most frequently due to myointimal hyperplasia of the vein conduit, is the most common cause of intermediate graft failure.[18, 19] Approximately 20% of all vein graft conduits will develop a region of stenosis. Nearly 80% of vein graft stenosis occurs within the first 18 months, most between 4 and 12 months.[20] The stenosis most often presents as a localized stricture in the midgraft, or in the region of the anastomoses.[21, 22] The distal segment of the harvested saphenous vein appears to be the most vulnerable to this degenerative process, with stenosis developing most frequently within 4 cm of the proximal anastomosis in the reversed vein graft and in the mobilized distal segment of the in situ bypass graft.[22, 23] Occasionally, the stenotic process is diffuse and involves long segments of, or even the entire, vein conduit.[6, 20, 24, 25] Although some have suggested that this is unrelated to the valve sites, tributaries, clamp injury, or residual competent valve leaflets in the in situ vein,[21] the more typical findings suggest at least some association with these sites (Fig 1).[26, 27] Abnormal valves can produce increased stress and turbulence with intimal hyperplasia and eventual graft stenosis.[28] Occasionally, improper tunneling of the graft leads to entrapment and partial compression, with repeated trauma at the entrapment site resulting in a hyperplastic response with graft stenosis and even complete occlusion.[7, 10]

In addition to the altered hemodynamics in the arterialized vein,[20, 25] recent experimental and clinical experience suggests that the method of vein preparation may also play a vital role in the development of intimal hyperplasia and stenosis, and the durability of the vein graft conduit. Factors investigated include the pH, composition and temperature of the irrigation fluid, duration of storage, mechanical distension, and prevention of spasm.[29-32] Although only severe and extensive physical damage to the vein graft may create a sufficiently thrombogenic surface to produce an acute occlusion, less severe forms of injury may be the critical factor in the development of intimal hyperplasia and localized vein graft stenosis and failure within the first postoperative year.[31]

Late vein graft failure, after 2 or more years, is most commonly associated with advancing atherosclerosis, especially in the native arteries of the outflow tract.[6] Stenosis due to significant atherosclerotic disease of the conduit itself accounts for graft failure in only ±24% of vein graft conduits.[33, 34] Although fibrous plaques and lipid infiltration are commonly identified in vein grafts within the first 2 years of implantation,

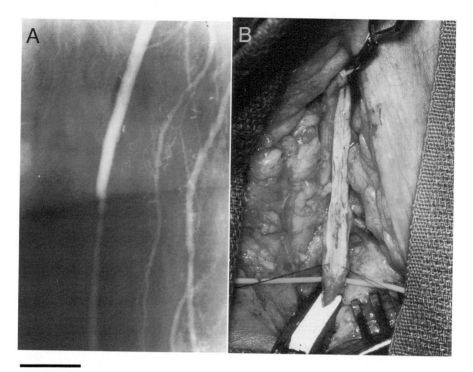

FIGURE 1.

Failing above-knee femoropopliteal saphenous vein bypass graft with a region of stenosis. **A,** preoperative angiogram demonstrates a segmental stenosis at the junction of proximal and mid-thirds of the graft. **B,** the intimal hyperplasia appears to start at the site of a previously lysed valve. The irregular thickening of the walls with significant reduction of luminal area is well seen.

severe, clinically significant atherosclerotic degeneration with stenosis usually develops slowly, after 5 or more years.[25]

Vein graft conduits do dilate over time and may even develop focal or diffuse aneurysmal changes. However, these changes rarely reach a size that results in rupture or graft thrombosis.[27, 33−35]

ANATOMY AND SOURCE OF AUTOGENOUS VEIN

Although the anatomy may have some influence on the durability of the graft, factors related to the indication for surgery and runoff appear to be more significant than the anatomy alone. Patency of grafts performed for claudication with a patent popliteal and tibial outflow tract is in general better than that of grafts performed for limb salvage.[36−39] More controversial are the source and the configuration of the vein.

Autogenous saphenous vein from the ipsilateral or contralateral leg is generally regarded as the best conduit. Other common sources of autogenous vein include the lesser saphenous[40−42] and arm veins.[43−52] The use of the superficial femoral vein, popliteal vein, and deep femoral vein is another alternative source championed by some.[53−56] The results of a direct comparison of the efficacy and durability of the various alternative vein sources have not been reported, certainly not in any prospectively randomized fashion. The various indications for surgery and reasons for the unavailability of suitable saphenous vein would make such a study complex and difficult to perform, requiring large numbers of cases to attain sufficient statistical power for meaningful analysis of the results.

In recent studies of infrainguinal bypass grafts, the use of alternative vein is most frequently associated with reoperative or revision bypass surgery and not due to "inadequate" or inferior vein.[52, 57] In a study of 109 consecutive arm vein bypasses, almost 80% of the patients lacked saphenous vein because of use in previous bypass surgery—infrainguinal bypass in 60.6% and coronary artery bypass in 18.3%. Inadequate or inferior saphenous vein after surgical exploration or harvesting in this series accounted for 13.8%, and previous varicose vein stripping accounted for only 7.3%.[57]

Patency of infrainguinal arm vein bypass grafting, particularly primary patency, has varied considerably.[45–47, 51, 57] The primary patency rate at 1 year varies from 46% to 71%, and the secondary patency at 3 years ranges from 50% to 66%.[51, 57, 58] Despite results inferior to those with the greater saphenous vein, easy accessibility and long lengths of available autogenous vein have made the arm veins an attractive alternative when greater saphenous vein is unavailable. With selection of optimal-quality arm vein segments or endoluminal correction of abnormalities,[57, 58] or the use of routine postoperative Duplex ultrasound surveillance,[59] long-term patency with arm vein as the alternative conduit to saphenous vein has improved significantly.

The lesser saphenous vein, because of its shorter length, has been less favored as a suitable conduit for femorodistal revascularization. This is due in part to the lack of visual clues on physical examination as to its presence and size, as well as the awkwardness in harvesting the vein in the supine patient. The caliber, diameter, quality, wall thickness, and suturability compare favorably with the greater saphenous vein.[40, 42] Most lesser saphenous veins can be used for short, single bypasses, such as femoral above-knee popliteal, popliteal-tibial, and tibiotibial reconstructions. It is possible to attain sufficient conduit for the longer femorodistal reconstructions by using the lesser saphenous vein from both legs. Harvesting the vein through a medial incision by entering the subfascial plane posteriorly and using an additional lateral incision for harvesting the lateral plantar vein is another way to increase the length of a lesser saphenous vein conduit. In addition, an in situ technique for popliteal-distal bypasses has been described.[40, 42] The reported patency for a lesser saphenous vein conduit is similar to that of arm vein (72%–77% at 1 year and 55%–60% at 3 years).[41, 42]

CONFIGURATION OF THE VEIN

No significant differences in graft patency could be demonstrated in a retrospective analysis[2, 4, 5, 60] or a randomized prospective trial[61, 62] comparing in situ with reversed greater saphenous vein bypass grafts. Even though Ku and colleagues[63] have suggested that the intact valves in the reversed vein show a higher resistance to flow than in the cut, incompetent valves of the in situ or nonreversed translocated vein, no study comparing reversed and nonreversed translocated vein in the various infrainguinal bypasses has been reported. Nonreversed and in situ vein have the advantage of better anastomotic size match, simplifying the anastomotic suture and increasing significantly the use of the vein conduits of smaller diameter.[2, 64, 65]

VEIN QUALITY

It is now well recognized that vein quality is the single most important determinant of the success of vein bypass grafting in the lower extremity.[50, 57, 66] However, the criteria for an inferior vein remain poorly defined.[9, 19, 57, 67] Previously, the single most important criterion and determinant of vein quality was size. Vein less than 4 mm in external diameter was considered inferior and unsuitable for bypass grafting.[18, 67, 68] Such veins were routinely discarded. The presence or absence of intraluminal pathology was not much discussed in these early studies, although strictures, thrombi, and synechiae within the vein were recognized. With the increasing use of in situ and nonreversed vein graft bypass techniques, and the almost exclusive use of autogenous vein for all distal bypass grafts, veins as small as 2 mm were found to be of little significance in graft patency, provided vein quality was good and surgical technique proficient.[69–74] Until the introduction of angioscopy, little attention was paid to the acute intraluminal injury invariably associated with valvulotomy or the presence of endoluminal pathology. Routine angioscopy during vein graft preparation and completion monitoring has changed the appreciation of these findings and helped redefine the concept and criteria of vein quality.[9, 15, 57, 75]

CLINICAL EXPERIENCE WITH ANGIOSCOPY

INDICATIONS AND TECHNIQUES

Our indications and techniques for angioscopy have been previously described in detail (Fig 2).[15, 49, 75–79] We have found angioscopes with ex-

Angioscopy Directed Valvulotomy

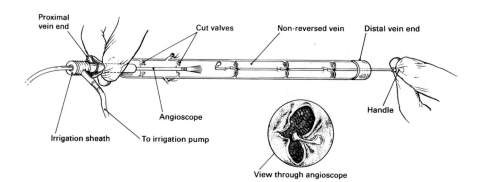

FIGURE 2.

The technique of angioscopy for directed valvulotomy in nonreversed vein grafts. (From Stonebridge P, Miller A, Tsoukas A, et al: *Ann Vasc Surg* 5:170–175, 1991. Used by permission.)

ternal diameters of 1.4 mm (Olympus Corp.) to be the most useful size of angioscope for routine angioscopy during infrainguinal bypass grafting. Depending on the vein and native artery size, we also use angioscopes with external diameters of 2.2 mm and 0.8 mm. We have found larger angioscopes (>2.5 mm outside diameter) and those with irrigating channels too rigid and large for routine use, particularly for completion angioscopy where the entire vein conduit, distal anastomosis, and runoff artery are routinely examined.

Proper technique, especially in irrigation and obtaining a clear visual field, is critical to successful application of angioscopy.[77, 80] The experience required to consistently produce highly successful studies is generally underestimated. In addition to proper technique, familiarity with the ancillary angioscopic equipment is critical to success. Finally, interpretation of the findings remains somewhat problematic, particularly because the angioscope is a qualitative instrument. The accurate assessment of size of the angioscopic image on the video monitor is currently not possible. Magnification of the image changes with the distance of the angioscope lens to the object; the closer the object to the lens, the larger the image.[81]

Indications and use during infrainguinal bypass depend to a large extent on the individual surgeon and his or her own ingenuity. During vein harvesting, a preliminary endoscopic examination of the undissected vein may alter the extent of the dissection and determine which vein to expose. This is not unusual in the arm veins, where the incidence of intraluminal disease is very high.[57] In the failing or failed graft, early use of the angioscope may localize the cause of graft failure and allow assessment of the quality of the graft and the volume of residual thrombus within the graft after thrombectomy or thrombolysis. These factors are critical in deciding whether salvage of the graft is worthwhile or if a new bypass is necessary.[58]

ENDOLUMINAL PATHOLOGY OF AUTOGENOUS VEINS

Our early experience[9, 15, 78] showed that angioscopy was useful in detecting both unsuspected intraluminal pathology and technical imperfections resulting in unexpected graft failure. Angioscopic findings correlating with graft failure from these studies are listed in Table 2. Of all the findings, recanalization of the vein (Fig 3) is the most common and the most significant with regard to graft failure. Although the phenomenon of recanalization within thrombosed veins is well known and has been well described, its etiology, its incidence in the various veins, and its relationship to vein graft failure have not been documented prior to routine use of angioscopy during vein preparation.

The angioscopic appearance of recanalization varies with the amount of previous thrombus formation within the vein. Fine intraluminal strands or bands are seen where the previous thrombus was minimal. With more extensive thrombus, a weblike appearance, with multiple intraluminal channels, is noted (Figs 4,A and B). These may be sparse, allowing passage of the angioscope or valvulotome, or so dense that neither can be passed through the vein. The length of the segment involved varies. It may be extremely short, or the process may involve the entire

TABLE 2.
Endovascular Findings Associated With Graft Failure*

Vein Graft
    Residual competent valve leaflets (uncut/partially cut)
    Unligated tributaries (AV fistula)
    Valvulotome-induced injury
    Thrombosis and recanalization (webs, bands, strands)
    Thrombus (organized, platelet, fresh)
    Intimal hyperplasia
    Mural sclerosis
    Atherosclerotic degeneration
Anastomosis
    Intimal flaps/residual valve leaflet on hood
    Distorted or small apex or outflow tract
    Irregular suture line
    Thrombus (organized, platelet, fresh) on suture line/hood/floor
    Arterial/vein wall pathology
Artery
    Intimal flap/dissection
    Clamp injury
    Thrombus (organized, platelet, fresh)
    Atherosclerotic disease (?plaque characteristics)

*From Miller A, Stonebridge P, Kwolek C: The role of routine angioscopy for infrainguinal bypass procedures, in Moore W, Ahn S (eds): *Endovascular Surgery*. Philadelphia, WB Saunders, 1992, pp 58–69. Used by permission.
AV = arteriovenous.

vein. Bands and strands are usually easily disrupted or cut with the valvulotome, but the dense webs may be tenacious and elastic and usually cannot be adequately cut with the valvulotome.

A consistent angioscopic finding associated with the recanalization process is a large increase in the number of vasa vasorum in the diseased segment of the vein. The vasa vasorum are easily recognized endoscopically by the multiple fine streams of blood flowing into the clear irrigation fluid. This is most frequently seen in the undissected recanalized in situ vein. A similar increased concentration of vasa vasorum occurs at the needle-stick sites of the autogenous arteriovenous fistula used for vascular access.[82]

The incidence of recanalization in the different veins varies and is probably related to the etiology. In series of 53 consecutive greater saphenous vein conduits extending from the groin to the inframalleolar region of the foot, recanalization was noted in only 13.5% of the veins.[75] In the arm vein conduit used for infrainguinal reconstruction, the incidence is significantly increased and ranges from 60% to 70%.[49, 57] The more accessible the veins to needle-sticks for phlebotomy and infusion, the higher the incidence of recanalization (Fig 5). The inaccessible upper arm basilic vein has only an 11% incidence of segmental recanalization, quite similar to that of the greater saphenous vein. The low incidence of re-

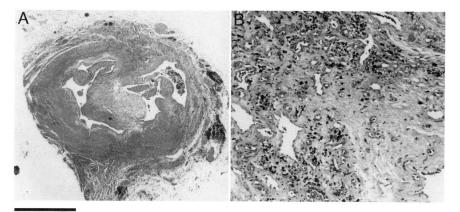

FIGURE 3.

Partially occluded saphenous vein due to recanalized organized thrombus. **A,** low-power photomicrograph of vein cross section demonstrating residual webs from recanalization of vessel. **B,** high-power photomicrograph demonstrating neovascularization with both large and small blood channels, chronic inflammation, and hemosiderin pigment indicative of organized thrombus. Hematoxylin and eosin: **A,** ×20; **B,** ×150. (From Miller A, Jepsen S, Stonebridge P, et al: *Arch Surg* 125:749–755, 1990. Used by permission.)

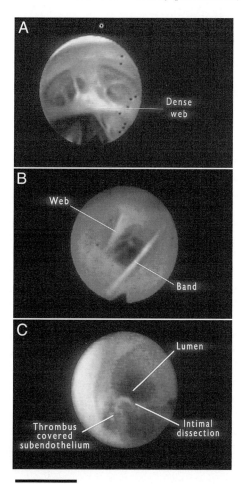

FIGURE 4.

A, dense webs in a segment of saphenous vein. **B,** sparse webs in a segment of saphenous vein. **C,** localized intimal injury following "blind" retrograde valvulotomy. (Part B from Miller A, Jepsen S, Stonebridge P, et al: *Arch Surg* 125:749–755, 1990. Used by permission.)

Segmental Pathology: Incidence and Distribution

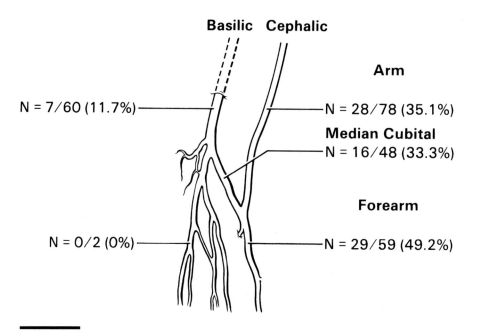

FIGURE 5.

The incidence and distribution of the segmental pathology detected with angioscopic preparation and monitoring of 113 arm veins harvested for infrainguinal bypass conduits is illustrated. (From Marcaccio E, Miller A, Tannenbaum G, et al: *J Vasc Surg* 17:994–1004, 1993. Used by permission.)

canalization in both these veins suggests that the etiology of recanalization in these veins is due to a phlebitic process rather than the iatrogenic trauma of phlebotomy or intravenous infusion.

Clinically, it is important to appreciate that the recanalization process with its multiple channels is more frequently than not undetectable at surgery by external inspection and palpation alone, even with the vein fully exposed. Flushing the vein with saline or blood is always possible unless the vein is completely obstructed. Flow through the vein does not exclude the presence of a region of recanalization. The recanalized segment of vein may act as a filter with acute thrombosis and early graft failure, or it may be the site for development of localized vein stenosis and stricture, probably as the result of "intimal hyperplasia," and cause graft failure within the first year or two after bypass surgery. The stimulus and propensity for these localized regions of diseased vein to stricture are still uncertain. Use of good-quality vein without any evidence of recanalization significantly improves graft patency.[57]

PREPARATION OF THE OPTIMAL QUALITY VEIN CONDUIT

The preparation of an optimal vein conduit requires a meticulous vein preparation technique as well as a conduit free of all endoluminal disease. Vein configuration may influence the quality of the final conduit. Reversed vein requires less intraluminal manipulation than nonreversed or in situ vein. We,[75] as well as others,[83–85] have described the techniques and benefits of angioscopically directed valvulotomy versus the usual "blind" valvulotomy techniques. We have shown that angioscopically directed valvulotomy almost completely eliminates the previously unappreciated high incidence of endoluminal vein injury, as well as the problem of leaving competent valve leaflets (Fig 4C, Table 3). Furthermore, the routine inspection of the final vein conduit, irrespective of the vein configuration, accurately localizes various intraluminal lesions and pathologies so that precise and directed interventions to correct or eliminate them can be performed. Inspection also documents any residual intraluminal pathology or technical deficits and provides a reliable method to document the quality of the vein conduit, whether it is minimally, moderately, or severely diseased.

We,[9, 57] as well as others,[19] have shown that vein conduit quality correlates closely with graft patency. More important, we have shown the value of upgrading the quality of the vein conduit by elimination of grossly abnormal vein segments, web disruption, cutting of fine strands and bands, removal of intraluminal thrombus, and patch angioplasty of stenotic segments. In a series of 109 arm veins,[57] 71 veins were found to be abnormal. Eighty-three angioscopically directed interventions were performed in 68 (95.8%) of the abnormal vein grafts. In the remaining 3 vein grafts, although significant disease was noted, further intervention was not performed because of constraints with regard to conduit length. Angioscopically directed interventions resulted in upgraded vein conduit in 47 (66.1%) of the 71 abnormal grafts. Primary patency for grafts with normal and upgraded conduit was similar in both primary and redo bypass procedures. Overall, the early (<30-day) patency rate for all grafts with normal or upgraded conduits was 85 (95.5%) of 89 grafts. This was considerably better than 14 (70%) of 20 conduits whose quality remained "inferior" despite attempted angioscopic correction ($P = .0024$, two-sided Fisher's exact test). Life-table analysis showed that this difference in early patency rates persisted through 1 year of follow-up (Fig 6). A 3-year follow-up of these grafts and an additional 150 arm vein grafts prepared angioscopically shows that this difference persists.[86] In our series, splic-

TABLE 3.

Ratio of Valvulotome-Induced Injury Per Number of Cut Valves*

	Mean No. of Valves Per Vein	No. of Injured Veins	No. of Cut Valves (A)	No. of Injured Areas (B)	B/A
BRV (n=53)	7.3	45 (84.9%)	389	190	0.49
ADV (n=32)	7.8	5 (15.6%)	250	5†	0.02

*From Miller A, Stonebridge P, Tsoukas A, et al: *J Vasc Surg* 13:813–821, 1991. Used by permission.
†Including one transsected vein.
BRV = blind retrograde valvulotomy; ADV = angioscopically directed valvulotomy.

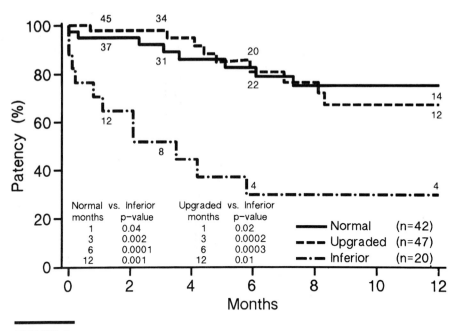

FIGURE 6.

Comparison of primary graft patency for the 109 infrainguinal arm vein bypass grafts as determined by life tables with comparisons of "normal" vs. "upgraded" vs. "inferior" quality arm vein grafts. (From Marcaccio E, Miller A, Tannenbaum G, et al: *J Vasc Surg* 17:994–1004, 1993. Used by permission.)

ing of multiple segments of good-quality vein to attain adequate length had little influence on patency. Patency was similar to that of single lengths of arm vein conduit.[57, 86]

In an attempt to improve postoperative patency, routine surveillance of vein grafts has been advocated by some.[59] The use of intraoperative angioscopy to select optimal segments of vein conduit may obviate the need for routine postoperative graft surveillance. In fact, it strongly suggests that selective surveillance based on the angioscopic quality of the final graft conduit may be a much more cost-effective method of graft surveillance.

COMPARISON WITH OTHER METHODS OF VEIN CONDUIT QUALITY ASSESSMENT

Although attempts to determine vein quality preoperatively continue, they remain unreliable. Preoperative venography is useful in determining length and continuity of available vein but is a poor determinant of vein quality.[87, 88] Furthermore, it is an invasive procedure associated with patient discomfort and occasional contrast sensitivity, phlebitis, and renal impairment. Duplex scanning and vein mapping are noninvasive and safe.[89–94] Although the presence of usable vein and its continuity are reliably determined, size and accurate localization of endoluminal pathology, unless severe and occlusive, are more problematic. They are time-consuming and technologist-dependent.

With the refinement of Duplex technology, intraoperative monitoring is possible,[95] with residual defects identified in 13% to 18% of a miscellaneous graft of arterial reconstructions, highest for infrainguinal vein bypass grafts.[96] Routine intraoperative Duplex examination is hindered by the complexity of instrumentation as well as the difficulties in accurate interpretation. Familiarity with the instrumentation and the pitfalls of color-flow Doppler imaging, including recognition of artifacts, aliasing, improper Doppler angle, and assignment of sample volume placement, is critical for interpretive accuracy. In a blinded comparison of intraoperative Duplex ultrasound, intraoperative angiogram, and angioscopy, Gilbertson and colleagues[97] showed that angioscopy is far more sensitive and specific in detecting residual competent valves in the in situ vein bypass graft, residual unligated tributaries, and technical deficits than are the other methods. This is particularly so in situations where flow hemodynamics are minimally altered.

The insensitivity of the "gold-standard" intraoperative angiogram to accurately delineate endoluminal abnormalities intrinsic to the native vessels and surgical technique has been well documented.[8, 16, 97, 98] In a prospectively randomized study comparing 122 cases of completion angiography with 128 cases of angioscopy, only 7 interventions were performed in the angiography group as compared with 32 in the angioscopy group (Table 4). Most significant, there was only a single finding in the vein conduit in the intraoperative angiogram group—a residual competent valve—as compared with 28 findings resulting in intervention in the conduit of the angioscopy group.

This was not clearly reflected in the overall results of the study, which showed only a statistical trend favoring angioscopic monitoring in the early (<30-day) graft patency. However, with subgroup analysis and the exclusion of a group of 11 plantar artery bypasses that had a 35% early

TABLE 4.
Relevant Findings and Clinical Decisions Resulting in 39 Interventions in 36 Bypass Grafts During the Completion Monitoring of 250 Infrainguinal Bypass Grafts*

Intervention (N = 36 Bypass Grafts)		
	Angioscopy	**Angiogram**
Vein conduit	28	1
Residual competent valve	9	1
Vein preparation/selection	6	0
Tributary ligation	13	0
Anastomosis	3	5†
Distal artery	1	1
Total	32	7

*Modified from Miller A, Marcaccio E, Tannenbaum G, et al: *J Vasc Surg* 17:382–398, 1992. Used by permission.
†Two of these five findings were false-positive.

failure rate, this difference achieved statistical significance (Fig 7). Determination of vein quality based on intraoperative angiogram alone is not feasible unless significant hemodynamic and obstructive changes are present.

Others have attempted to define vein conduit quality by examination of vein wall characteristics, both dynamic and histopathologic. Davies and associates[28] studied vein wall compliance preoperatively to predict vein grafts at risk for failure in patients undergoing infrainguinal revascularization. This group showed that vein conduits with a higher incidence of graft failure were less compliant and, on histologic examination, showed increased intramural fibrosis at the time of insertion. Marin and colleagues[99] examined discarded segments of harvested vein subsequently used for bypass grafting. This study showed that veins with thick and calcified walls or hypercellular intima at the time of grafting were at increased risk of developing intragraft lesions and graft failure.

Both studies suggest that vein quality may be determined by study of only a short segment of the vein conduit. Our own results, where "upgraded" arm veins have similar patency to angioscopically normal arm veins, do not entirely support this hypothesis (see Fig 6). Rather, our re-

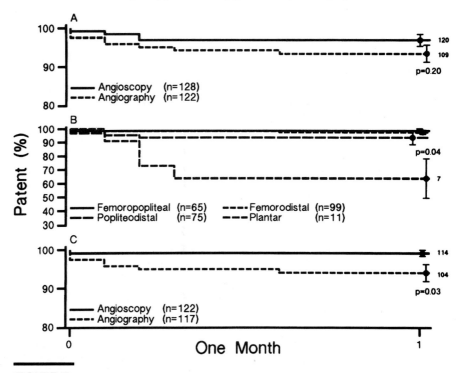

FIGURE 7.

Life-table analysis to 1 month comparing the proportions of primary graft failure. **A,** failure of the angioscopy and angiogram groups. The difference at 1 month is not statistically significant ($P = .2$). **B,** failure of the 11 bypasses to the plantar arteries and the remaining 239 bypasses in the study. At 1 month the difference is statistically significant ($P = .04$). **C,** failure of the angioscopy and angiogram groups with the 11 plantar arteries excluded. The difference at 1 month is statistically significant ($P = .03$). (From Miller A, Marcaccio E, Tannenbaum G, et al: *J Vasc Surg* 17:382–398, 1992. Used by permission.)

sults suggest that vein pathology resulting in graft failure is frequently segmental. Abnormalities detected in one segment of the vein conduit do not reflect the quality of the entire length of vein conduit selected. Thus, for clinical purposes, irrespective of configuration (reversed, nonreversed, or in situ), angioscopic examination of harvested vein conduit and removal or repair of angioscopically recognized endoluminal pathology is the simplest and most reliable method to accurately assess and optimize the final quality of the vein conduit used. Routine angioscopic examination would improve vein graft patency and could also provide a firm basis for selective postoperative graft surveillance.

THE IMPACT OF ANGIOSCOPY ON THE FAILING AND FAILED BYPASS GRAFT

The incidence of reoperation for failing or failed infrainguinal bypass grafts increases with time. These revision or redo operations are difficult, tedious, and frustrating. Often, despite extensive preoperative evaluation and prolonged surgery, the exact cause of failure remains elusive. Direct angioscopic evaluation at the time of surgery has proved effective not only in identifying the cause of graft failure but also in monitoring the adequacy of thrombectomy or thrombolysis. Most important of all, angioscopy provides a means of assessing the adequacy of the vein conduit after all interventions.

A review of 79 failing or failed grafts showed that the angiogram consistently underestimates the amount of residual thrombus in the graft or native vessel.[58] We[9, 58] and others[100, 101] have consistently shown that angioscopy remains the most sensitive method to evaluate the amount of residual thrombus after thrombectomy and thrombolysis. The more residual thrombus within the graft conduit, anastomosis, and runoff artery at the end of the reoperation, the poorer the early and long-term patency (Fig 8). This may explain the consistent finding that despite an initial high "success" rate of 48% to 86% for preoperative thrombolysis, and even with correction of underlying lesions, the long-term patency of failed grafts is disappointing at 20% to 77% at 1 year.[102–106]

Because of these results of attempted graft salvage, some recommend abandonment of the old graft and establishment of a new graft if sufficient autogenous vein is available.[107] The fate of graft endothelium and intimal surfaces after thrombosis is unknown, but it has been suggested that ischemic or inflammatory changes occur during the time of thrombosis until resumption of arterial blood flow can be achieved, revitalizing the endothelium.[108] Others have suggested intimal "injury" attributed to balloon thrombectomy or some unknown direct action of the thrombolytic agents to the endothelial cells as the critical factor in graft durability. The angioscopic appearance of the graft luminal surface after thrombolysis and thrombectomy may provide a clue to the "health" of the vascular endothelium. Grafts that cannot be adequately cleared of adherent thrombus may contain large areas of dead or dysfunctional endothelium, whereas grafts with intact cellular linings can resist the adherence of thrombus through the action of their surface anticoagulant glycoproteins or other unknown mediators.

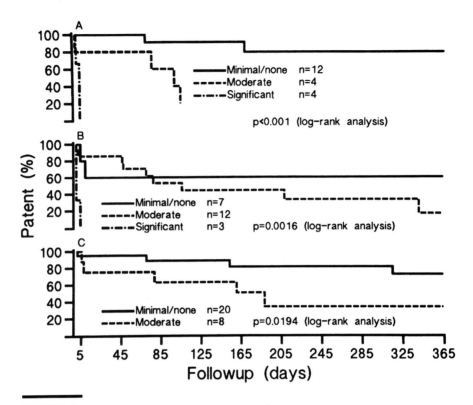

FIGURE 8.

Graft patency by life-table analysis within subgroups defined by residual thrombus within the graft. **A,** early graft failure (P < .001, log-rank analysis). **B,** late failed grafts (P = .0016, log-rank analysis). **C,** late failing grafts (P = .0194, log-rank analysis). (From Hölzenbein T, Miller A, Tannenbaum G, et al: *Ann Vasc Surg* 8:74–91, 1994. Used by permission.)

CONCLUSIONS

With modern surgical techniques, lower-extremity revascularization, even to the most distal arteries in the foot, is not only feasible but effective, with a dramatic lowering of the primary amputation rate.[109] For these distal bypasses, autogenous vein conduit remains the conduit of choice. The single most important factor influencing the durability of infrainguinal vein graft bypass grafts remains the intrinsic quality of the vein conduit. Routine endoscopy of these vein conduits at the time of surgery has resulted in the recognition of previously unsuspected incidences of endoluminal pathology within the autogenous vein and an appreciation of their impact on graft failure.[9, 15, 78] This new awareness has resulted in a search for reliable methods to detect these abnormalities before, during, and even after the bypass surgery.

We,[16] as well as others,[97, 98] have shown that unlike intraoperative angiography and Duplex ultrasound, direct intravascular visualization by angioscopic examination is a simple method to reliably and accurately assess the quality of the autogenous venous conduit. It allows the surgeon to select the best available conduit, or, when the conduit is diseased, to optimize the available autogenous conduit by directed interventions.

Although routine postoperative surveillance of all grafts has been advocated by some,[59] we have shown that the intraoperative detection and correction of any conduit pathology results in improved outcomes with significant savings in the cost of routine surveillance.[57, 86] Our results suggest that routine angioscopic examination of the vein conduit allows an accurate assessment of vein quality and may allow a selective surveillance for that group of "inferior" quality grafts at highest risk. Such an approach could significantly reduce the burden of routine surveillance of all vein bypass grafts with its excessive costs and time for both the patient and the medical team. Investment in the necessary angioscopic equipment and training would be more than offset by such savings.

The technical difficulties for the occasional angioscopist in achieving reliable, high-quality angioscopic examinations must be recognized and addressed. Like all other endoscopic techniques, proficiency is obtained only by routine and repeated application. Unlike other endoscopic techniques, angioscopy requires the removal of all blood from the visual field for successful endoluminal visualization. This complicates the procedure and increases the learning curve.

Finally, the benefits of angioscopy for the modern vascular surgeon may not be confined to the assessment of vein quality or the optimization of the technical aspects of bypass surgery. With the development of new instrumentation, the goal of minimally invasive bypass surgery with complete endoluminal preparation of the vein conduit will be realized.[110] The combination of endoluminal visualization with other developing modalities that assess the structure and histochemistry of the vein conduit,[111] or even alter the cellular function of the vein conduit, may eventually allow better definition of vein quality and the selection of the truly optimal vein graft conduit.[112, 113] Such autogenous vein conduits, free not only from macroscopically recognized disease but also from functional abnormalities, will provide the most reliable and durable bypass grafts.

REFERENCES

1. Kunlin J: Le traitement de l'arterite obliterante par la greffe veineuse. *Arch Mal Coeur* 42:371–374, 1949.
2. Leather R, Shah D, Chang B, et al: Resurrection of the in situ vein bypass: 1000 cases later. *Ann Surg* 208:435–442, 1988.
3. Bandyk D, Kaebnick H, Bergamini T, et al: Hemodynamics of in situ saphenous vein arterial bypass. *Arch Surg* 123:477–482, 1988.
4. Taylor L, Edwards J, Porter J: Present status of reversed vein bypass: Five year results of a modern series. *J Vasc Surg* 11:207–215, 1990.
5. Donaldson M, Mannick J, Whittemore A: Femoral-distal bypass with in situ greater saphenous vein. Long-term results using the Mills valvulotome. *Ann Surg* 13:457–465, 1991.
6. Donaldson M, Mannick J, Whittemore A: Causes of primary graft failure after in situ saphenous vein bypass grafting. *J Vasc Surg* 15:113–120, 1992.
7. Gutierrez I, Barone D, Currier C, Makula P: Iatrogenic entrapment of the femoropopliteal bypass. *J Vasc Surg* 2:468–471, 1985.
8. Stept L, Flinn WR, McCarthy W, et al: Technical defects as a cause of early graft failure after femorodistal bypass. *Arch Surg* 122:599–604, 1987.

9. Miller A, Jepsen S, Stonebridge P, et al: New angioscopic findings in graft failure after infra-inguinal bypass grafting. *Arch Surg* 125:749–755, 1990.

10. Carpenter J, Lieberman M, Schlansky-Goldberg R, et al: Infrageniculate bypass graft entrapment. *J Vasc Surg* 18:81–89, 1993.

11. Craver J, Ottinger L, Darling R, et al: Hemorrhage and thrombosis as early complications of femoropopliteal bypass grafts: Causes, treatment and prognostic implications. *Surgery* 74:839–845, 1973.

12. Towne J, Bernhard V, Hussey, et al: Antithrombin III deficiency: A cause of unexplained thrombosis in vascular surgery. *Surgery* 89:735–742, 1981.

13. Taylor LJ, Phinney E, Porter J: Present status of reversed vein bypass for lower extremity revascularization. *J Vasc Surg* 3:288–297, 1986.

14. Bandyk D, Kaebnick H, Stewart G, et al: Durability of the in situ saphenous vein arterial bypass: A comparison of primary and secondary patency. *J Vasc Surg* 5:256–268, 1987.

15. Miller A, Stonebridge P, Jepsen S, et al: Continued experience with intraoperative angioscopy for monitoring infrainguinal bypass grafting. *Surgery* 109:286–293, 1991.

16. Miller A, Marcaccio E, Tannenbaum G, et al: Comparison of angioscopy and angiography for monitoring infrainguinal bypass grafts: Results of a prospective randomized trial. *J Vasc Surg* 17:382–398, 1992.

17. Mills J, Fujitani R, Taylor S: The contribution of routine intraoperative completion arteriography to early infrainguinal bypass patency. *Am J Surg* 164:506–511, 1992.

18. Imparato A, Bracco A, Kim G, et al: Intimal and neointimal fibrous proliferation causing failure of arterial reconstruction. *Surgery* 72:1007–1017, 1972.

19. Panetta T, Marin M, Veith F, et al: Unsuspected preexisting saphenous vein disease: An unrecognized cause of vein bypass failure. *J Vasc Surg* 15:102–112, 1992.

20. Mills J, Fujitani R, Taylor S: The characteristics and anatomic distribution of lesions that cause reversed vein graft failure: A five-year prospective study. *J Vasc Surg* 17:195–206, 1993.

21. Moody A, Edwards P, Harris P: The etiology of vein graft strictures: A prospective marker study. *Eur J Vasc Surg* 6:509–511, 1992.

22. Berkowitz H, Fox A, Deaton D: Reversed vein graft stenosis: Early diagnosis and management. *J Vasc Surg* 15:130–142, 1992.

23. Varty K, London N, Brennan J, et al: Infragenicular in situ vein bypass graft occlusion: A multivariate risk factor analysis. *Eur J Vasc Surg* 7:567–571, 1993.

24. Whittemore A, Donaldson M, Polak J, et al: Limitations of balloon angioplasty for vein graft stenosis. *J Vasc Surg* 14:340–345, 1991.

25. Mills J: Mechanism of vein graft failure: The location, distribution, and characteristics of lesions that predispose to graft failure. *Semin Vasc Surg* 6:78–91, 1993.

26. Whitney D, Kahn E, Estes J: Valvular occlusion of the arterialized saphenous vein. *Am Surg* 42:879–887, 1976.

27. Fuchs J, Mitchener J, Po H: Postoperative changes in autogenous vein grafts. *Ann Surg* 188:1–12, 1978.

28. Davies A, Magee T, Baird R, et al: Pre-bypass morphological changes in vein grafts. *Eur J Vasc Surg* 7:642–647, 1993.

29. Abbott W, Wieland E, Austen W: Structural changes during preparation of autogenous venous grafts. *Surgery* 76:1030–1040, 1974.

30. LoGerfo F, Quist W, Crawshaw H, et al: An improved technique for preservation of endothelial morphology in vein grafts. *Surgery* 90:1015–1024, 1981.

31. Sottiurai V: Saphenous vein preparation, in Bunt T, (ed): *Iatrogenic Vascular Injury.* Mount Kisco, New York, 1990. Futura, 73–101.

32. Quist W, LoGerfo F: Prevention of smooth muscle cell phenotypic modulation in vein grafts: A histomorphometric study. *J Vasc Surg* 16:225–231, 1992.

33. Szilagyi D, Elliott J, Hageman J, et al: Biologic fate of autogenous vein implants as arterial substitutes. *Ann Surg* 178:232–239, 1973.

34. Reifsnyder T, Towne J, Seabrook G, et al: Biologic characteristics of long-term autogenous vein grafts: A dynamic evolution. *J Vasc Surg* 17:207–217, 1993.

35. Peer R, Upson J: Aneurysmal dilation in saphenous vein bypass grafts. *J Cardiovasc Surg* 31:668–671, 1990.

36. Hobson RI, O'Donnell J, Jamil Z, et al: Below-knee bypass for limb salvage. *Arch Surg* 115:833–837, 1980.

37. Cranley J, Hafner C: Revascularization of the femoropopliteal arteries using saphenous vein, polytetrafluoroethylene and human umbilical vein grafts. *Arch Surg* 117:1537–1539, 1982.

38. Yeager R, Hobson RI, Lynch TG, et al: Analysis of factors influencing patency of polytetrafluoroethylene prostheses for limb salvage. *J Surg Res* 32:499–506, 1982.

39. Hall R, Coupland G, Lane R, et al: Vein, Gore-tex or composite graft for femoropopliteal bypass. *Surg Gynecol Obstet* 161:308–312, 1985.

40. Shandall A, Leather R, Corson J, et al: Use of short saphenous vein in situ for popliteal-to-distal artery bypass. *Am J Surg* 154:240–244, 1987.

41. Weaver F, Barlow C, Edwards W, et al: The lesser saphenous vein: Autogenous tissue for lower extremity revascularization. *J Vasc Surg* 5:687–692, 1987.

42. Chang B, Paty P, Shah D, et al: The lesser saphenous vein: An underappreciated source of autogenous vein. *J Vasc Surg* 15:152–157, 1992.

43. Kakkar V: The cephalic vein as a peripheral vascular graft. *Surg Gynecol Obstet* 128:551–556, 1969.

44. Campbell D, Hoar C, Gibbons G: The use of arm veins in femoral-popliteal bypass grafts. *Ann Surg* 190:740–742, 1979.

45. Schulman M, Badhey M: Late results and angiographic evaluation of arm veins as long bypass grafts. *Surgery* 92:1032–1041, 1982.

46. Harris R, Andros G, Dulawa L, et al: Successful long-term limb salvage using cephalic vein bypass grafts. *Ann Surg* 200:785–792, 1984.

47. Andros G, Harris R, Salles-Cunha S, et al: Arm veins for arterial revascularization of the leg: Arteriographic and clinical observations. *J Vasc Surg* 4:416–427, 1986.

48. Balshi J, Cantelmo N, Menzoian J, et al: The use of arm veins for infrainguinal bypass in end-stage peripheral vascular disease. *Arch Surg* 124:1078–1081, 1989.

49. Stonebridge P, Miller A, Tsoukas A, et al: Angioscopy of arm vein infrainguinal bypass grafts. *Ann Vasc Surg* 5:170–175, 1991.

50. Marcaccio E, Miller A, Tannenbaum G, et al: Can angioscopically directed intervention upgrade arm vein quality and improve early graft patency? (abstract) New England Vascular Society Meeting, Dixville Notch, New Hampshire, 1992.

51. Harward T, Coe D, Flynn T, et al: The use of arm vein conduits during infrageniculate arterial bypass. *J Vasc Surg* 16:420–427, 1992.

52. Londrey G, Bosher L, Brown P, et al: Infrainguinal reconstruction with arm vein, lesser saphenous vein, and remnants of greater saphenous vein: A report of 257 cases. *J Vasc Surg* 20:451–457, 1994.

53. Schulman M, Badhey M: Deep veins of the leg as femoropopliteal bypass grafts. *Arch Surg* 116:1141–1145, 1981.

54. Schulman M, Badhey M, Yatco R: An 11-year experience with deep leg veins as femoropopliteal bypass grafts. *Arch Surg* 121:1010–1015, 1987.

55. Schulman M, Badhey M, Yatco R: Superficial femoral-popliteal veins and reversed saphenous veins as primary femoropopliteal bypass grafts: A randomized comparative study. *J Vasc Surg* 6:1–10, 1987.

56. Coburn M, Ashworth C, Francis W, et al: Venous stasis of the use of the superficial femoral and popliteal veins for lower extremity bypass. *J Vasc Surg* 17:1005–1009, 1993.

57. Marcaccio E, Miller A, Tannenbaum G, et al: Angioscopically directed interventions improve arm vein bypass grafts. *J Vasc Surg* 17:994–1004, 1993.

58. Hölzenbein T, Miller A, Tannenbaum G, et al: Role of angioscopy in reoperation for the failing or failed infrainguinal vein bypass graft. *Ann Vasc Surg* 8:74–91, 1994.

59. Chalmers R, Hoballah J, Kresowik T, et al: The impact of color Duplex surveillance on the outcome of lower limb bypass with segments of arm veins. *J Vasc Surg* 19:279–288, 1994.

60. Bandyk D, Schmitt D, Seabrook G, et al: Monitoring functional patency of in situ saphenous vein bypasses: The impact of a surveillance protocol and elective revision. *J Vasc Surg* 9:286–296, 1989.

61. Harris P, How T, Joner DR: Prospectively randomized clinical trial to compare in situ and reversed saphenous vein grafts for femoropopliteal bypass. *Br J Surg* 74:252–255, 1987.

62. Harris P, Veith F, Shanik G, et al: Prospective randomized comparison of in situ and reversed infrapopliteal vein grafts. *Br J Surg* 80:173–176, 1993.

63. Ku D, Klafta J, Gewertz B, et al: The contribution of valves to saphenous vein graft resistance. *J Vasc Surg* 6:274–279, 1987.

64. Leather R, Shah D, Karmody A: Infrapopliteal arterial bypass for limb salvage: Increased patency and utilisation of the saphenous vein "in situ." *Surgery* 90:1001–1009, 1981.

65. Leather R, Shah D, Corson J, et al: Instrumental evolution of the valve incision method of in situ saphenous vein bypass. *J Vasc Surg* 1:113–123, 1984.

66. Plecha E, Seabrook G, Bandyk D, et al: Determinants of successful peroneal artery bypass. *J Vasc Surg* 17:97–106, 1993.

67. Szilagyi D, Hageman J, Smith R, et al: Autogenous vein grafting in femoropopliteal atherosclerosis: The limits of effectiveness. *Surgery* 86:836–849, 1979.

68. LoGerfo F, Corson J, Mannick J: Improved results with femoropopliteal bypass grafts for limb salvage. *Arch Surg* 112:567–571, 1977.

69. Sonnenfeld T, Cronestrand R: Intraoperative blood flow related to failure of femoropopliteal bypass grafts. *Scand J Thorac Cardiovasc Surg* 14:101–104, 1980.

70. LiCalzi L, Stansel H: Failure of autogenous reversed saphenous vein femoropopliteal grafting: Pathophysiology and prevention. *Surgery* 91:352–357, 1982.

71. Corson J, Karmody A, Shah D, et al: In situ vein bypass to distal tibial and limited outflow tract limb salvage. *Surgery* 96:756–761, 1984.

72. Abbott W, Megerman J, Hasson J, et al: Effect of compliance mismatch upon vascular graft patency. *J Vasc Surg* 5:376–382, 1987.

73. Scott D, Beard J, Wyatt M, et al: In situ vein femorodistal bypass: Does vein size matter? *Br J Surg* 61:610, 1988.

74. Bandyk D: The effect of vein diameter on patency of in situ grafts. *J Cardiovasc Surg* 32:192–195, 1991.

75. Miller A, Stonebridge P, Tsoukas A, et al: Angioscopically directed valvulotomy: A new valvulotome and technique. *J Vasc Surg* 13:813–821, 1991.
76. Majeski J: Forearm arterial venous shunt for hemodialysis. *Am Surg* 51:630–631, 1985.
77. Miller A, Lipson W, Isaacsohn J, et al: Intraoperative angioscopy: Principles of irrigation and description of a new dedicated irrigation pump. *Am Heart J* 118:391–399, 1989.
78. Miller A, Campbell D, Gibbons G, et al: Routine intraoperative angioscopy in lower extremity revascularization. *Arch Surg* 124:604–608, 1989.
79. Miller A, Jepsen S: Angioscopy in arterial surgery. In Bergan J, Yao J, editors: *Techniques in Arterial Surgery*. Philadelphia, 1990. WB Saunders, pp 409–416.
80. Kwolek C, Miller A, Stonebridge P, et al: Safety of saline irrigation for angioscopy: Results of a prospective randomized trial. *Ann Vasc Surg* 6:62–68, 1992.
81. Spears R, Marais H, Serur J, et al: In vivo coronary angioscopy. *J Am Coll Cardiol* 5:1311–1314, 1983.
82. Hölzenbein T, Miller A, Gottlieb M, et al: The role of angioscopy in vascular access surgery. *J Endovasc Surg*, 2:10–25, 1995.
83. Fleisher HI, Thompson B, McCowan T, et al: Angioscopically monitored saphenous vein valvulotomy. *J Vasc Surg* 4:360–364, 1986.
84. Matsumoto T, Yang Y, Hashizume M: Direct vision valvulotomy for nonreversed vein graft. *Surg Gynecol Obstet* 165:181–183, 1987.
85. Mehigan J: Angioscopic preparation of the in situ saphenous vein for arterial bypass: Technical considerations, in White G, White R (eds): *Angioscopy: Vascular and Coronary Applications*. St Louis, Mosby, 1989, pp 72–75.
86. Hölzenbein T, Pomposelli F, Miller A, et al: Arm veins for infrainguinal bypass: The first alternative to ipsilateral saphenous vein grafts? *J Vasc Surg* 21:586–594, 1995.
87. Veith F, Moss C, Sprayregen S, et al: Preoperative saphenous venography in arterial reconstructive surgery of the extremity. *Surgery* 85:253–256, 1979.
88. Moseley J, Manhire A, Raphael M, et al: An assessment of long saphenous vein before in situ bypass. *Br J Surg* 70:673–674, 1983.
89. Leopold P, Shandall A, Corson J, et al: Initial experience comparing B mode imaging and venography of the long saphenous vein before in situ bypass. *Am J Surg* 6:107–113, 1986.
90. Ruoff B, Cranley J, Hannan L, et al: Duplex ultrasound mapping of the greater saphenous vein before in situ infrainguinal revascularization. *J Vasc Surg* 6:107–113, 1987.
91. Seeger J, Schmidt J, Flynn T: Preoperative saphenous and cephalic vein mapping as an adjunct to reconstructive surgery. *Ann Surg* 205:733–739, 1987.
92. McShane M, Field J, Smallwood J, et al: Early experience with B mode ultrasound mapping of the long saphenous vein prior to femorodistal bypass. *Ann R Coll Surg* 70:147–149, 1988.
93. Bagi P, Schroeder T, Sillesen H, et al: Real time B-mode mapping of the greater saphenous vein. *Eur J Vasc Surg* 3:103–105, 1989.
94. Leopold P, Shandall A, Kupinski A, et al: Role of B-mode venous mapping in infrainguinal in situ vein arterial bypasses. *Br J Surg* 76:305, 1989.
95. Bandyk D, Jorgensen R, Towne J: Intraoperative assessment of in situ saphenous vein arterial grafts using pulsed Doppler spectral analysis. *Arch Surg* 121:292–299, 1986.

96. Bandyk D, Zierler R, Thiele B: Detection of technical error during arterial surgery by pulsed Doppler spectral analysis. *Arch Surg* 119:421–427, 1984.

97. Gilbertson J, Walsh D, Zwolak R, et al: A blinded comparison of arteriography, angioscopy, and Duplex scanning in the intraoperative evaluation of in situ saphenous vein bypass grafts. *J Vasc Surg* 15:121–129, 1992.

98. Baxter B, Rizzo R, Flinn W, et al: A comparative study of intraoperative angioscopy and completion arteriography following femorodistal bypass. *Arch Surg* 125:997–1002, 1990.

99. Marin M, Veith F, Panetta T, et al: Saphenous vein biopsy: A predictor of vein graft failure. *J Vasc Surg* 18:407–415, 1993.

100. White G, White R, Kopchok B, et al: Angioscopic thrombectomy: Preliminary observations in a recent technique. *J Vasc Surg* 7:318–325, 1988.

101. Segalowitz J, Grundfest W, Treiman R, et al: Angioscopy for intraoperative management of thromboembolectomy. *Arch Surg* 125:1357–1362, 1990.

102. Durham J, Geller S, Abbott W, et al: Regional infusion of urokinase into occluded lower-extremity bypass grafts: Long term clinical results. *Radiology* 172:83–87, 1989.

103. v. Breda A, Robinson J, Feldman L, et al: Local thrombolysis in the treatment of arterial graft occlusions. *J Vasc Surg* 1:103–112, 1984.

104. McNamara T, Fischer R: Thrombolysis of peripheral arterial and graft occlusions: Improved results using high-dose urokinase. *AJR* 147:621–626, 1985.

105. Graor R, Risius B, Young J, et al: Thrombolysis of peripheral arterial bypass grafts: Surgical thrombectomy compared with thrombolysis. *J Vasc Surg* 7:347–355, 1988.

106. Gardiner G, Harrington D, Koltun W, et al: Salvage of occluded arterial bypass grafts by means of thrombolysis. *J Vasc Surg* 9:426–431, 1989.

107. Edwards JE, Taylor LM Jr, Porter JM: Treatment of failed lower extremity bypass grafts with new autogenous vein bypass grafting. *J Vasc Surg* 11:136–145, 1990.

108. Cox J, Chiasson D, Gottlieb A: Stranger in a strange land: The pathogenesis of saphenous vein graft stenosis with emphasis on structural and functional differences between veins and arteries. *Prog Cardiovasc Dis* 34:45–68, 1991.

109. LoGerfo W, Gibbons G, Pomposelli F, et al: Evolving trends in the management of the diabetic foot. *Arch Surg* 127:617–621, 1992.

110. Rosental D, Herring M, O'Conovan T, et al: Endoluminal in situ femoropopliteal bypass: Will this replace a classical procedure? *Angiology, International Congress V* (suppl) 43:274–275, 1992.

111. Baraga JJ, Feld MS, Rava RP: In situ optical histochemistry of human artery using near infrared Fourier Transform Raman spectroscopy. *Proc Natl Acad Sci USA* 89:3473–3477, 1992.

112. Nabel EB, Plautz G, Nabel GJ: Site-specific gene expression in vivo by direct gene transfer into the arterial wall. *Science* 249:1285–1288, 1990.

113. Ohno T, Gordon D, Sam H, et al: Gene therapy for vascular smooth muscle cell proliferation after arterial injury. *Science* 265:781–784, 1994.

The Role of Cryopreserved Vein Allografts in Infrainguinal Reconstructions

Gian Luca Faggioli, M.D.
Research Physician, University of Bologna, Bologna, Italy

John J. Ricotta, M.D.
Professor of Surgery, Director, Division of Vascular Surgery, SUNY at Buffalo, Millard Fillmore Hospital, Buffalo, New York

HISTORICAL BACKGROUND

Venous homografts and xenografts were first described by Yamamouchi[1] and Carrel,[2] who used these materials in experimental settings. Linton[3] and Dye and colleagues[4] reported the first clinical experiences with fresh venous homografts. Barner, DeWeese, and Schenk[5] proposed the idea of preserving the venous allografts in the late 1960s. In 1970, a clinical series of eight vein homografts preserved at −50°C was used for grafting or patching by Tice and Zerbino.[6] Two years later, 46 procedures had been performed in the same institution with an early patency rate of 72%.[7] After this, a number of experimental studies appeared evaluating both graft and host modification as mechanisms to improve patency. Small clinical series, using venous homografts in both the peripheral and coronary circulations, have continued to appear. Until recently, techniques of cryopreservation were not standardized. Within the last several years, graft preservation has evolved into a commercial process, permitting some quality control comparisons. However, patient selection and adjuvant therapies remain poorly defined.

THE POTENTIAL ROLE FOR CRYOPRESERVED VEIN ALLOGRAFTS

The autologous saphenous vein is unanimously considered the conduit of choice in infrainguinal reconstructions, with 3-year patency rates in the range of 77% to 86% for below-knee bypasses.[8] However, in as many as 20% of patients, this vein is not suitable for reconstruction, and in 10% of the cases, another possible vein conduit (i.e., lesser saphenous vein, arm veins) cannot be used.[9] The use of alternate vein conduits often requires extensive dissection, prolongs operative time, and may be associ-

Advances in Vascular Surgery®, vol. 3

ated with increased wound complications. It has become increasingly clear that the quality of the conduit is the prime determinant of graft patency, and alternate conduits are more often of inferior quality. Results with alternatives to greater saphenous veins, and even composite veins, have been inferior to results with ipsilateral saphenous vein arterial reconstructions.[10, 11] Many surgeons are reluctant to use an arm vein because of the necessity of tedious preparation and because of poor handling characteristics. Currently available alternatives, such as the human umbilical vein graft or synthetic prostheses, have significantly lower patency rates than autogenous veins.[8, 12] Although the human umbilical vein may perform better than other prosthetics, it is more difficult to handle and sew and is prone to late aneurysmal degeneration.[12] The cryopreserved vein has potential appeal because of its handling characteristics, which are singular to autogenous vein and its status as a biologic graft. It has been shown to resist infection[13] and might be expected to retain the antithrombotic properties of autogenous grafts. The prospect of developing an "off the shelf" arterial conduit has fueled the persistent interest in cryopreserved veins.

In the past, the use of homologous veins has been limited by scarce availability of fresh tissue and inadequacy of preservation techniques. However, progress in biotechnology in the last decade has resulted in the technical possibility of maintaining viable cells and tissues through exposure of the specimens to ultra-low temperatures, such as that of liquid N_2, in the presence of appropriate freezing media.[14] The major obstacle to the wide availability of homologous veins has therefore been overcome, and several companies now supply homologous veins for both cardiac and peripheral vascular use. It is worthwhile to review the current status of these conduits. Two factors need to be considered separately: the effect of the cryopreservation process itself and the changes associated with allograft placement.

CRYOPRESERVATION-INDUCED MODIFICATIONS OF THE VENOUS WALL

Mechanism of Cryoprotection

Cryopreservation will result in significant cell damage unless appropriate precautions are taken. The extracellular matrix freezes at 0°C, whereas the cytoplasm remains liquid at this temperature.[14] As a result, there is a vapor pressure gradient from the intracellular to the extracellular compartments. When the cooling process is slow, there is extracellular migration of water and cell dehydration. This is accelerated by rapid cooling, resulting in membrane disruption. Cryoprotectants function by entering the cytoplasm and reducing the vapor pressure gradient between intracellular and extracellular components. Examples of cryoprotective agents include ammonium acetate, glycerol, and dimethyl sulfoxide (DMSO).

The most commonly used cryoprotectant is DMSO at 10% to 17% dilution. There is no clear difference in effectiveness of cryoprotection within this range.[14] Cryopreserved tissues are currently stored at −102°C to −196°C. The rate of freezing is a matter of debate. Our recent experience suggests that rapid freezing (−5°C/sec) is most effective in preserving endothelial morphology.[14] As will be discussed below, duration of cryopreservation may also be important.

INTIMAL EFFECTS.—Overall, the morphology of the endothelial layer is maintained after appropriate cryopreservation of the venous wall.[15–26] Brockbank and associates[26] showed that although a significant number of endothelial cells are lost after cryopreservation, overall endothelial integrity is preserved, along with a normal fibrinolytic capacity and prostacyclin production.[19, 24, 27] Preservation of antithrombotic properties after appropriate freezing and thawing is further demonstrated by the fact that platelet adhesion to cryopreserved veins is similar to that of the fresh controls in the dog model.[21, 28] Although vessel architecture is initially preserved, high flow in the arterial system causes endothelial cell detachment and dehydration of the cryopreserved vein surface.[24] Endothelial cell detachment occurs in both cryopreserved autografts and allografts, but significant re-endothelialization occurs only in autografts (Figs 1 and 2).[20, 29] Whereas short-term cryopreservation results in morphologic and functional endothelial integrity,[20, 30] prolonged (i.e., 2 to 3 months) cryopreservation leads to both morphologic and functional alterations. Malone and colleagues[19] demonstrated that fibrinolytic activity is present in veins preserved short-term, but this is not the case for specimens stored longer than 3 months. In the same way, the endothelium-dependent relaxation response to acetylcholine, thrombin, and calcium ionophore A23187 in coronary arteries cryopreserved for 1 day is maintained, but it is significantly decreased after 7 days of cryopreservation.[31] Low-density lipoprotein (LDL)-cholesterol is accumulated more rapidly in cryopreserved saphenous veins as compared with fresh control in an ex-vivo system.[32] Our own data have shown ultrastructural alterations after 3 months of cryopreservation.[20, 22, 23]

EFFECTS ON THE MEDIA.—Smooth muscle cells (SMCs) are morphologically well preserved after storage in liquid nitrogen.[15, 25, 26, 30] However, these cells seem to be activated by exposure to arterial flow, as suggested by their conversion to a synthetic phenotype.[20, 23] Cryopreserved venous autografts appear to have a viable media,[20, 23] albeit with decreased secretory capacity, as demonstrated by a significant reduction in collagen synthesis.[26] Contraction induced by norepinephrine, KCl, and serotonin is not altered in cryopreserved veins,[26] and overall contractile capacity is maintained.[28] However, SMC reactivity to PGF_{2a} is increased in these conduits, and nitric oxide–induced relaxation is attenuated, resulting in an overall functional change.[28] This is confirmed by additional data from Thompson and associates[33] showing a decreased response to norepinephrine, histamine, and acetylcholine in cryopreserved rabbit arteries. The elastic lamina is not modified after long-term cryopreservation and subsequent implantation in the arterial system.[20, 23] The compliance and the elastic modulus[34] of cryopreserved grafts are initially maintained. However, Showalter and co-workers[25] found a significant loss of compliance in cryopreserved veins after implantation.

The fate of the SMCs depends on whether the vein is implanted as an allograft or as an autograft. Cryopreserved autografts implanted in the

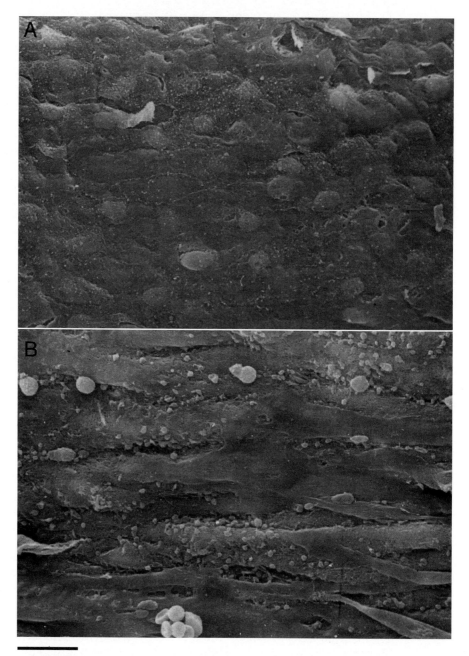

FIGURE 1.

Rabbit cryopreserved vein before **(A)** and 2 days after **(B)** implantation in the arterial system **(A).** A morphologically intact endothelial layer with minimal changes is depicted by scanning electron microscopy. **B,** two days after implantation in the arterial system, the vein surface appears to be denuded, with evident exposition of the subendothelial matrix and platelet adhesion. (Part A from Faggioli GL, Gargiulo M, Giardino R, et al: *Cardiovasc Surg* 2:259–265, 1994. Used by permission.)

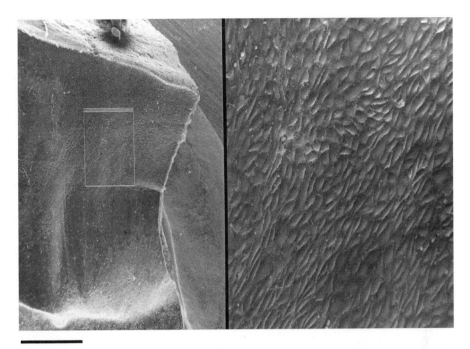

FIGURE 2.

Cryopreserved vein autograft 1 month after implantation in the arterial system. The anastomotic line is shown on the left. The area in the rectangle is illustrated at a higher magnification on the right and shows complete re-endothelialization of the surface. (From Faggioli GL, Gargiulo M, Giardino R, et al: *Cardiovasc Surg* 2:259–265, 1994. Used by permission.)

arterial system show morphologically intact, viable SMCs,[20, 23] whereas several reports suggest that the viability of SMCs is lost in cryopreserved allografts.[5, 29, 30, 35–37] Fresh and frozen venous allografts behave similarly in the dog model.[38–40] Overall, the media is subject to fibrotic changes that do not seem to depend on the changes in flow, because similar changes occur in both the arterial and the venous system.[41] SMCs show diminished responsiveness to several contractile agents, such as KCl, phenylephrine, endothelin, and UK 14304, in canine cryopreserved vein allografts.[42] Inflammatory infiltration and fibrotic changes of the media occur also in fresh allografts.[38] Therefore, these changes appear to result from an immunologically mediated rejection rather than the cryopreservation process *per se*. In humans, only anecdotal data are available on allografts; they suggest that SMCs are replaced by a fibrotic network a few months after implantation.[43–45] In our clinical series we were able to examine only one specimen of a patent graft a few months after implantation (Figs 3 through 6). Overall, the media showed a tendency toward fibrotic degeneration, although some SMCs still appeared to be present and viable; elastic fibers were disrupted (Figs 5 and 6).[46] In contrast, Piccone and colleagues[47] showed that two of three cryopreserved venous allografts implanted as angioaccess retained their cellular component. Perhaps random immunologic matching occurred in Piccone's patients, or the patients presented some degree of immunologic deficiency due to their renal disease. Frozen-irradiated allografts did not

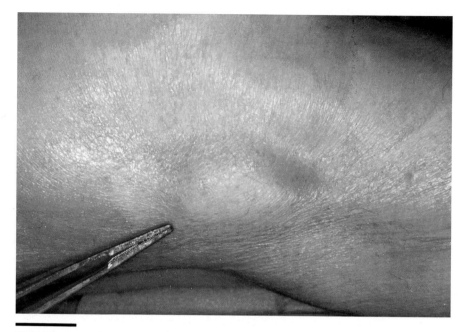

FIGURE 3.

Clinical presentation of an aneurysmal cryopreserved vein allograft 5 months after the patient was first seen. Venous graft dilation is evident through the skin.

cause either inflammatory or fibrotic changes in the experiment by Giordano and associates[48] in a canine model.

From all these data, one can conclude that although cryopreservation alone does not damage the overall media structure and viability, the immunologic allogeneic reaction leads to significant degenerative medial changes.

ANTIGENICITY OF CRYOPRESERVED VEIN ALLOGRAFTS

Early investigators postulated that homologous veins are weakly antigenic, and that cryopreservation is able to further reduce this antigenicity. This theory was based on the observation by Schwartz and coworkers[49] that implantation of a vein allograft did not accelerate subsequent skin rejection, the suggestion that allograft patency was not dependent on histocompatibility,[50] and the observation that the patency of cryopreserved vein allografts is superior to that of fresh controls.[16]

No immunologic data support those observations. On the contrary, more recent data have led to the conclusion that the cells of the venous wall (i.e., endothelial cells, smooth muscle cells, and fibroblasts) can express both class I and class II antigens, especially when they interact with activated T cells and lymphokines.[51–53] Moreover, it is now clear that cryopreservation does not decrease allograft antigenicity. This was demonstrated by the work of Calhoun and colleagues,[29] who found that the patency rate of cryopreserved allografts was dependent on host-donor histocompatibility in a dog model, and by other experiments in which both fresh and cryopreserved allografts provoked allogeneic skin rejection.[54–56] Several studies have also shown that immunosuppressive treatment was necessary to achieve acceptable patency with either fresh or

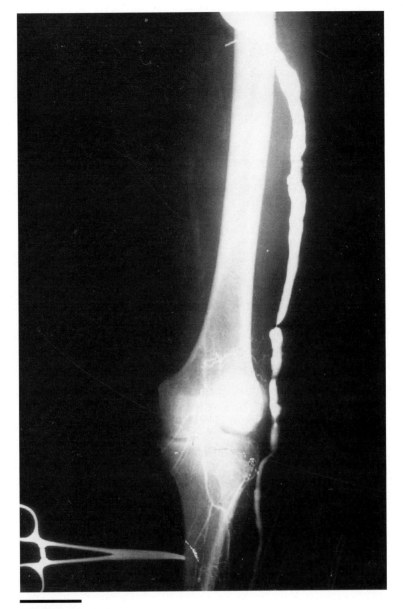

FIGURE 4.

Angiography in the same case shown in Figure 3. The cryopreserved vein appears to be diffusely dilated.

cryopreserved allografts in the dog model.[42, 57, 58] These results have not been conclusive, however, because azathioprine[59] and low-dose cyclosporine[42, 57, 58, 60] resulted in improved patency rates in some series but not in others.[61] Galumbeck and associates[62] suggest that loss of the endothelial cell layer may reduce antigenicity of venous allografts.

The most convincing evidence for an immune response is the reproducible characteristic inflammatory infiltrate, which is found in 70% to 80% of allografts in virtually every reported clinical or laboratory series. The fact that it does not occur in all cases may be due to chance matching of important immunologic loci. However, it is clear that this immu-

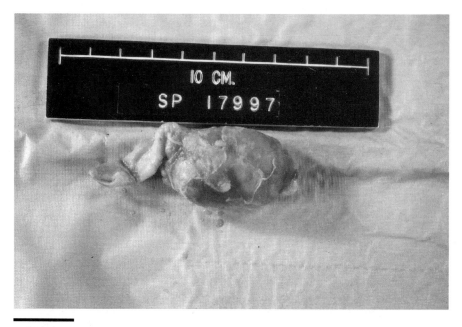

FIGURE 5.

Operative specimen of the same case shown in Figures 3 and 4. Vein enlargement appears as a true aneurysm 3.5 cm in transverse diameter.

nologic reaction represents the largest hurdle to be overcome before cryopreserved allografts become a practical alternative.

In summary, one can conclude that functional vascular integrity may be maintained for periods of 1 to 2 months with appropriate cryopreservation. However, cryopreservation does not alter the graft immunogenicity, which remains a significant clinical problem after implantation of these conduits. Some advances in histocompatibility or immune modulation will be required to overcome this barrier.

CLINICAL RESULTS

Clinical experiences with cryopreserved venous allografts for either coronary surgery or peripheral vascular reconstructions have been published sporadically in the literature since the first experiences of Tice and Zerbino in 1970[6, 7, 45–47, 63–72] (Table 1). Most of those series used non-standardized cryopreservation methods (e.g., cryopreservation at −50°C without cryoprotectant). Initial results were satisfactory, but long-term patency has been poor. Recent clinical trials have been undertaken on the basis of the renewed enthusiasm resulting from modern cryopreservation techniques. Experiments using grafts cryopreserved with modern techniques have demonstrated preservation of both endothelial and smooth muscle cell function.[26–28, 31, 32] Short-term and midterm clinical results are now available in the literature.[73] Many of these studies used veins obtained commercially; therefore, these modern data reflect experiences with conduits prepared and stored in a more standardized fashion. The short-term results are generally acceptable. Early patencies are not significantly different from those of other biologic conduits, such as umbili-

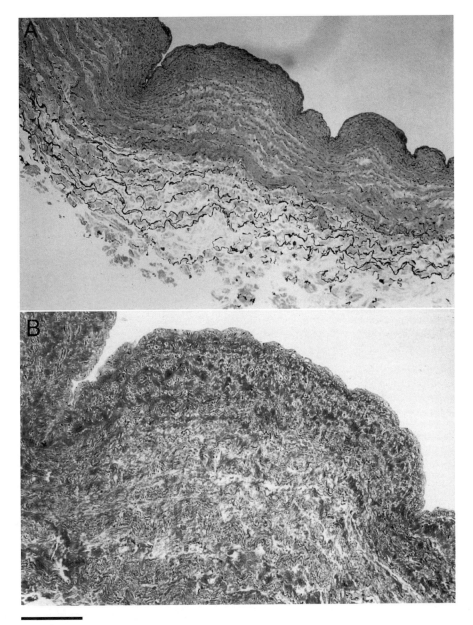

FIGURE 6.

A, histologically, the vein wall appears to be composed of a thickened media with fragmented elastic fibers and abundant collagen fibers (van Gieson elastic stain), **(B)** while few smooth muscle cells are retained (trichromic Masson stain). Few endothelial-like cells can be observed.

cal veins, while the cryopreserved grafts exhibited superior handling and sewing characteristics. However, midterm graft failure continues to be a problem with many of these implants. A review of the more recent series will serve to highlight areas for continued investigation.

Four series using cryopreserved allografts in intrainguinal reconstruction have been reported.[45, 46, 70, 71] Fujitani and colleagues[45] in 1992 re-

TABLE 1.

Results of Infrainguinal Reconstructions With Cryopreserved Vein Allografts

Author	Year	No. of Grafts	Patency Rate (%)			
			Periop	6 Mos	12 Mos	18 Mos
Tice and Zerbino[7]	1972	23	68	(48% at follow-up 0–3 years)		
Ochsner, Lawson, Eskind, et al.[65]	1984	75	82	—	50	40 (24 mos)
Selke, Meng, Rossi, et al.[67]	1989	6	67	50	50	—
Trotter, Painter, Casini, et al.[68]	1991	17	82	76	76	—
Fujitani, Bassiouny, Gewertz, et al.[45]	1992	10	90	90	90	—
Harris, Schneider, Ardros, et al.[71]	1993	25	87	42	6	—
Walker, Mitchell, McFadden, et al.[70]	1993	9	67	43	28	14
Walker, Mitchell, McFadden, et al.[70]	1993	9	87	61	46	3
Shah, Faggioli, Mangione, et al.[46]	1993	43	95	83.5	65.5	53.5
Gournier, Adham, Favre, et al.[72]	1993	27	92.5	(arterial allografts—mean follow-up: 8.7 mos)		

*Secondary patency.

ported a series of 10 cryopreserved allografts implanted in infected fields. The indication for infrainguinal grafting was limb salvage in the presence of prosthetic graft infection or local sepsis. Secondary graft patency was 90% at a mean follow-up of 9.5 months with no evidence of recurring infection.[45] In the series of 39 lower extremity bypasses reported by Walker and associates,[70] primary patency rates were disappointingly low (28% and 14% at 12 and 18 months, respectively). Secondary patency was also poor, with a 37% rate at 18 months,[70] indicating an underlying problem with the conduit itself, which did not allow successful graft salvage. Similarly, a secondary patency of 36% at 1 year was reported by Harris and co-workers[71] in a series of 25 revascularizations. Our reported results are slightly more favorable, with a 66% primary patency rate at 1 year.[46] This probably reflects a difference in indications rather than a better performance of the conduit in our hands. In fact, whereas most patients in the series conducted by Harris and Walker (79% and 87%, respectively) received the vein allograft as a secondary procedure, in our series of 45 cases, 55% were primary procedures.[46, 70, 71] Also, more than one half of the distal anastomoses were performed to the popliteal artery in our series,[46] whereas in more than 90% of patients in the other two series, bypasses were performed more distally.[70, 71] In Walker's series, many bypasses (40%) were constructed as composite grafts with adjunctive prosthetic material.[70] All of these technical differences are important in infrainguinal revascularization and may contribute to differences in mid-term and long-term results. Primary operations were associated with significantly better results in our series[46]; although this is not a consistent finding in all series, many other factors, such as ABO compatibility, might interact with individual variables in determining the result (Table 2). Patency rates in our series[46] were not influenced by postoperative anticoagulation; this suggests that poor results may be caused by changes in the properties of the media of the conduit (compliance and elasticity) rather than by modifications of luminal characteristics (thrombogenicity). The presence of significant medial changes is further supported by observations of aneurysmal degeneration.[46]

In our series, five variables were tested to identify possible predictors of late results[46]; secondary operations and use of more than one cryopreserved vein segment were significantly associated with increased risk of failure by logistic regression analysis, whereas the site of distal anastomosis, the quality of the outflow, and the use of postoperative oral anticoagulation did not significantly influence graft failure (see Table 2). This may suggest that the cryopreserved vein does provide a nonthrombogenic conduit, and that late failures are due to changes in the media, such as fibrosis or aneurysmal dilation. Graft dilation was common in our patients (mean diameter of 5–6 mm compared with implantation of 3–4 mm), and we documented three cases of frank aneurysmal degeneration (see Figs 3 through 6).

Histologic and immunohistochemical analysis showed generalized disruption of elastic fibers with some preservation of smooth muscle cells and endothelium (see Figs 5 and 6). The residual function of these elements is unknown. Such aneurysmal degeneration has been seen with arterial homografts[74] and human umbilical veins[12] but has not been reported with venous allografts. Intimal hyperplasia may be increased after

TABLE 2.
Variables Found to Decrease Mid-term Patency in Cryopreserved Vein Allografts

Variable	Harris, Schneider, Andros, et al.[71]	Walker, Mitchell, McFadden, et al.[70]	Shah, Faggioli, Mangione, et al.[46]
Diabetes	—	No	—
ABO incompatibility	—	No	—
Limited outflow	—	No	No
Tibial anastomosis	—	No	No
>1 Vein segment required	—	No	Yes
Orientation of vein (i.e., reversed vs nonreversed)	—	No	—
Secondary operation	—	No	Yes
Composite grafts	—	No	—
Anticoagulation	No	—	No

TABLE 3.
Reported Changes in Cryopreserved Venous Allografts After Implantation

	Fujitani, Bassiouny, Gewertz, et al.[45]	Harris, Schneider, Andros, et al.[71]	Walker, Mitchell, McFadden, et al.[70]	Shah, Faggioli, Mangione, et al.[46]
Aneurysmal disease	No	—	No	Yes
Intimal hyperplasia	—	Yes	No	—
SMC necrosis	Yes	—	—	Yes

SMC = smooth muscle cell.

cryopreservation, but this matter has not been systematically investigated, and only anecdotal reports exist[71] (Table 3). At present we do not know whether the poor long-term patency rates that have been observed reflect the increased risk of developing typical intimal hyperplasia or an intrinsic problem with the cryovein itself as a conduit.

Although the role of immunologic rejection in the high failure rate is yet to be defined, experimental data suggest that the only means of improving results in vein allografts is either a better histocompatibility matching between graft and host or some type of immunosuppressive treatment. Currently, only AB0 and Rh matching are recommended by cryopreserved vein allograft suppliers, and this has been the protocol followed in the series published to date, including ours.[45, 46, 70, 71] We are not aware of any clinical experience using either human leukocyte antigen (HLA) matching or host immunosuppression, but this will probably be required to improve on current results.

In evaluating the utility of cryopreserved grafts, one must address the issue of cost. The price of each segment of cryopreserved vein is over $3,000 in the United States, and multiple segments are needed in approximately one fifth of cases (8 of 43 in our series).[46] The current expense of allograft bypasses is therefore much higher than that of prosthetic replacement, and at present they do not show any advantage in terms of patency rates. This issue of cost will continue to be a major barrier to the use of this conduit unless clear benefits over other alternatives can be demonstrated.

The use of low-dose immunosuppression in patients receiving cryopreserved vein allografts has been proposed and could lead to better patency rates if the experimental data are applicable in the clinical situation. However, this kind of treatment is not suitable for patients with extensive or infected gangrenous areas and would further limit the use of this conduit. No clinical studies exist in this regard.

The capacity for complete re-endothelialization and media remodeling of these conduits is unknown. This is an important issue in a graft that is most often to be used in low-flow conditions. If the SMCs are damaged, or their viability is lost, intimal hyperplasia and late aneurysmal formation are both potential causes of failure of this graft, as we have noted earlier.

Not every cryopreserved vein allograft is subject to aneurysmal degeneration or early failure, and each clinical series showed that a small number of patients retain patent grafts for a long time period. This finding could be related to random host-graft immunologic matching. Further research should be directed to identify predictors of long-term success.

CURRENT INDICATIONS

Improved results reported by several investigators using alternate conduits and technical refinements directed at the site of distal anastomosis (arteriovenous fistulas, vein patches, and cuffs), together with the discouraging midterm results with the use of cryopreserved veins described above, have greatly limited the indications for the use of this conduit. Subsequent to our initial reported experience, we have not used a cryopreserved vein in more than 3 years, although some of our colleagues continue to use them selectively. The data from the literature and our experience support their use only in infected fields.[13, 45, 46, 70, 71, 73, 74] When autologous veins are not available for limb salvage procedures in patients with limited (i.e., <2 years) life expectancy, our experience can be used to support the placement of cryopreserved veins. However, comparisons with other conduits, particularly with modifications such as the Taylor patch,[75] are necessary before this position can be endorsed. The significant expense of cryopreserved tissue has dampened our enthusiasm for its use at present.

Although long-term results are unknown, it appears that only a very restricted group of patients may benefit from currently available cryopreserved allografts, and a better knowledge of host-graft interactions has to be pursued to improve the unsatisfactory results.

FUTURE DIRECTIONS

Modern improvements in cryopreservation techniques have increased the availability of homografts but have not significantly improved their long-term results. The initial hope that cryopreservation might reduce antigenicity, or that vessels would be significantly less antigenic than whole organs (which are, after all, lined with endothelium), seems naive in light of our present knowledge. It is clear that chronic rejection of these conduits is a problem that must be overcome before they can be considered for use in any but the most extreme circumstances.

Recent observations are beginning to draw attention away from the intima and toward the media. A number of experimental and clinical observations suggest that a thromboresistant intima can be maintained despite the loss of graft endothelium. It is likely that the ultimate failure of these conduits results from changes in the media leading to either hyperplasia or aneurysmal degeneration.

Any further clinical application of these prostheses will need to address the immunologic phenomena surrounding their implantation. There are currently no data on the length of time that these conduits remain immunogenic. This is an area that deserves further study. A second area of potential interest is development of novel strategies for immunomodulation of these conduits, perhaps by blocking antigen expression. Future clinical studies will need to consider improved histocompatibility matching and development of strategies for immunosuppression.

REFERENCES

1. Yamamouchi H: Uber die zirkularan gofassnohte and Arterlen-Venen Anastomosen sowie uber die Gefasstneansplantantionen. *Dtsch Z Chir* 112:1–118, 1911.
2. Carrel A: Ultimate results of aortic transplantations. *J Exp Med* 15:89–92, 1912.
3. Linton RR: Some practical considerations in the surgery of blood vessel grafts. *Surgery* 8:817–824, 1955.
4. Dye WS, Grove WJ, Olwin JH, et al: Two to four year behavior of vein grafts in the lower extremities. *Arch Surg* 72:64–68, 1956.
5. Barner HB, DeWeese JA, Schenk EA: Fresh and frozen homologous venous grafts for arterial repair. *Angiology* 17:89–91, 1966.
6. Tice DA, Zerbino VA: Clinical experience with preserved human allografts for vascular reconstruction. *Surgery* 67:49–58, 1970.
7. Tice DA, Zerbino VA: Clinical experience with preserved human allografts for vascular reconstruction. *Surgery* 72:260–267, 1972.
8. Dalman RL, Taylor LM: Basic data related to infrainguinal revascularization procedures. *Ann Vasc Surg* 4:9–12, 1990.
9. Kent KC, Whittemore AD, Mannick JA: Short term and midterm results of an all-autogenous tissue policy for infrainguinal reconstruction. *J Vasc Surg* 9:107–114, 1989.
10. Sesto MD, Sullivan TM, Hertzer NR, et al: Cephalic vein grafts for lower extremity revascularization. *J Vasc Surg* 15:543–549, 1992.
11. Donaldson MD, Whittemore AD, Mannick JA: Further experience with an all autogenous tissue policy for infrainguinal reconstruction. *J Vasc Surg* 18:41–48, 1993.
12. Dardik H, Miller N, Dardik A, et al: A decade of experience with the glutaraldehyde-tanned human umbilical cord vein graft for revascularization of the lower limbs. *J Vasc Surg* 7:6–46, 1988.
13. Snyder SO, Wheeler JR, Gregory RT, et al: Freshly harvested cadaveric venous homografts as arterial conduits in infected fields. *Surgery* 101:283–291, 1987.
14. Ricotta JJ, Faggioli GL: Strategies to improve the patency of homograft veins. In D'Addato M, Stilla A, editors: *Vein graft in vascular surgery.* Bologna, 1990, Ed Grasso, pp 291–295.
15. Lindenauer SM, Ladin DA, Burkel WE, et al: Cryopreservation of vein grafts in biologic and synthetic vascular prostheses. In Stanley JC, Burkel WE, Lindenauer SM, et al, editors: New York, 1982, Grune & Stratton, pp 97–422.
16. Ladin DA, Lindenauer SM, Burkel WE, et al: Viability, immunological reaction and patency of cryopreserved venous allografts. *Surg Forum* :460, 1982.
17. Dent TL, Weber TR, Lindenauer SM, et al: Cryopreservation of vein grafts. *Surg Forum* 25:241, 1974.
18. Weber TR, Lindenauer SM, Dent TL, et al: Long term patency of vein grafts preserved in liquid nitrogen in dimethylsulfoxide. *Ann Surg* 184:709–712, 1976.
19. Malone JM, Moore WS, Kischer CW, et al: Venous cryopreservation: Endothelial fibrinolytic activity and histology. *J Surg Res* 29:209–222, 1980.
20. Faggioli GL, Gargiulo M, Giardino R, et al: Long term cryopreservation of autologous veins in rabbits. *Cardiovasc Surg* 2:259–265, 1994.

21. Street DI, Russ GA, Ricotta JJ: Platelet avidity of cryopreserved veins: Thrombogenicity of cryopreserved veins. *J Surg Res* 45:6–917, 1988.
22. Faggioli GL, Ricotta JJ, Baier RE: Modifications of venous wall after cryopreservation. In D'Addato M, Stella A, editors: *Vein graft in vascular surgery*. Bologna, 1990, Ed Grasso, pp 280–290.
23. Pasquinelli G, Faggioli GI, Preda P, et al: Are long term cryopreservation and patency of cryopreserved venous allografts truly achievable? *Cells and Materials* 3:305–314, 1993.
24. Sachs SM, Ricotta JJ, Scott DE, et al: Endothelial integrity after venous cryopreservation. *J Surg Res* 2:218–227, 1982.
25. Showalter D, Durham S, Sheppeck R, et al: Cryopreserved venous homografts as vascular conduits in canine carotid arteries. *Surgery* 106:652–659, 1989.
26. Brockbank KGM, Donovan TJ, Ruby St, et al: Functional analysis of cryopreserved veins. Preliminary report. *J Vasc Surg* 11:94–102, 1990.
27. Ts'ao C, Ng AS, Holly CM: Increased production of PG12-like activity by frozen-thawed rat aorta. *Prostaglandins* 16:503–512, 1978.
28. Elmore JR, Gloviczki P, Brockbank KGM, et al: Cryopreservation affects endothelial and smooth muscle function of canine autogenous vein grafts. *J Vasc Surg* 1:584–592, 1991.
29. Calhoun AD, Bauer GM, Porter JM, et al: Fresh and cryopreserved venous allografts in genetically characterized dogs. *J Surg Res* 22:687–696, 1977.
30. Balderman SC, Montes M, Schmartz K, et al: Preparation of venous allografts. A comparison technique. *Ann Surg* 200:117, 1984.
31. Ku DD, Willis WL, Caulfield JB: Retention of endothelium-dependent vasodilatory responses in canine coronary arteries following cryopreservation. *Cryobiology* 27:511–520, 1990.
32. Ligush J, Berceli SA, Moosa HH, et al: First results on the functional characteristics of cryopreserved human saphenous vein. *Cells and Materials* 1:59–68, 1991.
33. Thompson L, Duckworth J, Bevan J: Cryopreservation of innervation endothelial and vascular smooth muscle function of a rabbit muscular and resistance artery. *Blood Vessels* 26:157–164, 1989.
34. L'Italian GJ, Maloney RD, Abbott WM: The preservation of the mechanical properties of venous allografts by freezing. *J Surg Res* 27:239–243, 1979.
35. Bank H, Schmerhl MK, Warner R, et al: Transplantation of cryopreserved canine venous allografts. *J Surg Res* 50:57–64, 1991.
36. Wright CB, Hobson RW, Swan KG: Autografts and homografts in canine femoral venous reconstruction: A double-blind study. *Surgery* 74:654–659, 1973.
37. Boren CH, Roon AJ, Moore WS: Maintenance of viable arterial allografts by cryopreservation. *Surgery* 83:382–391, 1978.
38. Henderson VJ, Cohen RG, Mitchell RS, et al: Biochemical (functional) adaptation of arterialized vein grafts. *Ann Surg* 203:339–345, 1986.
39. Earle AS, Horsley JS, Villavicencio JL, et al: Replacement of venous defects by venous autografts. *Arch Surg* 80:119–124, 1960.
40. Kraeger RR, Lagos JA, Barner HB: Long term evaluation of allogenic veins as arterial grafts. *Vasc Surg* 10:121–127, 1976.
41. Sitzman JV, Imbembo AL, Ricotta JJ, et al: Dimethylsulfoxide treated cryopreserved venous allografts in the arterial and venous system. *Surgery* 95:154–159, 1984.
42. Miller VM, Bergman RT, Gloviczki P, et al: Cryopreserved venous allografts: Effects of immunosuppression and antiplatelet therapy on patency and function. *J Vasc Surg* 18:216–226, 1993.
43. Ochsner JL, DeCamp PT, Leonard GL: Experience with fresh venous allografts as an arterial substitute. *Ann Surg* 176:933–939, 1971.

44. Stephen M, Sheil GR, Wong J: Allograft vein arterial bypass. *Arch Surg* 113:591–593, 1978.

45. Fujitani RM, Bassiouny HS, Gewertz BL, et al: Cryopreserved saphenous vein allogenic homografts: An alternative conduit in lower extremity arterial reconstruction in infected fields. *J Vasc Surg* 15:519–526, 1992.

46. Shah RS, Faggioli GL, Mangione SA, et al: Early results with cryopreserved saphenous vein allografts for infrainguinal bypass. *J Vasc Surg* 18:965–971, 1993.

47. Piccone VA, Sika J, Ahmed N, et al: Preserved saphenous vein allografts for vascular access. *Surg Gynecol Obstet* 147:385–390, 1978.

48. Giordano JM, Lamoy RE, Wright CB, et al: A comparison of autografts and frozen, irradiated homografts in canine femoral venous reconstruction. *Surgery* 81:100–104, 1977.

49. Schwartz SI, Kutner FR, Neistadt A, et al: Antigenicity of homografted veins. *Surgery* 61:471–477, 1967.

50. Harjola PT, Scheinn TM, Tilikainen A: Factors affecting early patency of human venous allografts in arterial reconstruction. *J Surg Res* 1:169–176, 1969.

51. Vetto RM, Burger DR: The identification and comparison of transplantation antigens on canine vascular endothelium and lymphocytes. *Transplantation* 11:374–377, 1971.

52. Burger DR, Vetto RM: Vascular endothelium as a major participant in T-lymphocyte immunity. *Cell Immunol* 70:357–361, 1982.

53. Pober JS, Gimbrone MA, Collins T, et al: Interactions of T-lymphocytes with human vascular endothelial cells: Role of endothelial surface antigens. *Immunobiology* 168:483–494, 1984.

54. Thiede A, Engerman R, Korner H, et al: Comparison of the immunologic reactions of arterial transplants in the arterial system and of venous transplants in the venous system using inbred strains of rats. *Transplant Proc* 11:603–606, 1979.

55. Axtheim SC, Porter JM, Strickland S, et al: Antigenicity of venous allografts. *Ann Surg* 180:290–293, 1979.

56. Cochran RP, Kunzelman KS: Cryopreservation does not alter antigenic expression of aortic allografts. *J Surg Res* 46:597–599, 1989.

57. Augelli NV, Lupinetti FM, Khatib HE, et al: Allograft vein patency in a canine model. *Transplantation* 52:466–470, 1991.

58. Bandlien KO, Toledo-Peryra, Barnhart MI, et al: Improved survival of venous allografts in dogs following graft pretreatment with cyclosporine. *Transplant Proc* 15(suppl 1):3084–3091, 1983.

59. Perloff LJ, Reckard CR, Rowlands DT, et al: The venous homograft: An immunological question. *Surgery* 72:961–970, 1982.

60. Schmitz-Rixen T, Megerman J, Colvin RB, et al: Immunosuppressive treatment of aortic allografts. *J Vasc Surg* 7:82–92, 1988.

61. Ricotta JJ, Collins GJ, Rich NM, et al: Failure of immunosuppression to prolong venous allograft survival. *Arch Surg* 115:99–101, 1980.

62. Galumbeck M, Sanfilippo FP, Hagen PO, et al: Inhibition of vessel allograft rejection by endothelial removal. Morphologic and ultrastructural changes. *Ann Surg* 206:757–764, 1987.

63. Tice DA, Zerbino VR, Isom OW, et al: Coronary artery bypass with freeze-preserved saphenous vein allografts. *J Thorac Cardiovasc Surg* 71:378–382, 1976.

64. Bical O, Bachet J, Laurian C, et al: Autocoronary bypass with homologous saphenous vein: Long-term results. *Ann Thorac Surg* 30:550–557, 1980.

65. Ochsner JL, Lawson JD, Eskind SJ, et al: Homologous veins as an arterial substitute: Long-term results. *J Vasc Surg* 1:306–313, 1984.

66. Gelbfish J, Jacobowitz IJ, Rose DM: Cryopreserved homologous saphenous vein: Early and late patency in coronary artery bypass surgical procedures. *Ann Thorac Surg* 42:70–73, 1986.
67. Selke FW, Meng RL, Rossi NP: Cryopreserved saphenous vein homografts for femoral-distal vascular reconstruction. *J Cardiovasc Surg* 30:838–842, 1989.
68. Trotter MC, Painter MW, Casini MP, et al: Cryopreserved allografts for limb salvage. Presented at the 20th World Congress ISCVS, Amsterdam, 1991.
69. Saunders CR, Tedesco DJ, Yee ES: Reverse saphenous vein homografts as bypass conduits: A preliminary report. *Vascular Surgery* 26:562–568, 1992.
70. Walker PJ, Mitchell RS, McFadden PM, et al: Early experience with cryopreserved saphenous vein allografts as a conduit for complex limb salvage procedures. *J Vasc Surg* 18:561–569, 1993.
71. Harris RW, Schneider PA, Andros G, et al: Allograft vein bypass. Is it an acceptable alternative for infrapopliteal revascularization? *J Vasc Surg* 18:553–560, 1993.
72. Gournier JP, Adham M, Favre JP, et al: Cryopreserved arterial homografts: Preliminary study. *Ann Vasc Surg* 7:503–511, 1993.
73. Faggioli GL, Ricotta JJ: Cryopreserved vein allografts for lower limb revascularizations. *(Review) Eur J Vasc Surg* 1994 (in press).
74. Kieffer E, Bahnini A, Koskas F, et al: In situ allograft replacement of infected infrarenal aortic prosthetic grafts: Results in forty-three patients. *J Vasc Surg* 17:349–356, 1993.
75. Taylor RS, Loh A, McFarland RJ, et al: Improved technique for polytetrafluoroethylene bypass grafting: Long-term results using anastomotic vein patches. *Br J Surg* 79:348–354, 1992.

Venous Patches, Collars, and Boots Improve the Patency Rates of Polytetrafluoroethylene Grafts

John H. N. Wolfe, M.S., F.R.C.S.
Consultant Vascular Surgeon, St. Mary's Hospital, London, England

M. R. Tyrrell, F.R.C.S., F.R.C.S.(Ed.)
Senior Registrar, Department of Surgery, Guy's Hospital, London, England

A pproximately 30% of patients with critical ischemia require either a femorocrural bypass or primary amputation. Because there is little doubt that autologous vein is currently the best conduit available, the surgeon should look assiduously for adequate lengths of vein in either the long or short saphenous vein or in the cephalic or basilic systems in the arm. For some surgeons this will completely preclude the need for a prosthetic femorocrural graft. There is, however, a cohort of patients in many surgeons' practices in whom adequate lengths are unavailable because of our increasingly interventional approach to arterial disease; many patients have undergone previous coronary artery bypass grafting or femorodistal reconstruction with the result that veins have been used for grafts or have been thrombosed as a result of infusion lines. Because critical ischemia is estimated to affect 500 to 1,000 people per million population each year,[1] this group of patients is not an inconsiderable problem. The mortality rate in this group of patients is approximately 18% within 1 year and 33% after 3 years,[2] but the aim of the vascular surgeon is, nevertheless, to maintain dignity and independence by avoiding amputation. Immobility and incarceration of a patient destroys his or her quality of life and is a drain on diminishing health resources.

When polytetrafluoroethylene (PTFE) became available there was a natural tendency to turn to "the graft on the shelf" rather than rely on the more demanding vein harvesting techniques, but there is now conclusive evidence that PTFE is inferior to vein. In fact, prosthetic grafts perform so badly in the infrapopliteal segment that many surgeons believe these operations should not be performed in the absence of vein.

The reasons for the discrepancy between vein and prosthetic graft patency at the crural level are complex and controversial but must include the increased thrombogenicity of the prosthetic material. In addition, anastomosing the rigid, large-diameter PTFE to a small-diameter tibial vessel is demanding of both surgeon and material. These factors cause

Advances in Vascular Surgery®, vol. 3
© 1995, Mosby–Year Book, Inc.

early failure, but the attrition rate for PTFE grafts remains high throughout the first 2 years. This is partly attributable to the formation of stenotic myointimal hyperplasia, and it has been suggested that this process is greater in PTFE grafts than in vein grafts.[3]

In the absence of adequate vein there are three options: primary amputation, development of a more successful prosthetic graft, and improvement in the patency of a PTFE graft.

PRIMARY AMPUTATION

There is little doubt that mobility after primary amputation is significantly impaired despite our best efforts with artificial prostheses. It has been suggested that only 50% of amputees are considered for the fitting of a prosthesis and remobilization.[1] Of these, many will find the prosthesis a burden and will use it only on outpatient visits to their surgeon. However, our own results of full-length PTFE grafts (from the common femoral artery to the crural vessel at the ankle) were so poor that secondary amputation seemed an almost inevitable outcome; therefore, a reconstructive policy could not be justified.

DEVELOPMENT OF A MORE SUCCESSFUL PROSTHETIC GRAFT

Human umbilical vein enjoyed a vogue and remains a useful graft, but it has patency rates that are roughly equivalent to those of PTFE[4] and has the added long-term problem of aneurysm formation.[5] Polyurethane grafts have been unsuccessfully tried in the past, and a new compliant polyurethane graft has not yet established a role in our armamentarium. Other grafts derived from animal tissue have not lived up to their early promise and have not made a dramatic impact on our practice.

IMPROVEMENT IN THE PATENCY OF A PTFE GRAFT

Various methods have been used, including composite sequential PTFE vein grafts, the Linton patch, the Taylor patch, the Miller collar, arteriovenous fistulae, and our adaptation of the Miller collar—the venous boot. Composite vein grafts are used to avoid PTFE across the knee joint.[6] However, there is a problem at the prosthetic-vein junction, which may kink when the knee is flexed. There is also the problem of the development of myointimal hyperplasia at this relatively narrow anastomosis. Consequently, the results of this technique do not differ significantly from those of PTFE alone. Various authors, therefore, championed the composite sequential graft wherein the vein graft to a crural artery is piggybacked onto the PTFE graft to the popliteal vessel.[7] These results seem to be an improvement over the composite grafts but require a patent popliteal segment, and in some cases the distal vein graft occludes because of diversion of the graft flow through the intermediate anastomosis into the popliteal artery.

LINTON PATCH

The Linton patch is a well-established technique but is, in the experience of the author, of no value on small crural arteries (Fig 1). Inserting a

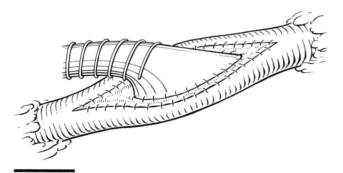

FIGURE 1.

Linton patch. (From Wolfe JHN: Polytetrafluoroethylene (PTFE) femorodistal bypass, in Jamieson CW, Yao JST (eds): *Vascular Surgery.* London, 1994, Chapman & Hall, pp 330–340. Used by permission.)

vein patch onto a 2-mm vessel and then anastomosing a PTFE graft to this patch is technically very demanding, and the distance between the two suture lines seems too narrow to be of benefit.

ARTERIOVENOUS FISTULAE

Another approach is to reduce the peripheral resistance to increase graft flow. A distal prosthetic graft has the inevitable problem of a large-diameter tube with an artificial and alien flow surface, which is anastomosed to a small vessel with a high resistance and low runoff capacity. The volume of blood carried by this graft, and its velocity, tend to be low, and there is a thrombotic "threshold" at which occlusion is likely to occur. The thrombotic threshold of PTFE is much lower than that of vein, rendering the conduit much more likely to thrombose. A second factor is the exposure of blood to the flow surface, which is increased by a high-circumference cross-sectional area ratio and is therefore greater in tubes of smaller diameter. Thus, the wider-diameter graft has a lower velocity, which falls below the thrombotic threshold and occludes, whereas the narrower, higher-velocity graft is at risk because of the greater exposure of blood to the artificial flow surface. If higher flow can be maintained in a wider-diameter graft, then the chances of patency are enhanced. Dardik and colleagues[8] introduced the distal arteriovenous fistula to reduce resistance and thus increase graft flow. There are good reasons to believe that a distal arteriovenous fistula will improve graft patency, but a disproportionate amount of the distal blood supply may bypass the distal vascular bed.

TAYLOR PATCH

The Taylor patch has been shown to be an extremely useful technique. This might be attributed to both the very long anastomosis and the segment of vein interposed as a diamond into the toe of the graft (Fig 2).[9] Taylor's results are exceptionally good, but the one theoretic drawback of the technique is the direct PTFE-to-artery anastomosis along the proximal part of the anastomosis and at the heel. As a result, the inevitable myointimal hyperplasia will impinge on the recipient artery and may preclude any proximal retrograde flow in the crural vessel. This proximal flow may be important because the calf musculature requires a blood sup-

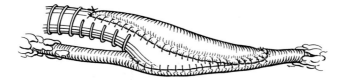

FIGURE 2.

Taylor patch. (From Wolfe JHN: Polytetrafluoroethylene (PTFE) femorodistal by-pass, in Jamieson CW, Yao JST (eds): *Vascular Surgery*. London, 1994, Chapman & Hall, pp 330–340. Used by permission.)

ply that may not be obtained easily by way of an incomplete pedal arch. Furthermore, this proximal flow significantly reduces peripheral resistance.

MILLER COLLAR

The venous collar was popularized by the late Justin Miller from Adelaide, Australia. Like Robert Taylor in London, he was able to publish remarkably good results (Fig 3).[10] The theoretical disadvantage of this technique is the rather ugly oval cushion that lacks the hemodynamic elegance of the Taylor patch. The considerable turbulence in the collar probably predisposes the graft to intermediate failure. We therefore attempted to develop a technique that would harness the advantages of both the Taylor patch and the Miller collar.[11]

VENOUS BOOT

Technique

The proximal end of the 6-mm PTFE graft is anastomosed to the common femoral artery with 6-0 polypropylene sutures. The graft is then tunneled directly to the lower third of the calf *without* a counterincision by use of a specially constructed long Meadox tunneler. A segment of either arm or leg vein is then slit along its length to form a rectangle (Fig 4).

The depth of the boot should be approximately 3 to 4 mm, and any redundant width should be removed (this is rarely necessary). The arteriotomy in the crural vessel should be at least 2 cm long, and we have

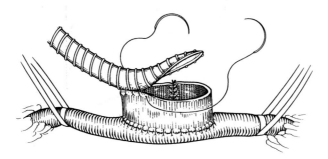

FIGURE 3.

Miller collar. (From Wolfe JHN: Polytetrafluoroethylene (PTFE) femorodistal by-pass, in Jamieson CW, Yao JST (eds): *Vascular Surgery*. London, 1994, Chapman & Hall, pp 330–340. Used by permission.)

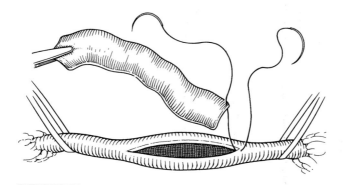

FIGURE 4.

A segment of vein has been split open longitudinally, and one corner is anastomosed to the apex of the arteriotomy. (From Tyrrell MR, Wolfe JHN: *Br J Surg* 78:1016, 1991. Used by permission.)

recently resorted to even longer anastomoses because we believe that this is an important factor in the success of the procedure. There should be an excess of vein so that mosquito forceps can be applied to one end of the vein to anchor and control this segment while the anastomosis is being performed.

Magnification loops are essential, and the distal edge of the vein is anastomosed along one side of the arteriotomy using the shorter end of a double-ended 7-0 polypropylene suture (Fig 5). The distal edge of the venous sheet is then draped around the arteriotomy and sewn down with the longer end of the suture (Fig 6). Great care must be taken to ensure that there is no nipping at the heel of the suture line, because proximal flow may be as important as distal flow in these very distal grafts.

By positioning the mosquito forceps correctly, it is possible to align the vein along the anastomosis without difficulty so that the assistant can concentrate on the anastomosis itself. The venous sheet is then anastomosed along the anterior edge until the venous anastomosis to the artery is complete. The suture is tied to the initial stitch, thus anchoring this anastomosis. Redundant vein is then resected using a pair of Pott's scis-

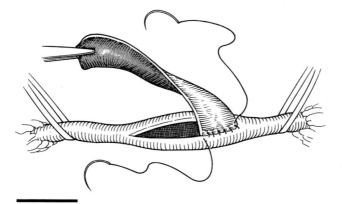

FIGURE 5.

The distal leading edge is anastomosed along the side of the arteriotomy. (From Tyrrell MR, Wolfe JHN: *Br J Surg* 78:1016, 1991. Used by permission.)

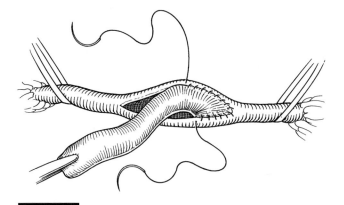

FIGURE 6.

The longitudinal length of vein is then anastomosed around the arteriotomy. (From Tyrrell MR, Wolfe JHN: *Br J Surg* 78:1016, 1991. Used by permission.)

sors, and the anastomosis is continued so that the terminal edge of the vein boot is sewn to the side of the vein near the apex (Figs 7 and 8).

The boot is completed by cutting back the heel to allow the PTFE graft to be anastomosed to the collar at a 30% angle to the artery (see Fig 8). Once the boot has been completed, the anastomosis between PTFE and vein is quite simple (Fig 9).

Results

Taylor[9] obtained primary patency rates of 74% and 58% at 1 and 3 years, respectively, by using his distal anastomotic vein patch technique. Miller's[10] earlier results were similarly encouraging; but our own early results cannot match these data.[12] The indications for using PTFE, however, vary from one series to the next, as do the level of anastomosis and the degree of ischemia. It is therefore perhaps more appropriate to compare PTFE grafts with the crural vessels with in situ vein grafts to the crural vessels carried out by the same surgeons. In our own unit, PTFE grafts constitute 8% of all infrainguinal grafts but 18% of all femorocrural grafts. The results of PTFE with the venous boot are approximately 20% to 25% worse

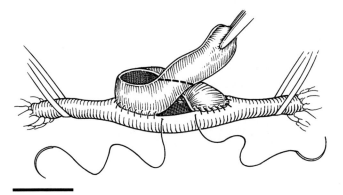

FIGURE 7.

A collar is formed and the redundant vein can be removed. The proximal edge of the vein collar is then anastomosed to the longitudinal edge. (From Tyrrell MR, Wolfe JHN: *Br J Surg* 78:1016, 1991. Used by permission.)

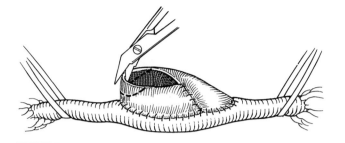

FIGURE 8.

A segment of posterior collar is incised to increase the size of the anastomosis between PTFE and vein collar. (From Tyrrell MR, Wolfe JHN: *Br J Surg* 78:1016, 1991. Used by permission.)

than those of in situ vein.[13] This is probably a better indicator of efficacy, or lack of it, than comparing series from disparate units.

The Joint Vascular Research Group (JVRG) in Great Britain has now completed a randomized comparison between above-knee and below-knee PTFE grafts with and without a venous collar.[14] There was no significant difference for above-knee grafts, but the grafts with a venous boot fared significantly better when the distal anastomosis was located in the below-knee popliteal segment. There are at least two other ongoing randomized studies in Europe; one is in Scandinavia (randomizing PTFE crural grafts to a venous collar or direct anastomosis), and another is a JVRG study comparing the venous collar and the Taylor patch for below-knee and crural PTFE grafts.

Postulated Reasons for Improved Results

Having had some clinical success, we performed some bench experiments to establish the reasons for this success and perhaps make further improvements.[15] We first examined the venous elastic properties of 16 specimens of normal vein and 9 specimens containing a short interposed segment of reoriented vein. We then assessed the elastic properties of the wall by measuring strain as a function of distending pressure. To do this, two pressure reservoirs were set up to instantly deliver a preset pressure that distended the segment of vein at the end of the delivery tube. Dimensional changes of the vein were then measured. Each specimen was inflated to a baseline pressure of 10 mm Hg and then to 150 mm Hg for 5 minutes. The relative strains in the longitudinal and circumferential dimensions were measured, and the longitudinal strain was, on average,

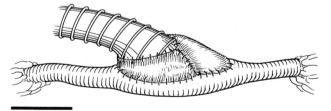

FIGURE 9.

The completed anastomosis. (From Tyrrell MR, Wolfe JHN: *Br J Surg* 78:1016, 1991. Used by permission.)

7.2 times the circumferential strain. We concluded that vein is anisotropic, so that by reorienting the vein as a collar around the distal anastomosis, its compliant characteristics are maximized.

In a second study we examined the flow through the end-to-side anastomosis. A segment of PTFE was anastomosed to fresh cadaveric internal mammary artery with and without an interposition vein collar. A double-headed pinch roller pump simulated pulsatile flow. Flow was then measured out of the proximal and distal limb of the internal mammary artery. All specimens were perfused under conditions of pulsatile flow (pressure, 120/80 mm Hg; pulse rate, 100 per minute). We found that there was no significant difference in total flow because the overriding feature of this model was the diameter of the internal mammary artery. We reconsidered our results and found that with the vein collar the flow was directly proportional to the diameter of the internal mammary artery. However, this was not true for direct PTFE-to-artery anastomoses. This suggested that there was resistance within the direct PTFE-to-artery anastomosis that was removed by the interposition vein collar.

In the third experiment, casts were made of the anastomoses that confirmed an inevitable distortion of the artery when direct PTFE-to-artery anastomoses were performed. This oval distortion has a deleterious effect on flow.

These studies gave us some insight into the reasons for improving the early results of PTFE grafts, but they did not fully explain the long-term improvement. The major component of success appears to be related to the process of myointimal hyperplasia. This occurs at the interface between PTFE and autologous tissue. By moving this interface away from a delicate, narrow anastomosis on a 2-mm artery to a point where there is an 8-mm-diameter reservoir, the same amount of myointimal hyperplasia will have a less deleterious effect. Suggs and colleagues[16] suggested in their in vivo studies and in an animal model that myointimal hyperplasia was reduced by the interposition of a venous collar. Our clinical evidence does not support this hypothesis, but the site of occurrence of the myointimal hyperplastic lesion may be all-important.

Vein remains the graft of choice, but there is now sufficient evidence to consider vein boots with PTFE if all sources of vein have been exhausted.

REFERENCES

1. Dormandy J, Thomas P: History of a critical ischaemic patient with and without his leg, in Greenhalgh R, Jamieson C, Nicolaides A (eds): *Limb salvage and amputation for vascular disease*. London, 1988, WB Saunders, pp 11–26.
2. Tyrrell MR, Wolfe JHN: Critical leg ischaemia: An appraisal of clinical definition. *Br J Surg* 80:177–180, 1993.
3. Taylor RS, McFarland RJ, Cox MI: An investigation into the cause of failure of PTFE grafts. *Eur J Vasc Surg* I:335–343, 1987.
4. McCollum C, Kenchington G, Alexander C, et al: PTFE or HUV for femoropopliteal bypasses: A multicentre trial. *Eur J Vasc Surg* 5:435–443, 1991.
5. Dardik H, Ibrahim IM, Sussman B, et al: Biodegration and aneurysm forma-

tion at umbilical vein graft: Observations and a realistic strategy. *Ann Surg* 199:61–68, 1984.

6. DeLaurentis DA, Freedman P: Sequential femoro-popliteal bypasses: Another approach to the inadequate saphenous vein problem. *Surgery* 71:400, 1972.
7. Flynn WR, Flanigan DP, Verta MH Jr, et al: Sequential femoro-tibial bypass for severe limb ischemia. *Surgery* 88:357, 1980.
8. Dardik H, Sussman B, Ibrahim IM, et al: Distal arteriovenous fistula as an adjunct to maintain arterial and graft patency for limb salvage. *Surgery* 94:478–486, 1983.
9. Taylor RS, Loh A, McFarland RJ, et al: Improved technique for polytetrafluoroethylene bypass grafting: Long term results using anastomotic vein patches. *Br J Surg* 79:348–354, 1992.
10. Miller JH, Foreman RK, Fergusson L, et al: Interposition vein cuff for anastomosis of prosthesis to small artery. *Aust NZ J Surg* 54:283–285, 1984.
11. Tyrrell MR, Wolfe JHN: New prosthetic venous collar anastomotic technique: Combining the best of other procedures. *Br J Surg* 78:1016–1017, 1991.
12. Tyrrell MR, Grigg MJ, Wolfe JHN: Is arterial reconstruction to the ankle worthwhile in the absence of autologous vein? *Eur J Vasc Surg* 3:429–434, 1989.
13. Cheshire NJW, Wolfe JHN, Noone MA, et al: The economics of femorocrural reconstruction for critical leg ischemia with and without autologous vein. *J Vasc Surg* 15:167–175, 1992.
14. Stonebridge P, for the Joint Vascular Research Group. Randomised trial comparing PTFE graft patency with and without a "Miller cuff." Presented at The Vascular Surgical Society of Great Britain and Ireland, November 1994. *Br J Surg* 82:555–556, 1995.
15. Tyrrell MR, Chester JF, Vipond MN, et al: Experimental evidence to support the use of interposition vein collars/patches in distal PTFE anastomoses. *Eur J Vasc Surg* 4:95–101, 1990.
16. Suggs WD, Henriques HF, DePalma RG: Vein cuff interposition prevents juxta-anastomotic neointimal hyperplasia. *Ann Surg* 207:717–722, 1988.

Lower Limb Reconstruction With Combined Distal Vascular Bypass Surgery and Microsurgical Free Tissue Transfer

Lawrence B. Cohen, M.D.
Associate Professor, Department of Plastic and Reconstructive Surgery, Eastern Virginia Medical School, Norfolk, Virginia

Craig Rubinstein, M.B.M.S. (Melb.), F.R.A.C.S.
Department of Plastic and Reconstructive Surgery, Eastern Virginia Medical School, Norfolk, Virginia

Jack Cronenwett, M.D.
Professor of Surgery, Chief, Section of Vascular Surgery, Dartmouth Medical School, Dartmouth-Hitchcock Medical Center, Lebanon, New Hampshire

OVERVIEW

Approximately 30,000 major lower extremity amputations are performed in the United States yearly. These patients usually have significant peripheral vascular disease and intractable ulceration, often related to diabetes mellitus.[1] Of the 10 million Americans who have diabetes, 15% (1.5 million) will develop foot ulcers. Approximately 20% of all diabetic patients who enter the hospital are admitted for foot problems, and 50% to 70% of amputations performed in the United States occur in the diabetic population.[2] Once an amputation has been performed, the incidence of a contralateral limb amputation approaches 50% within 2 years.[3–5]

In the absence of peripheral ischemia, plastic surgeons have successfully used free tissue transfer techniques to obtain soft-tissue coverage of large defects in the leg and foot.[6] These large wounds result from trauma, from extirpative surgery, and after debridement of bone or soft-tissue infection. Vascularized flaps have been shown to increase local antibiotic delivery to the wound, improve oxygen tension of the wound, augment neutrophil activity within the wound, and generally assist in the treatment of chronic infections in ischemic regions.[7] During the past decade,

Advances in Vascular Surgery®, vol. 3
© 1995, Mosby–Year Book, Inc.

significant advances in reconstructive surgery, coupled with improvements in the management of diabetes mellitus and peripheral vascular disease, have generated a "new" patient population for the plastic and reconstructive surgeon. As refinements in vascularized tissue transfer, both as pedicle and free flaps, have been realized, parallel advances have been made within the specialty of vascular surgery, leading to improved patency rates of infrapopliteal bypass procedures. Newer revascularization techniques have allowed for the routine use of bypass grafts to the level of the ankle and foot.[8–12] Plastic surgeons are now faced with the challenge of reconstructing complex foot wounds in patients who previously would have undergone below-the-knee amputations. When patients are carefully selected, lower extremity bypass surgery in combination with free tissue transfer by use of microvascular techniques may be an alternative to amputation.[13–18] Because the need for close cooperation between the vascular surgeon and the plastic surgeon is mandatory, this technique represents an exciting frontier in the continuing advances in the treatment of ischemic extremities.

The traditional indications for distal arterial reconstruction in the ischemic leg have included rest pain, severe claudication, and ulceration. More recent indications include patients who have wounds secondary to trauma, previous surgery, or neuropathy, have monophasic blood flow at the ankle, and require free tissue transfer to reconstruct these wounds. In these patients, distal ischemic tissue loss may not even be present, but because they do not have adequate arterial inflow at the infrapopliteal level, revascularization will be required to ensure a successful outcome from a free flap procedure. Similarly, large ulcers that fail to heal in the face of adequate inflow after bypass grafting may be ideal for reconstruction with free tissue transfer techniques. In some of these patients, even if the level of amputation can be converted from an above-knee to a below-knee by efforts at reconstruction, the chances of successful ambulation are increased. It is well known that the amount of additional energy expenditure required by the patient for ambulation on an above-knee amputation is about twice that for the below-knee level.[19]

An alternative to below-knee amputation is combined revascularization and free tissue transfer. The indications for this procedure include diabetic, neurotrophic ulcers; post-traumatic, infected ulcers; open midfoot amputations; and the provision of isolated, nutrient flaps. Numerous reports in the vascular surgery and plastic surgery literature during the past decade support these concepts.[14, 18, 20, 21] Further evidence in the vascular surgical literature has shown that limb salvage is generally less costly than amputation.[22] These techniques are of most utility in diabetic patients who present with severe infrapopliteal occlusive disease[23] and coexistent large neuropathic ulcers, often on the weight-bearing plantar surface.[24] These wounds are usually proximal to the metatarsal heads, exposing tendon and bone, and are frequently accompanied by chronic infection. Even though vein bypass grafts to the distal tibial and pedal arteries might be technically feasible,[9] these patients have traditionally undergone below-knee amputations. This is because such extensive tissue loss means that primary wound healing cannot be anticipated, even after a successful arterial reconstruction. It is here that combined revascularization and free tissue transfer often provide the best option for the patient. Although there are many contraindications for combined revascularization and free tissue transfer, they are of varying significance, and some "traditional" contraindications are now being questioned.

The goal of lower limb reconstruction in vascular patients is to maintain bipedal ambulation. Skin grafts, limited amputations, and local tissue transfer procedures are simpler techniques than free tissue transfer, and should always be considered first. Despite the many advances in fasciocutaneous flaps, musculocutaneous flaps, and microsurgical free tissue transfer, reconstruction of the foot remains a complex problem. Certain principles must be followed to ensure a satisfactory result. Technical considerations for free tissue transfer include the size and type of defect to be repaired, the likely donor site morbidity, and the return of function anticipated with "successful" surgery. The presence of severe peripheral vascular disease strongly influences the type of reconstruction that can be accomplished. Almost all of the local flaps suitable for plantar foot reconstruction are based upon antegrade blood flow through the posterior tibial artery and its medial and lateral plantar branches. Patients who have undergone recent distal vascular bypass procedures to either the anterior tibial or peroneal vessels at the level of the ankle may not be suitable candidates for reconstruction with these flaps. As such, wound closure will require free tissue transfer using the revascularized vessel for inflow into the flap. When distal vascular bypass surgery has been performed, direct arterial anastomosis to the bypass graft is always preferred. If, however, the revascularization is performed to the popliteal artery, the more distal vasculature must be evaluated for its suitability as a recipient for the transplanted tissues. In planning the reconstruction, the underlying bony framework and its weight-bearing characteristics also need to be considered, because recurrent ulceration is more likely with gait abnormalities caused by bone and joint deformity, especially in the neuropathic foot.

This chapter will review the indications, contraindications, and techniques of lower limb reconstruction in vascular disease patients using the combination newer distal revascularization techniques and microsurgical free tissue transfer.

INDICATIONS FOR COMBINED REVASCULARIZATION AND FREE TISSUE TRANSFER

The goal of any reconstructive procedure performed on the foot should be the maintenance of bipedal ambulation. Combined revascularization plus free tissue transfer has achieved long-term ambulation in more than 80% of patients who, in our experience, would previously have been candidates only for major amputation. Close collaboration of plastic and vascular surgeons has made these results possible and reproducible in a number of tertiary centers. This technique represents an important advance in improving limb salvage and ambulation for selected patients with leg ischemia combined with extensive tissue loss.

Distal revascularization combined with free tissue transfer is applicable only to a small group of patients who are seen with lower extremity tissue loss. Even in a tertiary referral center, the need for free tissue transfer is infrequent, being required after fewer than 5% of infrainguinal arterial revascularizations.[6] The reasons for this include the following:

1. Most patients develop ischemic tissue loss or gangrene of the toes or forefoot, which is readily treated by toe or transmetatarsal amputation.
2. Patients with heel and hindfoot ulcers usually are seen early, when tissue loss is minimal, such that primary healing can occur after revascularization, possibly aided by split-thickness skin grafts.
3. Some patients are seen with severe gangrene and infection, or without a suitable distal target artery, such that primary, major amputation is mandatory.

In addition, there is a high potential for perioperative morbidity and mortality, and these patients may already have a short life expectancy. Patients who benefit from revascularization combined with free tissue transfer may be categorized as follows: those with peripheral vascular disease and ulceration (including post-traumatic, infected ulcers), patients with diabetic/neurotrophic ulcers, patients with open midfoot amputations, individuals who may benefit from isolated nutrient flaps, and possibly patients with severely calcified tibial arteries without ischemia.

PERIPHERAL VASCULAR DISEASE WITH ULCERATION, INCLUDING POST-TRAUMATIC, INFECTED ULCERS

These patients, who may not have diabetes, usually have chronic infection in a severely ischemic limb and large soft-tissue defects resulting from trauma, previous surgery, or burns. Multiple attempts at closure have usually been undertaken, but these have been unsuccessfully completed because of exposed bone or tendon and the associated chronic infection. In these patients, it is necessary to perform aggressive debridement of the infected soft tissue and bone. This is best performed after the extremity is revascularized so that adequate assessment of tissue viability may be performed. The resulting larger soft-tissue defect may then present a defect unsuitable for skin grafting. There may have been temptation to do a lesser debridement to simplify wound closure; however, the option of using free tissue techniques to close any wound permits adequate debridement and assists in the eradication of chronic infection, as well as supplies well-vascularized tissue coverage (Fig 1).

DIABETIC, NEUROTROPHIC ULCERS

More than 85% of our patients who require a combined vascular and plastic surgical approach are diabetic and are seen with large, chronic, con-

---

FIGURE 1.

A, medial malleolar ulcer with bone and tendon involvement. Patient had undergone aortobifemoral bypass grafting and femoropopliteal bypass grafting in preparation for lower extremity reconstruction. Note great toe tip necrosis. **B,** intraoperatively, after superficial temporal fascial free flap transfer with the revascularized fascia being perfused via anastomoses of the superficial temporal artery with the posterior tibial artery and the superficial temporal vein with the posterior tibial vein. **C,** one year after surgery. The superficial temporal fascia was covered with a split-thickness skin graft.

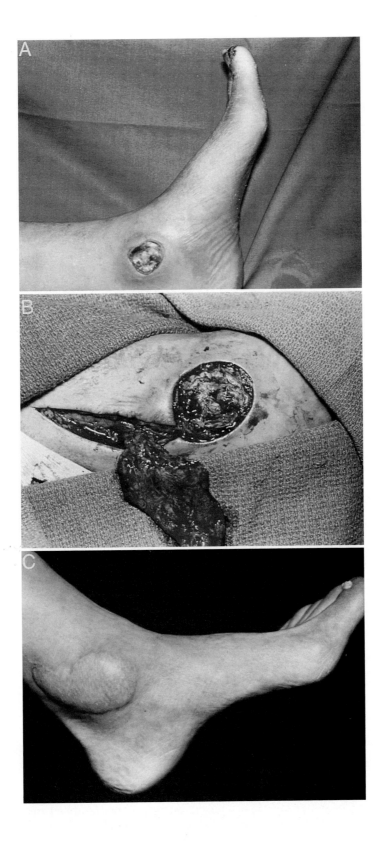

taminated, neurotrophic ulcers. Most of these neurotrophic ulcers are located on the weight-bearing surface of an insensate foot, where the reconstructive options are limited. Debridement and split-thickness skin grafts are usually not successful, and most local flaps, on the basis of antegrade blood flow through the posterior tibial artery and its medial and lateral plantar branches, may be jeopardized by marginal blood flow, even after revascularization, if the distal bypass was performed to the dorsalis pedis or peroneal vessels. In these cases, free tissue transfer may provide an effective alternative to amputation.

It must be emphasized that the transferred free flap is insensate. Because the remainder of the diabetic foot is also neuropathic, adherence to the usual diabetic foot precautions is mandatory to "protect" the free flap as well as the remainder of the foot. Recurrent ulcers have been reported in diabetic patients with free flaps transferred to the plantar surface; however, these occurred only after several years of walking on the flap and may be repaired with a small revision or a second free flap.[17, 18] The occurrence of flap ulceration on the plantar surface of the foot is multifactorial. Many recurrences may be avoided by meticulous inset of the flap at the time of reconstruction to avoid flap redundancy and the excessive shear forces that result. Despite this, diabetic patients who develop large ulcers on the weight-bearing heel should be candidates for free tissue transfer only if they are well motivated to practice careful diabetic foot care postoperatively. Even nondiabetic patients who undergo free tissue transfer must observe similar precautions (Fig 2).

OPEN MIDFOOT AMPUTATIONS

Free tissue transfer may also be useful to obtain closure of open guillotine-type midfoot amputations because there is often extensive bone exposure at the amputation site precluding skin graft coverage. These wounds would require either Syme's or below-knee amputations to obtain primary healing if free tissue transfer is not used. Free tissue transfer may be a better alternative to a more proximal, major amputation. This is especially useful in patients who have previously had a contralateral amputation (Fig 3).

ISOLATED, NUTRIENT FLAPS

When there is severe, advanced peripheral vascular disease, the placement of a free tissue transfer may provide a "nutrient flap" to the distal extremity if the tissue is vascularized by a bypass graft from a proximal vessel. This option is available when no target artery is present in the distal leg. Several successful cases have been reported where distal bypass grafts were performed only to supply blood flow to a free flap, because no large target arteries were present in the adjacent foot.[25, 26] Our experience indicates that the inherent blood flow of the adjacent foot is very important for initial flap healing and incorporation. A "nutrient" free flap may remain viable but may not provide collateral circulation to the adjacent foot within the first month of transfer. Several cases have been reported in which a below-knee amputation was required despite a viable pedal free flap because the adjacent foot remained severely is-

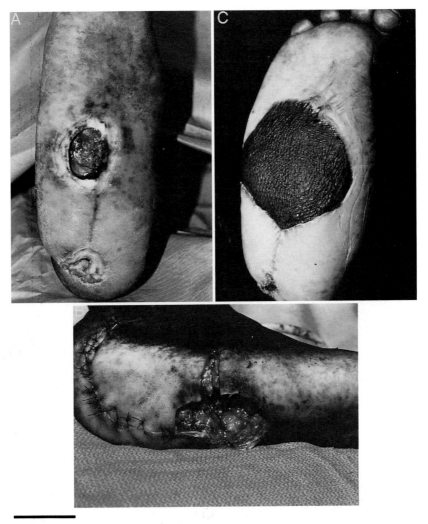

FIGURE 2.

A, diabetic with neurotrophic ulceration of the heel and midfoot exacerbated by infection and infrapopliteal arterial occlusive disease. This patient had undergone contralateral below-the-knee amputation several years earlier because of plantar abscess formation. **B,** one week after popliteal to dorsalis pedis bypass grafting, the wounds are debrided and the heel is reconstructed with "local" tissue. The midfoot wound, now larger, is prepared for closure with a serratus anterior muscle transplant (covered with split-thickness skin graft) with vascular anastomoses being performed between the thoracodorsal artery and the distal bypass graft. Venous outflow from the flap was directed into a deep vein traveling with the dorsalis pedis artery. **C,** three years after the reconstruction there is "stable" coverage and no evidence of impending reulceration.

chemic.[15, 18] Thus, although blood flow through a free flap appears sufficient to maintain patency of a vein bypass anastomosed only to the free flap, ultimate success appears to require an otherwise viable foot adjacent to the soft-tissue defect being covered (Fig 4). In such cases, after free flaps have been in place for several years, there does appear to be neovascularization of the tissue adjacent to the free flap, as demonstrated by late arteriograms taken from selected patients.

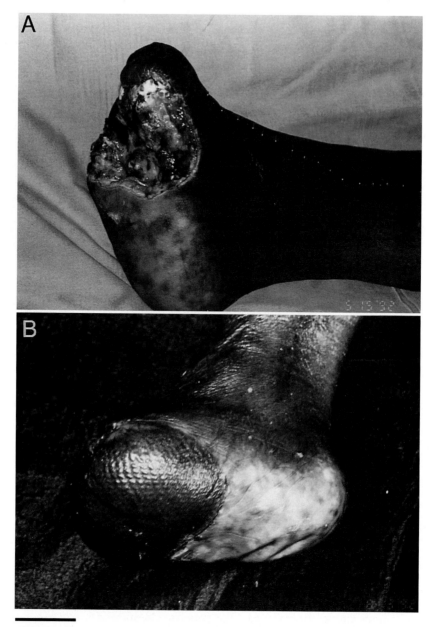

FIGURE 3.

A, open midfoot amputation with limb salvage afforded by popliteal to dorsalis pedis bypass grafting. **B,** three months after serratus anterior muscle transplantation. Coverage of the remaining, exposed plantar structures allowed preservation of a proximal transmetatarsal amputation. The alternative would have been either Syme's amputation or below-knee amputation.

SEVERELY CALCIFIED TIBIAL ARTERIES

The presence of severely calcified tibial arteries, though patent with biphasic blood flow, might jeopardize a successful free flap procedure. Attempts at performing microvascular anastomoses to such severely calcified arteries can lead to thrombosis of the anastomosis or even of the cal-

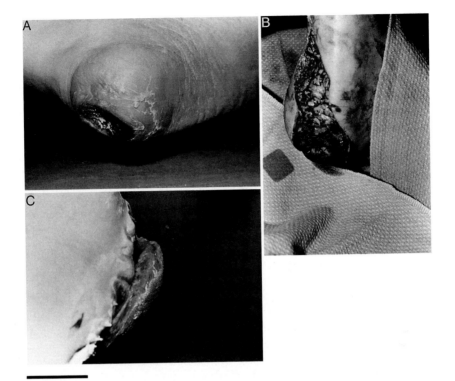

FIGURE 4.

A, lateral, posterior heel ulcer in a diabetic man with a contralateral above-knee amputation. During exploration for distal anastomosis of a femoral bypass graft, no suitable vessel was found. **B,** the wound was enlarged during debridement to provide for a larger flap that would supply additional outflow for the bypass graft and thereby maintain its patency. **C,** in spite of "successful" femoral to free flap bypass grafting, repeated dehiscence of the flap from the foot occurred. The forefoot became progressively more ischemic, and the decision for below-knee amputation was made.

cified vessel itself. In these patients, construction of a vein graft from a more proximal normal artery to either the free flap itself or to a distal target artery is an appropriate alternative. In our experience, most patients requiring free tissue transfer plus arterial reconstruction have required tibial-level vein bypass grafts, although some patients may be effectively treated with a proximal balloon angioplasty or bypass such that the free flap can be based on the "native" popliteal or tibial vessels.

CONTRAINDICATIONS FOR COMBINED REVASCULARIZATION AND FREE TISSUE TRANSFER

A negative fatalism has prevailed in the treatment of diabetic patients with peripheral neuropathy and a distal wound because it was thought that salvage of the limb was probably not advisable because of the rapid recurrence of ulceration secondary to poor sensibility. As such, many surgeons have advocated early proximal amputation. We have found this not to be true and, with education and proper precautions, have not found the problem of recurrent ulceration insurmountable. Likewise, it was previously believed that patients with disturbance of gait secondary to Charcot deformities or other arthritic disease would likely have reappearance of skin breakdown even after coverage. With appropriate tendon releases, midfoot fusions, and the use of orthotics, we have not found this to be the case. The contraindications to free tissue transfer with microvascular techniques range from absolute to relative and may be subclassified as general and local contraindications.

GENERAL MEDICAL CONTRAINDICATIONS

Patients requiring distal arterial reconstruction for extensive tissue loss may be unfit for anesthesia or a prolonged surgical procedure because they frequently have associated coronary artery disease and must be regarded as high-risk patients. These patients are often diabetic and may be unable to ambulate, which may mask the normal warning symptom of angina pectoris. The combination of free tissue transfer and distal arterial reconstruction, whether performed sequentially or as part of the same operation, can be associated with substantial morbidity and mortality because of the systemic complications of atherosclerosis. Thus, the major contraindication to undertaking revascularization plus free tissue transfer is severe associated coronary disease; primary amputation would be a lower-risk alternative. All of these patients need comprehensive preoperative medical assessment and stabilization. Because the purpose of free tissue transfer is to preserve limb length and ambulation, this procedure is not appropriate for nonambulatory patients; in these patients, primary amputation is equally efficacious and more cost-effective.

All patients must be able to manage their free flap postoperatively in a responsible fashion. This includes limb elevation to avoid edema, special protection to avoid trauma (particularly in the insensate foot), and progressive, supervised ambulation. Thus, a relative contraindication for this combined procedure is a nonmotivated patient or unintelligent patient, including individuals who have had a stroke, who cannot understand the importance of these special precautions. Free tissue transfer is not necessary for patients with small ulcers, especially those located on the toes or forefoot, where primary healing may occur or where they may be well managed by local amputation and/or a local flap to obtain bone coverage.[24]

Although some believe the presence of synthetic bypass grafts (polytetrafluoroethylene [PTFE] or Dacron) in a below-knee position may be a relative contraindication to distal free flap transfer because of their relatively poor long-term patency rates and thrombogenicity,[27] we do not be-

---

FIGURE 5.

A, lateral midfoot wound after resection of a bony prominence. **B,** after femoral to posterior tibial bypass grafting, debridement was performed and closure accomplished with a serratus anterior muscle transplant and split-thickness skin grafting. One month postoperatively, the bypass graft clotted. The flap appears cyanotic because the thoracodorsal artery supplying the flap was anastomosed to the saphenous vein bypass graft. **C,** two years after thrombectomy of the bypass graft. The flap is quite viable, even though the bypass graft clotted within 6 months of the thrombectomy procedure. Because there were no areas of impending tissue loss, no further vascular surgery was performed.

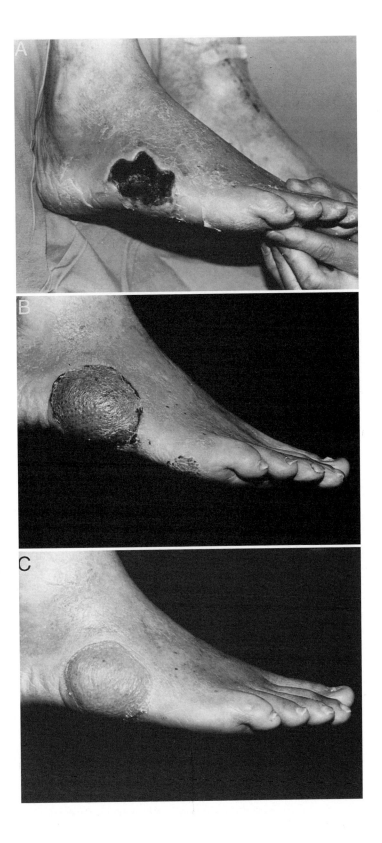

lieve this to be true. The distal bypass need only be patent until primary healing of the flap has occurred, especially if the primary etiology of the ulceration is neuropathy. Even with bypass graft occlusion, the foot will usually remain healed and the reconstruction will be successful (Fig 5).

PREOPERATIVE EVALUATION

Evaluation begins with a comprehensive clinical examination to determine the location and size of the wound, the status of the peripheral circulation, and the presence or absence of peripheral neuropathy. Gait abnormalities and anatomic foot deformities should also be noted. Regular laboratory investigations must include a thorough cardiac examination as well as assessment of the osseous structures of the foot. Plain x-ray films may be supplemented with high-resolution, three-dimensional computed tomography (CT) imaging to outline bony anatomy. Radionuclide scans, magnetic resonance imaging (MRI), and bone biopsy may also be indicated, depending on the specific clinical problem.

VASCULAR EVALUATIONS

When a patient presents with extensive lower extremity tissue loss, evaluation of the arterial circulation is indicated. Arteriography can be used to demonstrate vessel patency, levels of occlusion, which vessels have adequate outflow distally, location of arterial stenoses, and potential sites for microvascular anastomosis. Arteriography may also disclose borderline disease in a patient without obvious ischemic symptoms, but with chronic tissue loss associated with osteomyelitis or previous trauma, who then warrants vascular reconstruction. Duplex ultrasound flow studies, which have been used extensively in the evaluation of carotid disease,[28] have proved valuable in the evaluation of flow in the distal extremities before free flap transfer.[29] It can provide accurate measurements of vessel diameter, screen for ischemia, confirm the presence of stenosis secondary to atherosclerosis, and be used to select potential sites for microvascular anastomosis. Direct imaging of potential recipient veins, including the deep veins, is possible, as is the ability to assess their size, patency, and valvular competency. Transcutaneous oxygen tension or toe pressure measurement may also be helpful in the diabetic patient with calcified, noncompressible tibial arteries. These values are particularly important when bypass grafting directly to a free flap (rather than a pedal vessel) is contemplated, because adequate $TcPO_2$ is necessary for healing of the flap to the recipient foot. On the basis of these investigations, arterial reconstruction before free tissue transfer may be indicated whenever the ankle brachial index is less than 0.7, the transcutaneous oxygen tension is less than 30 mm Hg, or biphasic Doppler waveforms are not present in the recipient artery.

TIMING

Free flap transfer may be delayed until after arterial reconstruction or performed during the same procedure. There are several reasons for delaying the free tissue transfer procedure.[14] If the arterial reconstruction is at all questionable, delaying the free tissue transfer is recommended to avoid the risk of early flap loss with early postoperative bypass graft occlusion. This might apply to patients with a marginal-quality vein graft, a poor distal target artery, or other suboptimal circumstances for arterial reconstruction. Delaying the free tissue transfer also permits confirmation of adequacy of debridement in patients with severe localized infection in whom extensive debridement is required at the time of the arterial reconstruction.

For some patients, however, simultaneous procedures may be optimal.[15, 30] A combined procedure is indicated if the soft-tissue defect encompasses the area where a vein graft will be placed, because immediate coverage of the arterial bypass graft will be necessary. In other circumstances, the flap may provide additional outflow for the bypass graft, thus potentially increasing graft patency in high-risk cases. Certain flaps also offer the benefit of a secondary outflow branch that may be used for distal revascularization. For example, the thoracodorsal artery of the latissimus flap offers the potential for revascularization of the foot by anastomosis of the serratus branch to the dorsalis pedis or posterior tibial artery (Fig 6). By combining the procedures, a second anesthetic may be avoided. Finally, simultaneous performance of the arterial reconstruction and free flap hastens rehabilitation, decreases length of hospital stay, and thereby reduces the total expense of the reconstruction. It should probably be reserved, however, for "good-risk" patients with an "optimal" arterial reconstruction, because the length of surgery is clearly increased if both procedures are performed during the same operation, and complications may increase because of prolonged general anesthesia.

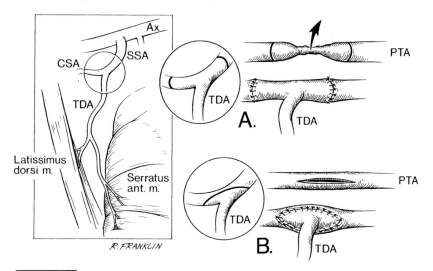

FIGURE 6.

The thoracodorsal artery (TDA) originates from the subscapular artery (SSA) at the location where the circumflex scapular artery (CSA) originates. **A,** a Carrel patch of vessel may be used to facilitate an end-to-side anastomosis of the thoracodorsal artery with the recipient artery. **B,** a segment of subscapular and circumflex scapular artery may be interposed in an end-to-end fashion to replace a localized area of stenosis.

RECONSTRUCTIVE TECHNIQUES

FOOT DORSUM

Free flap coverage is rarely necessary on the dorsum of the foot because split-thickness skin grafting or local flap coverage is generally adequate. Large areas of exposed bone and tendons on the dorsal foot have historically been covered with a cross-leg flap. In these circumstances, free composite tissue transplantation is preferable because of the shortened immobilization time, the ease of a one-stage, two-team procedure, and the aesthetics of the donor and recipient sites. If only extensor tendon exposure is evident on the foot dorsum, excision with split-thickness skin grafting of the underlying periosteum is the most prudent alternative.

PLANTAR FOREFOOT

Free flap coverage of this anatomic site after distal revascularization is rarely performed because limited amputation or local flap transfers are often adequate to maintain bipedal ambulation. In most patients, it is preferable to perform a transmetatarsal amputation or a more proximal resection of the metatarsals in their entirety (amputation of Lisfranc) rather than a free tissue transfer procedure, because stable biomechanics of ambulation are preserved with relatively simple operative procedures. During the past 10 years, we have not used free tissue transfer techniques for repair of forefoot wounds in patients requiring revascularization procedures.

PLANTAR MIDFOOT

The midfoot is usually a non–weight bearing surface; hence, split-thickness skin grafts are usually adequate. In diabetic patients, however, where neuroarthropathy has caused the collapse of the transverse and longitudinal arches of the foot, the midfoot becomes weight bearing, and skin grafts are no longer sufficient. The tarsal and the metatarsal bones are involved in almost 60% of patients with Charcot deformities. Wounds larger than 4 to 6 cm will usually require free flap reconstruction or midfoot amputation to obtain stable wound closure. It is important to try to maintain foot length at the midfoot level so that orthotics rather than prostheses may be used for ambulation. Resection of the metatarsals in their entirety (amputation of Lisfranc) and amputation through the midtarsal joints (at the level of Chopart) allow for weight-bearing ambulation without the need for a prosthesis. Free tissue transfer to close a midfoot amputation will permit maintenance of a Lisfranc or Chopart amputation, thereby avoiding the need for a more proximal amputation that would require the use of a prosthetic device. The combination of distal revascularization and free tissue transfer has had a profound effect on limb salvage in patients with midfoot ulceration. A recent study reports an 83% incidence of below-knee amputation in this subgroup of patients. No free tissue transfer techniques were used in this retrospective review.[31] When free transfer combined with revascularization is selectively used for this group of patients, we have lowered the incidence of below-knee amputation to 2%.[32]

WEIGHT-BEARING HINDFOOT (HEEL PAD)

There is no perfect technique of reconstructing the thick durable heel pad when undertaking the closure of wounds in this region. Small wounds of the hindfoot, in patients with normal arterial anatomy, may be closed with numerous regional flap techniques. However, except for the lateral calcaneal artery flap, all local tissue transpositions require antegrade flow in the posterior tibial artery and its distal branches. Defects in patients without antegrade adequate flow in these vessels, such as after bypass grafting to the distal peroneal or dorsalis pedis arteries, or with large plantar hindfoot wounds (greater than 6 cm), should usually be reconstructed with microsurgical composite free tissue transfer. In general, muscle flaps covered with skin graft are the tissues of choice for reconstructing defects in this area. Fasciocutaneous flaps tend to slide over the calcaneus during walking, creating shear stress and recurrent ulceration.

POSTERIOR HINDFOOT (ACHILLES TENDON)

The posterior hindfoot, unlike the plantar hindfoot, requires thinner, more pliable flap coverage than the thicker coverage required for the weight-bearing portions of the heel. Suitable flaps include the radial and ulnar forearm flaps as well as a variety of thin fascial flaps that may be covered with a skin graft.

FLAP SELECTION

After distal revascularization, multiple factors should be considered in the selection of the appropriate donor flap. These include the specific characteristics of the flap (dimensions, pedicle length, vessel size, donor site morbidity), defect size, wound location, the vessel revascularized in the foot, the status of "runoff" in the foot, and the vascular resistance of the flap. Flaps harvested above the waist reduce the likelihood of atherosclerotic involvement of the pedicle artery and are therefore preferred. The serratus anterior muscle flap has been our flap of choice because of the long pedicle length it affords. Based on the thoracodorsal artery, it can easily be anastomosed in an end-to-side fashion to an in situ saphenous vein bypass graft in those patients who have previously undergone revascularization to the anterior tibial or dorsalis pedis artery, and can still reach the plantar surface of the foot. When wounds larger than 150 cm^2 require closure, the latissimus dorsi muscle is usually used. Scapular fascia or fasciocutaneous flaps are useful for small defects in patients who have been bypassed to the posterior-tibial vessels at the ankle. Because of the shear forces acting on the skin portion of the scapular flap during ambulation (when placed on the plantar surface), we have been reluctant to routinely use this tissue for plantar defects. The rectus abdominis muscle provides large amounts of donor tissue with a long vascular pedicle (the deep inferior epigastric vessels); however, preoperative assessment with duplex scanning should be performed to make sure there is no atherosclerotic involvement of the pedicle vessels. Free muscle transfer and split-thickness skin graft are optimal for patients with documented osteomyelitis because this technique has proved effective in the definitive treatment of bone infection for the reason that muscle tissue can adequately fill the irregular contours of an adequately performed bone debridement. Ulcers without osteomyelitis may be covered with fascial, muscle, or fasciocutaneous flaps, with the specific choice dictated by the length of the vascular pedicle required as well as the size and location of the defect.

If flap thinness is a primary consideration, cutaneous flaps may have some advantage. Thin free flaps are most useful for dorsal foot reconstruction and coverage of the exposed Achilles tendon or malleoli. The forearm flaps have great utility in this regard because they are often thin enough to allow the patient to wear a normal shoe. These donor tissues are best used for shallow wounds with no underlying bone infection. When avoiding general anesthesia is a concern, the forearm flaps permit tissue dissection under axillary block and transfer to the recipient area with epidural anesthesia. Fascial flaps with overlying skin graft provide another alternative for thin donor tissue. The choice of temporalis fascia, scapular fascia, forearm fascia, or lateral arm fascia depends on the wound size and location. The temporalis fascia flap is relatively small with a short vascular pedicle, in contrast to the scapular fascial flap, which is larger in size and has a longer pedicle length.

Many neurosensory flaps have been described for microvascular transplantation as an attempt to provide sensation to plantar reconstructions. Two usual donor sites include the deltoid and the lateral arm flaps. These flaps are thin and have reliable neurovascular anatomy. If a suitable recipient nerve is present, flap innervation is possible with microneural coaptation. The role of neurosensory flaps, however, remains controversial, especially in patients with diabetic peripheral neuropathy. At least equally as important in flap longevity is the surgical technique used, including meticulous flap inset, removal of underlying bony prominences, patient education, and the judicious use of custom-made orthotics postoperatively.

PERIOPERATIVE CONSIDERATIONS

Arterial revascularization combined with free tissue transfer requires a carefully coordinated effort by vascular and plastic surgeons. The arterial reconstruction must be performed with consideration for the planned anastomotic site of the free flap pedicle. Whenever possible, the free flap is best anastomosed directly to the distal vein graft; thus, the distal anastomosis of the bypass graft must be sufficiently near the soft-tissue defect to accommodate the length of the flap pedicle.

A two-team approach is recommended for free tissue transfer to simultaneously dissect the flap, debride the wound, and expose the recipient vessels, if this is not done during the same operation as a distal arterial bypass. Microvascular anastomoses are performed with an operating microscope and usually interrupted 9-0 polypropylene suture.

We do not use a pneumatic tourniquet in a patient who has vascular disease and has undergone prior bypass. Veins placed for arterial conduits suffer a period of endothelial loss for up to 2 weeks,[33] and placement of a tourniquet around a graft could lead to thrombosis during this period. In situ grafts show less endothelial loss in the first 24 hours than reversed grafts,[34] but this probably does not make them safer in terms of tourniquet application. Even after this 2-week period we avoid use of a tourniquet for fear of damaging the graft and promoting thrombosis. In an attempt to further minimize thrombosis and to optimize flap pedicle patency, we routinely use pentoxifylline in the preoperative, intraoperative, and postoperative periods. Pentoxifylline, a methylxanthine derivative, alters the hemorheology of circulating blood in a manner that, theoretically, should improve the outcome from combined distal bypass and free flap surgery. Pentoxifylline has the ability to increase red blood cell deformability, decrease blood viscosity, decrease platelet aggregation, decrease red blood cell aggregation, and decrease white blood cell activation.[35-37] Some of these effects occur soon after the medication is begun; however, maximal benefit is reached after 8 weeks of treatment. Pentoxifylline should be started as soon as the patient is brought to the attention of either the vascular or plastic surgeon.

OPTIONS FOR ARTERIAL ACCESS

The recipient vessels for free flap transfer should ideally be adjacent to the area to be reconstructed. Only vessels with biphasic or triphasic flow should be used because monophasic flow may predispose to anastomotic thrombosis. End-to-side anastomosis is usually preferable to maintain important blood flow to the distal limb. When there is only a single vessel supplying the leg or when the saphenous bypass graft is used for arterial inflow, end-to-side anastomosis is the *only* acceptable anastomosis to perform. If more than one vessel supplies the foot and the area chosen for anastomosis is found to have intramural plaque, end-to-end anastomosis may be preferable to a difficult end-to-side anastomosis.

Although every attempt should be made to use "healthy" regions of recipient vessels, sometimes calcified vessels and areas of soft plaque in the media that are prone to intimal separation cannot be avoided. Application of vascular clamps may be quite difficult when recipient vessels are severely calcified. If standard clamping techniques are unable to occlude blood flow adequately, the placement of balloon occlusion catheters proximally and distally will be necessary. If a soft area of the vessel is identified, incision of this area with a No. 11 scalpel blade or micro-blade may be the best choice for gaining access to the recipient artery's lumen. Lateral arteriotomies in vessels with plaque or vessels that are heavily calcified may not be possible with micro-scissors, which may damage the vessel wall. Alternatives include a vascular punch that cuts a round hole in the recipient vessel, the diameter of which depends on the size of the anvil,[38] or small bony rongeurs that readily cut through calcification. Local removal of calcium plaques can be accomplished through the edges of the arteriotomy if necessary. Suture technique may also have to be modified by replacing the standard 100-μm-diameter microneedle with standard vascular suture in the 8-0 size range (with its proportionately larger needle) or using specialized calcium-cutting needles. When the recipient vessel is severely calcified, an additional option is to use a Carrel patch of subscapular artery/circumflex scapular artery, which may be obtained with the thoracodorsal artery that supplies either a serratus muscle or latissimus muscle flap (see Fig 6).

Occasionally, an end-to-side anastomosis cannot be completed. If the recipient vessel is nonessential to the distal limb viability, the anastomosis may be converted to an end-to-end repair to support the free flap. If the artery is necessary for distal limb viability, it may be patched with a vein patch graft, and an alternate site for flap anastomosis can be sought. On occasion, a segment of calcified vessel may be excised and replaced with an interpositional vein graft. The flap may now be anastomosed, end-to-side, to the vein graft. In a similar manner, a segment of recipient vessel may be resected and replaced with the confluence of the subscapular and circumflex scapular vessels. The thoracodorsal artery will take its origin from this confluence and supply either the serratus anterior flap or the latissimus dorsi flap (see Fig 6).

If long-vein grafting is required for arterial access, the in situ technique may be used. This has been widely used in peripheral vascular surgery, with patency rates comparable to those of standard vein grafting.[8, 11] Use of an in situ vein in microsurgical tissue transfer also has the advantage that the distal portion of the graft more closely matches pedicle vessels. If a reversed vein graft is used, there is frequently a size discrepancy between the larger proximal vein graft and the flap artery. Although the distal saphenous vein has a thicker wall diameter than it has proximally, this is less of a problem than the presence of an internal diameter mismatch. When this occurs, an end-to-side anastomosis to the vein graft (with oversew of the end of the graft) may be preferable. No reliable synthetic grafts exist at present for microvascular anastomotic purposes; however, recent work with small (2-mm) PTFE and other synthetics is encouraging and may offer an alternative to vein grafts in the future.[39] Intraoperative angiography is "standard" in the evaluation of anastomoses performed during limb revascularization. Such examinations are rarely indicated in the assessment of microvascular anastomoses because poorly performed arterial anastomoses will thrombose shortly after release of the vascular clamps.

OPTIONS FOR VENOUS ACCESS

The deep veins of the leg are the preferable sites for venous anastomosis for free flap transfer. Although vein preparation may be tedious because of the perivascular inflammatory changes that accompany atherosclerosis, the deep system will be less subject to impingement and occlusion from postoperative swelling or postsurgical dressings. The status of the deep system is readily assessed preoperatively by duplex imaging, and this system usually provides acceptable venous outflow. If, however, the patient has had a history of deep venous thrombosis, the superficial venous system should be chosen. The superficial system may have been harvested for cardiac or limb bypass. In these situations, the lesser saphenous system is usually satisfactory. If local veins are found to be unsuitable, vein grafting to the nearest open vessel may be necessary. It is helpful if this is anticipated preoperatively, because grafts can be harvested during flap dissection.

SPECIAL CONSIDERATIONS

For short segment vascular occlusions, reconstruction of the soft tissue defect and the diseased arterial segment may be performed with certain free flaps alone. The vascular anatomy of the latissimus muscle and the serratus muscle is such that the arterial reconstruction may be accomplished "with" the vascular pedicle to the flap (see Fig 6). The forearm free flaps may also be useful in this situation, providing for wound closure and distal revascularization with one procedure. Because the vascular conduits provided by these flaps are only 5 to 15 cm in length, their applicability is limited to short-segment vascular reconstructions and wounds that are immediately adjacent to the vascular reconstruction.

Each donor flap used for lower extremity reconstruction has an inherent vascular resistance.[40] Based on the nature of the blood supply in the recipient extremity and the way in which the limb has been revascularized, flap selection should take into account the vascular resistance of the available donor tissues. For example, when performing a flap transfer to a foot that has recently undergone distal bypass grafting, a very low resistance free flap (*i.e.*, the rectus abdominis muscle) may actually divert blood flow away from the foot and into the flap. This theoretically would jeopardize foot viability. A higher resistance flap may be a better choice (*i.e.*, fascial flaps or the serratus anterior muscle). Alternatively, a low-resistance flap may have a favorable effect on bypass graft patency rates if the outflow into the foot is inherently poor. When there is no acceptable target vessel in the foot for bypass grafting, the graft may be anastomosed directly into a low-resistance flap, which will be capable of sustaining graft patency and will set the stage for primary healing.

POSTOPERATIVE CARE

Because of the prolonged surgery and the high incidence of concomitant medical problems, we often monitor the patient in the intensive care unit or similar facility for at least 24 hours after free flap transfer. The medical status of the patient is managed by the medical unit, but the flap is monitored by the surgical team. Dextran and pentoxifylline are usually administered, and aspirin (81 mg *per os* daily) replaces the use of dextran once the patient is able to tolerate oral intake. In selected cases, the use of continuous epidural anesthesia may help to decrease vasospasm and improve microvascular anastomotic patency rates.[41] Low-dose continuous intravenous heparin (400–500 units per hour) is reserved for patients who exhibit anastomotic thrombosis intraoperatively.

All free flaps are initially insensate, and these patients, who often have diabetes, may also have other areas of decreased sensation. Pressure necrosis may occur without the patient being aware of pain. Therefore, where the extremity is splinted, great care must be taken to pad the limb appropriately, and close attention must be paid to the flap and its skin graft, if present. For heel flaps, the splint must not contact the flap directly at any point. In spite of all necessary care being exercised, these patients have a high incidence of local wound-healing problems.[42]

Patients are kept in bed with the leg elevated for 2 weeks and then gradually allowed to increase extremity dependency. Good team communication is required while the patient works closely with the physical therapist commencing ambulation during the third week. Full weight-bearing ambulation is usually possible by this time if flaps are on non–weight bearing positions of the foot. When plantar foot reconstruction is performed, partial weight bearing will be started during week 3, progressing to full weight bearing by 6 weeks.

Wound breakdown at the flap margins must be dealt with early to prevent infection and further tissue loss. Compressive elastic wrapping is worn whenever the leg is dependent, and this is continued for at least 6 months after surgery. Heat-molded shoe inserts are used to protect the operative site, and an orthotist may be consulted for fitting of custom footwear. As flap bulk subsides, modifications will be necessary.

When free flap reconstruction has not been successful, amputation may be a reasonable alternative to a second flap, because the second may prove more problematic than the first. Vascular disease is unfortunately a progressive disease, and despite initial success, further limb ischemia can occur with worsening proximal disease, occlusion of vascular grafts, or distal embolization. These events may preclude limb salvage even in the face of a viable flap. With recurrent complications, the patient may choose to abandon the flap and have an amputation. On some occasions, the flap may be used for conservation of length and stump coverage, or it may have to be discarded with the limb. It should be remembered, however, that amputation is irreversible, and that after careful consultation and consideration, limb salvage is still likely to be the better option.

The ultimate goal of managing patients with vascular disease is returning the patient to as near normal as possible. Close cooperation between the vascular surgeon and the plastic surgeon may provide the greatest opportunity to maximize functional restoration in these difficult patients. Support by endocrinologists, cardiologists, and podiatrists will further improve the likelihood for success.

REFERENCES

1. Barber CC, McPhail NV, Scobie TK, et al: A prospective study of lower limb amputations. *Can J Surg* 26:339–341, 1983.
2. A report of the National Diabetes Advisory Board. NIH publication number 81-2284. Bethesda, Md, 1980, p 25.
3. Kucan JO, Robson MC: Diabetic foot infections: Fate of the contralateral foot. *Plast Reconstr Surg* 77:439–441, 1986.
4. Bodily DC, Burgess EM: Contralateral limb and patient survival after leg amputation. *Am J Surg* 146:280, 1983.
5. Couch NP, David JK, Tilney NL, et al: Natural history of the leg amputee. *Am J Surg* 133:469, 1977.
6. Swartz WM, Mears DC: The role of free-tissue transfers in lower extremity reconstruction. *Plast Reconstr Surg* 76:364–373, 1985.
7. Eshima I, Mathes SF, Paty P: Comparison of the intracellular bacterial killing

activity of leukocytes in musculocutaneous and random pattern flaps. *Plast Reconstr Surg* 86:541–547, 1990.

8. Levine AW, Davis RC, Cingery RO, et al: In situ bypass to the dorsalis pedis and tibial arteries at the ankle. *Ann Vasc Surg* 3:205–209, 1989.

9. Magnant JG, Cronenwett JL, Walsh DB, et al: Surgical treatment of infrainguinal arterial occlusive disease in women. *J Vasc Surg* 17:67–78, 1993.

10. Matsumoto T, Rajyaguru V, Okamura T: Laser recanalization, laser assisted balloon angioplasty and laser angioplasty. *Surg Gynecol Obstet* 169:195–198, 1989.

11. Brinton MH, Stahler C, Cibbons C: Lower extremity revascularization with in situ saphenous vein for critical ischemia. *Am J Surg* 155:701–703, 1988.

12. Palmaz JC, Carcia OJ, Schatz RA, et al: Placement of balloon-expandable intraluminal stents in iliac arteries: First 171 procedures. *Radiology* 174:969–975, 1990.

13. Briggs SE, Banis JC Jr, Kaebnick H, et al: Distal revascularization and microvascular free tissue transfer: An alternative to amputation in ischemic lesions of the lower extremity. *J Vasc Surg* 2:806–811, 1985.

14. Colen LB: Limb salvage in the patient with severe peripheral vascular disease: The role of microsurgical free-tissue transfer. *Plast Reconstr Surg* 79:389–395, 1987.

15. Serletti JM, Hurwitz SR, Jones JA, et al: Extension of limb salvage by combined vascular reconstruction and adjunctive free-tissue transfer. *J Vasc Surg* 18:972–980, 1993.

16. Shestak KC, Fitz DC, Newton ED, et al: Expanding the horizons in treatment of severe peripheral vascular disease using microsurgical techniques. *Plast Reconstr Surg* 85:406–411, 1990.

17. Greenwald LL, Comerota AJ, Mitra A, et al: Free vascularized tissue transfer for limb salvage in peripheral vascular disease. *Ann Vasc Surg* 4:244–254, 1990.

18. Cronenwett JL, McDaniel MD, Zwolak RM, et al: Limb salvage despite extensive tissue loss. Free tissue transfer combined with distal revascularization. *Arch Surg* 124:609–615, 1989.

19. Malone JM, Coldstein J: Lower extremity amputation. In Moore WS, editor: *Vascular Surgery: A Comprehensive Review*. New York, 1983, Grune and Stratton.

20. Dabb RW, Davis RM: Latissimus dorsi free flaps in the elderly: An alternative to below-knee amputation. *Plast Reconstr Surg* 73:633–640, 1984.

21. Chowdary RP, Celani VJ, Goodreau JJ, et al: Free-tissue transfers for limb salvage utilizing in situ saphenous vein bypass conduit as the inflow. *Plast Reconstr Surg* 87:529–535, 1991.

22. Veith FJ, Cupta SK, Samson RH, et al: Progress in limb salvage by reconstructive arterial surgery combined with new or improved adjunctive procedures. *Ann Surg* 194:386–401, 1981.

23. Schneider JR, Walsh DB, McDaniel MD, et al: Pedal bypass versus tibial bypass with autogenous vein: A comparison of outcome and hemodynamic results. *J Vasc Surg* 17:1029–1040, 1993.

24. Morain WD, Dellon AL, MacKinnon SE, et al: Current concepts in plastic surgery for the diabetic. *Adv Plast Reconstr Surg* 4:1–36, 1987.

25. Mimoun M, Hilligot P, Baux S: The nutrient flap: A new concept of the role of the flap and application to the salvage of arteriosclerotic lower limbs. *Plast Reconstr Surg* 84:458–467, 1989.

26. Shestak KC, Hendricks DL, Webster MW: Indirect revascularization of the lower extremity by means of microvascular free-muscle flap. A preliminary report. *J Vasc Surg* 12:581–585, 1990.

27. McAuley C, Steed D, Webster M: Seven year follow-up of expanded polytetrafluoroethylene (PTFE) femoropopliteal bypass grafts. *Ann Surg* 199:57, 1984.

28. Spurk P, Angelkort B, Selter P: Incidence of arteriosclerotic lesions of the carotid arteries in chronic peripheral arterial disease and myocardial infarction. *Angiology* 40:39–44, 1989.

29. Colen L, Musson A: Preoperative assessment of the peripheral vascular disease patient for free tissue transfers. *J Reconstr Microsurg* 4:1–14, 1987.

30. Ciresi KF, Anthony JP, Hoffman WY, et al: Limb salvage and wound coverage in patients with large ischemic ulcers: A multidisciplinary approach with revascularization and free tissue transfer. *J Vasc Surg* 18:648–655, 1993.

31. Wieman TJ, Griffith GD, Polk HC: Management of diabetic midfoot ulcers. *Am J Surg* 215:627–632, 1992.

32. Colen LB: A ten year experience with the diabetic foot. Presented at the Annual Meeting of the American Association of Plastic Surgeons, San Diego, 1995.

33. Rao VK, Nightingale C, O'Brien BMcC: Scanning electron microscope study of microvenous grafts to artery. *Plast Reconstr Surg* 71:98–106, 1983.

34. Pederson WC, Barwick WJ, Serafin D: Loss of microsurgically transferred tissue: Critical review of 27 flap losses. Presented at the Fourth Annual Meeting of the American Society for Reconstructive Microsurgery, Baltimore, September 1988.

35. Mueller R, Lehrach F: Hemorheological role of platelet aggregation and hypercoagulability in microcirculation. Therapeutic approach with pentoxifylline. *Pharmacotherapeutica* 2:372, 1980.

36. Hamerschmidt DE, Kotasek D, et al: Pentoxifylline inhibits granulocyte and platelet function including granulocyte priming by platelet activating factor. *J Lab Clin Med* 112:254, 1988.

37. Schonharting M, Musikic P, Muller R: The hemorheological and antithrombotic potential of pentoxifylline (Trental): A review. *Pharmatherapeutica* 5:159, 1988.

38. Pederson WC, Barwick WJ: Use of the vascular punch in microsurgery. *J Reconstr Microsurg* 5:80, 1989.

39. Klitzman B, Serafin D: Denucleation of PTFE graft material and patency rates for microvascular prostheses. Presented at the Annual Meeting of the Plastic Surgery Research Council, 1993.

40. Sasmor MT, Reus WF, Straker DJ, et al: Vascular resistance considerations in free tissue transfer. *J Reconstr Microsurg* 8:195–200, 1992.

41. Weber S, Bennett CR, Jones NF: Improvement in blood flow during lower extremity microsurgical free tissue transfer associated with epidural anesthesia. *Anesth Analg* 67:703–705, 1988.

42. Pederson WC: Microsurgical management of lower extremity ulceration in the diabetic patient with peripheral vascular disease. Presented at the Annual Meeting of the American College of Surgeons, South Texas Chapter, Austin, Texas, January 26, 1990.

PART V

Portal Hypertension

Current Management of Variceal Hemorrhage: Problems, Priorities, and Perspectives

Richard J. Gusberg, M.D.

Professor and Chief, Vascular Surgery, Yale-New Haven Hospital, Yale University School of Medicine, Director, Yale Vascular Center, New Haven, Connecticut

A 45-year-old cirrhotic and reformed alcoholic with portal hypertension arrives in the emergency room following an episode of massive hematemesis. He is mildly confused, slightly jaundiced, and hypotensive. What are the problems and priorities in the management of this patient? What is the initial approach? What are the risks and benefits of the treatment options? What are the validated management guidelines? What are the unanswered questions? The controversies? This chapter will focus on these issues, discussing the current approaches to portal hypertension and variceal hemorrhage in the context of its pathophysiology and prognosis. It will attempt to clarify the role of shunt surgery in the modern context of both less invasive treatment options and liver transplantation.

BACKGROUND

Portal hypertension has long been recognized as a potentially lethal consequence of chronic liver disease. During the past decade, basic research has clarified both the pathophysiology and hemodynamic patterns of patients bleeding from esophageal varices. The portal hypertensive state in cirrhosis reflects high intrahepatic resistance and diffusely increased portal pressure that results in the development of portal-systemic collaterals, low vascular resistance (both systemic and splanchnic), and an elevated cardiac output. This sepsislike, hyperdynamic state increases the hemodynamic stress and appears to be mediated in large part by nitric oxide.

Furthermore, the hemodynamic basis for both the development and the natural history of varices has been better defined. In patients with portal hypertension on the basis of postsinusoidal obstruction, characteristic of alcoholic cirrhosis, portal pressures reliably reflect the difference between the wedged and free hepatic vein pressure. An hepatic venous

Advances in Vascular Surgery®, vol. 3
© 1995, Mosby–Year Book, Inc.

pressure gradient of 12 mm Hg defines the threshold above which varices develop and are likely to bleed. Higher pressures are associated with larger varices and a higher risk of both bleeding and death.[1]

Portal hypertension, then, is defined by the systemic and splanchnic hemodynamic consequences of chronic liver disease. The prognosis of these patients is linked to both the progression of their liver disease and risks associated with variceal hemorrhage. Any therapy advocated for the management of these patients must, therefore, be evaluated on the basis of its impact on both the liver disease and the bleeding.

THE SETTING

Variceal hemorrhage remains a significant cause of morbidity and mortality in patients with cirrhosis and is a significant challenge for the physicians who are treating them.

Varices develop in about 60% of cirrhotic persons and 30% of these patients with varices bleed from them; this occurs in most within the first 2 years after their discovery. After the initial episode of bleeding, approximately 20% of patients will re-bleed, most within the first year. About one third die within 6 weeks of an initial hemorrhage and another one third die within 1 year, which places a significant amount of stress on the patient, their caregivers, and the health care system.[2] Since the introduction of modern shunt surgery during the last half century, there has been significant progress in our understanding and management of these patients.

Who are most likely to bleed among portal hypertensive patients with documented varices? Several factors have been identified that appear to be associated with an increased risk.

1.   Multiple, large dilated varices documented by endoscopy. The risk of rupture probably relates to wall tension as described by Laplace's Law.
2.   "Cherry red spots" endoscopically identified on the varices.
3.   Co-existent esophageal and gastric varices.
4.   Prograde, as opposed to hepatofugal, portal flow.
5.   Alcoholism.
6.   Diminished hepatic functional reserve, as assessed by Child's criteria.
7.   A corrected hepatic vein wedge pressure greater than 12 mm Hg.

It is in this setting that the natural history of cirrhosis with portal hypertension should be considered and the risks and benefits of the management options should be evaluated.

THE PROBLEM AND PRIORITIES

Although the development of portal-systemic collaterals and varices is a common complication of cirrhosis, most patients with varices never bleed from them. The management of portal hypertension has focused, therefore, primarily on patients with documented bleeding. Although there is increasing evidence to support the prophylactic use of nonoperative interventions, no reliable criteria have been established to guide their application. Surgery, however, has no confirmed role in the prophylactic treatment of these patients. Nonselective shunts have been shown to have a deleterious effect on both short-term and long-term outcomes as compared with expectant medical therapy.[3] Although some have advocated selective shunts in selected patients with varices that have never bled,[4] the risks and costs appear to outweigh the potential benefit. The surgical treatment of portal hypertension is reserved, therefore, for the treatment of variceal hemorrhage.

In portal hypertensive patients who present with upper gastrointestinal hemorrhage, it is important to remember that a nonvariceal source exists approximately 30% to 50% of the time. Once bleeding from either varices or portal hypertensive gastropathy is documented, however, treatment directed at preventing recurrent hemorrhage is indicated. Without vigorous intervention, recurrent and lethal bleeding is highly likely. The selection of the most appropriate method of treatment, however, remains a challenge. Although Child's criteria reliably predict acute morbidity and mortality associated with treatment, these criteria are not useful for defining long-term outcomes.

Although management decisions must be tailored to the individual patient's status and stability, the initial approach to patients suspected of bleeding from varices should be guided by certain priorities.

1. Initial resuscitation and stabilization.
2. Emergency endoscopy to document bleeding site.
3. Endoscopic sclerotherapy or banding if active variceal bleeding is identified.
4. Adjunctive pharmacologic therapy with pitressin or somatostatin.
5. Balloon tamponade if previous methods fail.
6. Definitive treatment to prevent recurrent bleeding.

The timing of definitive intervention will be dictated by the patient's overall stability, hepatic reserve, coagulation profile, and degree of initial bleeding control. Any delay required to optimize the patient's status must be weighed against the risk of recurrent bleeding and further deterioration before such optimization can be achieved.

ACUTE CONTROL

Although acute variceal bleeding may be self-limited, several methods have been shown to be effective in providing acute control.

Sclerotherapy, either intravariceal or paravariceal, can be done at the time of initial endoscopy and has been reported to control the bleeding in 75% to 90% of cases.[5, 6] At present, it appears more useful in the acute management of variceal hemorrhage than in its long-term control.

Acute pharmacologic control has been advocated in the initial management of variceal hemorrhage for at least 40 years and a variety of vasoactive agents provide transient control in most patients. Their usefulness has been limited by both the transient nature of their effectiveness and their side effects. Intravenous vasopressin, a nonselective vasoconstrictor, remains widely prescribed, providing acute control in 60% to

70% of patients and can be initiated during initial endoscopy.[7-9] Terlipressin (a tricyclyl synthetic analogue of vasopressin with a longer duration of action and no cardiac side effects), somatostatin (which lowers azygous blood flow without causing systemic vasoconstriction), and octreotide (a longer acting synthetic analogue of somatostatin) have been shown in well-designed trials to provide acute bleeding control in 80% to 90% of patients, which is more effective than either placebo or vasopressin and associated with fewer complications.[10-14]

Balloon tamponade is generally reserved for patients who fail sclerotherapy and pharmacologic control because of significant associated risks. Several principles are important to minimize these hazards.

1. Esophageal tamponade should be instituted by experienced personnel.
2. Airway control with planned endotracheal intubation and adequate sedation are essential.
3. To minimize the risk of esophageal rupture, position of the gastric balloon must be confirmed by x-ray evaluation before inflation.
4. Esophageal suction, proximal to the gastric or esophageal balloon, must be established to reduce the significant risk of aspiration.

Although balloon tamponade can be effective, the significant associated morbidity and mortality rates require that it be applied with care under appropriate circumstances.

Once bleeding is controlled initially, the focus should turn toward preventing recurrence, and several premises should guide the interventional decisions. The indication for intervention is preventing recurrent hemorrhage, while minimizing any deleterious impact on the liver. All shunting procedures (including transjugular intrahepatic portosystemic shunt [TIPS]) should be considered palliative, because neither hepatic function nor patient survival will be enhanced. The benefits of bleeding control must be weighed against the acute operative and long-term risks: operative mortality and the impact of treatment on long-term survival, hepatic function, encephalopathy, cost, and quality of life. Furthermore, all treatment options should be considered in the context of the only definitive treatment for portal hypertension and cirrhosis: hepatic transplantation. The choice and timing of therapy should be dictated, in part, by the patient's potential as a transplant recipient.

CONTROL OF RECURRENT BLEEDING: THE OPTIONS

The treatment of portal hypertension is directed primarily at the 30% of patients in whom variceal hemorrhage develops. Interventional or operative approaches are rarely indicated in actively bleeding patients because these invasive approaches are associated with a substantial mortality rate when applied in the emergency setting. The various nonoperative measures (pharmacologic, endoscopic, or tamponade) temporarily control the bleeding in almost all patients. Nonselective shunts (e.g., end-side or side-side portocaval, central splenorenal, or mesocaval) can provide effective, immediate portal decompression and bleeding control but are associated with operative mortalities in the 30% to 50% range.[15] The best results with this approach have been reported by Orloff et al. using a prospective program in which emergency shunts were performed in all patients presenting with variceal hemorrhage. The operative mortality was 20% with a better than 50% 5-year survival.[16] Small caliber, interposition portacaval shunts, introduced by Rypins and Sarfeh,[17] may provide safer and comparably effective immediate decompression.

Selective shunts have been associated with good short-term and long-term results when applied in the elective setting. Although low operative mortalities have been reported in a series of good risk patients undergoing emergency distal splenorenal shunts,[18] the delayed decompression of the esophagogastric varices that follows this shunt, as pressures equalize between the variceal bed and the low pressure splenorenal anastomosis, limits its role in the management of the actively bleeding patient. The TIPS has been advocated as an alternative to shunt surgery in both the acute and chronic setting. Although this approach has been shown to achieve effective short-term bleeding control, the associated morbidity and mortality rates when applied in the acute setting are comparable to those of operative shunting.[19]

The initial priorities in portal hypertensive patients with suspected variceal hemorrhage are clear. Endoscopic documentation of the source and site should be followed by an organized attempt at immediate control with a combination of sclerotherapy and/or drug treatment, with balloon tamponade used for persistent bleeders. Interventional or operative options should be reserved, if at all possible, for the chronic control of bleeding in the stable patient.

LONG-TERM THERAPY

After initial control and stabilization, attention should be directed at achieving definitive and durable long-term control of recurrent bleeding while minimizing deleterious consequences for the chronically injured and compromised liver. Several treatments are available and appropriate selection should be guided by several factors.

1. The patient's overall condition, including age, stability, general status, and co-morbid conditions.
2. Hepatic histology (alcoholic vs. nonalcoholic cirrhosis) vs. extrahepatic causes of portal hypertension.
3. Hepatic status and functional reserve assessed according to Child's classification.
4. Likelihood of dense and hypervascular adhesions from previous surgery.
5. Caliber and patency of portal, splenic, and mesenteric veins.
6. Bleeding site (esophageal, gastric, or distal intestinal varices or portal hypertensive gastropathy).
7. Additional factors that might preclude adequate operative decompression such as elevated systemic or inferior vena cava (IVC) pressure or compartmentalization of the portal system by thrombus.

In evaluating the outcomes of the various available interventions and their relative cost-effectiveness, several principals apply. First, these treatments are costly. Second, in patients with alcoholic cirrhosis, no intervention confers a significant long-term survival advantage; there are, however, procedure-related differences in the incidence of encephalopathy and recurrent bleeding. Finally, there are differences in the procedure-related mortality rates, which generally reflect the patient's stability and the hepatic reserve.

The spectrum of treatments advocated for the long-term prevention of recurrent variceal hemorrhage range from drug therapy to liver transplantation.

β BLOCKERS

Beta blockade, usually established with propranolol, has been shown in numerous prospective trials to provide a modest reduction in the incidence of recurrent bleeding when compared with placebo.[20] The rate of recurrent bleeding, however, remains quite high (40% to 60%).[21, 22] Patient compliance, the cost of long-term drug administration, and the potentially adverse consequences of chronic beta blockade limit wide applicability and efficacy.

SCLEROTHERAPY

Although endoscopic sclerotherapy is effective in the acute management of variceal bleeding, its role in the long-term prevention of recurrent hemorrhage is less clear. First reported more than 50 years ago,[23] sclerotherapy has been widely advocated for variceal bleeding only in the last decade. Although several controlled trials have documented a reduction in rebleeding rates in patients undergoing sclerotherapy, this outcome is neither predictable nor durable[24–26] and there is no associated prolongation of survival.[27] Furthermore, successful control of varices requires complete obliteration, which necessitates multiple sessions and considerable patient compliance. Neither gastric varices nor portal hypertensive gastropathy can be successfully treated by sclerosis. Significant complications include esophageal ulcers, strictures, and extra variceal sclerosant escape, which causes splanchnic venous thrombosis.[28] This latter complication may be subtle in its presentation and result in a compartmentalization of the portal system, which limits options for surgical decompression. There is some evidence that endoscopic ligation or banding might provide comparable bleeding control with fewer associated complications and lower mortality.[29] Further studies are needed to confirm its role. Even with complete variceal obliteration without any sclerosis-related complications, about 40% to 60% of patients will bleed again.

Several controlled trials have compared shunt surgery with chronic sclerotherapy in the prevention of recurrent variceal bleeding in cirrhotics.[30–33] The selective distal splenorenal was the primary shunt used in most of these trials. A consistent finding was significantly better control of bleeding in the shunted patients (rebleeding rates 3% to 17%) vs. those undergoing long-term sclerotherapy (rebleeding rates 35% to 60%). There remains some controversy, however, about the procedure-related survival advantage. Two comparably designed studies document conflicting results and merit special attention. The Henderson et al.[31] reported improved survival in patients undergoing initial sclerotherapy one-third of whom were eventually shunted for recurrent and unremitting bleeding. The median follow-up time in this trial was 5 years, and 59% of the sclerotherapy patients were hospitalized for rebleeding. Nearly all of those who could not be easily controlled were successfully shunted. In the Rikkers et al. trial,[30] which also involved a group of predominantly alcoholic cirrhotic persons, there were 60 patients randomized and followed for a mean of 7 years. In this study, 60% of the sclerotherapy patients rebled, which is comparable to the Henderson et al. series; but, in contrast, most bled to death before an operation could be performed (consistent with all other trials). Most patients who fail sclerotherapy cannot be salvaged with shunt surgery. In the Rikkers trial, the long-term outcome of the shunted patients was significantly superior to that of those undergoing sclerotherapy in terms of both recurrent bleeding and survival.[30]

Although sclerotherapy clearly has a role in the chronic management of cirrhotics with variceal hemorrhage, the available data do not support unselected application. Its usefulness seems limited to poorly compliant patients, those without easy access to a major medical center, and patients bleeding from either gastric varices or portal hypertensive gastropathy. For the remainder, its appropriateness for any individual must be weighed against the risks and benefits of the alternatives.

DECOMPRESSIVE SHUNTS

During the fifty years since Whipple[34] and Blakemore[35] first reported their initial experiences with portacaval shunting in patients with portal hypertension and variceal bleeding, a variety of operative approaches have been advocated and refined. Improved understanding of the pathophysiology of variceal hemorrhage along with better initial resuscitation and bleeding control have allowed the more appropriate prioritization of definitive management decisions and optimization of the status of patients who might benefit from surgery. With advances in anesthesia, perioperative monitoring, and operative technique, shunt surgery has become safer and more broadly applicable. Furthermore, advances in immunobiology have enhanced the feasibility of transplantation in selected patients with variceal hemorrhage and end-stage liver disease.

As the experience with total portal-systemic shunts accumulated, early enthusiasm for their role in variceal bleeding became tempered as several prospective randomized controlled trials comparing shunts with expectant medical therapy in cirrhotic persons who had bled.[36-38] Patients in these trials consisted predominantly of alcoholic cirrhotic persons, and total portal-systemic decompression was provided with either end-side or side-side central portacaval shunts. Although these nonselective shunts appeared effective at controlling variceal bleeding and were associated with a somewhat improved survival, death from hemorrhage was replaced by death from hepatic failure and a significant percentage of the survivors had encephalopathy develop.

The evolving surgical experience with shunt surgery in the 1950s and 1960s confirmed both the feasibility of performing these complex vascular operations in a high risk population with poor prognosis and their effectiveness in controlling recurrent hemorrhage. New operative alternatives emerged during the following decades that were designed to reduce short-term risks and enhance the long-term outcomes in these challenging patients. Portal-systemic shunts for variceal decompression fall into four categories (Table 1).

1. Total portal-systematic shunts divert all portal flow away from the liver and are presumed to cause immediate variceal decompression.
2. Partial shunts reduce portal pressure below the bleeding threshold of 12 mm Hg but preserve some hepatopedal portal flow.
3. Selective shunts decompress the esophagogastric-splenic variceal bed while maintaining prograde portal flow and elevated mesenteric-portal vein pressures.
4. Percutaneous shunts are side-to-side shunts that may provide either total or partial decompression depending on their position and caliber.

TOTAL PORTAL-SYSTEMIC SHUNTS

Total portal-systemic shunts provide complete and immediate decompression of the esophagogastric varices, splenic bed, mesenteric and portal veins, and intrahepatic sinusoids. The prototypical total shunt is constructed with either an end-to-side or side-to-side portacaval anastomosis. Consistent variceal decompression requires complete patency throughout the portal system without partial or segmental obstruction that might limit or compartmentalize postshunt pressure changes and sufficiently low systemic pressure in an unobstructed IVC. Either anastomosis is usually performed by way of a right subcostal incision and requires full mobilization of the portal vein from its retropancreatic portion to its bifurcation. Care must be taken to avoid inadvertent injuries to the head of the pancreas, the common bile duct, or the coronary vein, which usually drains into the midposteromedial aspect of the main portal vein.

In the *end-to-side shunt* the distal portal vein is ligated; sometimes, in an effort to achieve more portal vein length, the right and left branches are individually ligated. The vein is divided, and the proximal portion is brought down to create an end-to-side anastomosis to the anteromedial aspect of the infrahepatic IVC using an elliptical opening to enhance shunt flow. Factors that may increase the difficulty of (or preclude) accomplishing this shunt include dense and highly vascular adhesions from previous surgery upon the right upper quadrant; pylephlebitis from previous partial portal vein thrombosis; previous pancreatitis that limits mobilization of the portal vein; and a large caudate lobe, which may interfere with vein mobilization or prevent accurate positioning of the anastomosis leading to compression or kinking. Previous surgery, portal vein thrombosis, and pancreatitis can be anticipated from a thorough preoperative history and evaluation. A large caudate lobe, interposed between the portal vein and IVC, can be partly resected if necessary. This shunt, if appropriately constructed, effectively and durably lowers variceal and portal pressure because the patency rate is high and the rate of recurrent bleeding is low. Operative mortality rates generally reflect the patients' Child's classification. With appropriate surgical expertise in a good risk patient (Child's class A and B) elective operative mortality rates under 3% can be achieved.[39] Even if the primary objective of bleeding control with a low operative mortality rate is achieved, these shunts pose several problems. Prograde portal flow is irretrievably lost, with potentially adverse consequences to hepatocyte integrity and function. The intrahepatic sinusoids are not maximally decompressed and ascites formation may persist. Finally, the portal dissection required may increase the difficulty and operative risk of subsequent hepatic transplant.

The *side-to-side portacaval shunt* maximally decompresses both the splanchnic venous bed and the intrahepatic sinusoids. Anastomosis of elliptically tailored venotomies at least 10 mm in length between the portal vein and IVC (or a tributary) should acutely lower the portal pressure to normal and provide total diversion of portal flow. Simultaneous decompression of both the splanchnic bed and the liver effectively controls both variceal hemorrhage and ascites. Technical challenges are similar to those associated with the end-to-side portacaval shunt but a tension-free, side-to-side portacaval anastomosis of adequate caliber can be difficult because maximal mobilization of both the portal vein and IVC is required. In view of the currently available alternatives, this shunt is rarely indicated for bleeding control because coincident, intractable ascites is infrequent. Aggressive medical therapy, including sodium and water restriction in combination with diuretics and/or intermittent large volume paracenteses, usually provides satisfactory control, and truly refractory ascites can be managed successfully with one of the peritoneovenous shunts.

The Budd-Chiari syndrome, which results from hepatic venous outflow obstruction, however, remains one indication for a total side-to-side shunt. Portal and sinusoidal decompression early in the course of the disease is the key to effective treatment, which limits hepatocyte necrosis and optimizes hepatic functional recovery. Portocaval, mesocaval, and mesoatrial shunts have all been advocated for this condition, the choice dictated by the status of the portal venous system and the level of IVC obstruction.[40–42]

The *mesocaval shunt* also provides total decompression and is occasionally indicated to control variceal bleeding in patients with portal hypertension from cirrhosis. Its successful accomplishment requires a patent superior mesenteric vein of sufficient length and an unobstructed IVC. At surgery, the superior mesenteric vein is identified at the root of the mesocolon just to the right of the pulsation from the superior mesenteric artery and is mobilized for a length of approximately 6 cm. A 12- to 16-mm prosthetic is anastomosed to the IVC just beneath the duodenum, which is mobilized superiorly. The length of the graft should be minimized as much as possible and then anastomosed to the SMV. Many surgeons now prefer an externally supported graft because its course is usually curvilinear. Although the long-term patency of this shunt has been considered inferior to that associated with more central shunts,[43] recent reports suggest more durable outcomes than previously described.[44] Its relative ease of performance, an operative field distant from the collateral-filled porta hepatitis, and immediate postshunt variceal decompression make it an appropriate option in selected urgent or emergent situations, particularly in potential transplant candidates.

The *central splenorenal shunt* provides total nonselective portal decompression. The central end of the mobilized and divided splenic vein is anastomosed to the anterior wall of the left renal vein, resulting in total decompression of the hepatic-mesenteric-esophagogastric beds. It offers no hemodynamic or metabolic advantage over the portacaval shunt, has been associated with a high shunt thrombosis rate (approximately 20%),[45] and offers no advantages over conventional portocaval shunts in terms of encephalopathy or long-term survival.[46, 47] It can, however, provide effective and immediate variceal decompression in patients with dense adhesions from any previous right surgery upon the upper quadrant and for those whose portal area should be preserved for any future transplant.

DISTAL SPLENORENAL SHUNT

All of the total shunts are conceptually similar hemodynamically and share common benefits and risks. In good risk patients, they can provide safe, effective, and durable portal decompression; they do so, however, at the expense of portal perfusion of the liver and are, therefore, associated with a significant incidence of encephalopathy and hepatic failure, particularly in alcoholic patients who continue to drink. In an effort to preserve the benefits of total shunt while minimizing its risks,[48] the distal splenorenal shunt (DSRS) was developed in 1967 to selectively decompress the esophagogastric varices while preserving prograde portal flow to minimize encephalopathy and hepatic failure. The accumulated experience has confirmed that this shunt achieves most of its hemodynamic and metabolic objectives. In several prospective randomized controlled trials it has been shown to be as effective as total shunts in controlling variceal bleeding and appears to be associated with fewer short-term and long-term risks including encephalopathy and recurrent hemorrhage.[49-51] These objectives are accomplished presumably by creating two distinct splanchnic venous compartments: a decompressed esophagogastric-splenic-pancreatic bed and a hypertensive, undecompressed hepatomesenteric bed. Several technical points are worth emphasizing. Adequate exposure by way of a generous mid-line or left-sided upper abdominal transverse incision is required. Central division of the splenic vein and adequate circumferential mobilization facilitates an unkinked, tension-free, end-to-side distal splenorenal anastomosis. Particular care must be taken in mobilizing the splenic vein from its retropancreatic junction with the portal vein and out toward the splenic hilum because multiple, high pressure pancreatic tributaries must be gently secured. Both the splenic and left renal veins should be mobilized sufficiently and the intervening tissue divided appropriately to ensure a tension-free, hemodynamically favorable anastomosis constructed with the use of atraumatic vascular clamps, an elliptical venotomy on the anterosuperior surface of the renal vein, and fine vascular sutures. The inferior mesenteric, left adrenal, and left gonadal veins are often divided. A compulsive attempt at portal-azygous disconnection must be made to promote durable prograde portal flow. This effect requires division of as many splenic vein tributaries as is technically feasible; secure ligation of the coronary vein (recognizing its variable drainage into the splenic and/or portal vein); ligation of the inferior mesenteric vein; ligation of the right gastric vein just superior to the pylorus; and division of potential portal-systemic collateral connections from the pylorus to the short gastric veins. Postoperative evaluation should include an attempt to verify the technical sufficiency of the procedure and might include Doppler ultrasound or magnetic resonance imaging. Transcaval shunt catheterization may be useful if shunt patency or adequate decompression remain uncertain. The accumulated experience with the DSRS confirms its low operative mortality, low rate of recurrent bleeding comparable to that achieved after total shunts, and relatively low incidence of postshunt encephalopathy.[52] There has been, however, a wide variability in the reported incidence of post-DSRS encephalopathy, particularly among alcoholics. Achieving a durable selective shunt with consistent maintenance of prograde portal flow appears to be of central importance in minimizing the risk of postshunt hepatic decompensation and/or encephalopathy, and possibly in prolonging survival.

Although the DSRS is based on a sound hemodynamic premise, its risks and benefits are a reflection of both uncontrollable progression of the hepatic disease and the postshunt changes in splanchnic hemodynamics. Because the route of decompression from the esophagogastric varices to the low pressure splenorenal anastomosis is somewhat circuitous through the short gastric veins, there is probably some delay in pressure equilibration and adequate postshunt reduction of variceal pressure. This shunt is not, therefore, the best option in the emergency setting with an actively bleeding patient. Although hypersplenism is virtually never an indication for portal decompression, its relief can be anticipated in most patients following DSRS.[53]

Although effective variceal decompression with continued prograde portal flow can be anticipated after DSRS, the degree of prograde flow appears to decline with time.[54] The juxtaposition of the high pressure hepatic-portal-mesenteric vascular bed and the decompressed esophagogastric-splenic bed leads to progressive development of portal-systemic collaterals with an increasing percentage of portal flow diverted away from the liver. The rapidity and extent of the reduction in hepatic flow appear to reflect both the nature and progression of the underlying liver disease and the completeness of the portal-azygous and splenopancreatic disconnection (SPD) at the time of surgery.[55, 56] Although as many as 90% of nonalcoholic persons maintain significant prograde portal flow, such is the case in only 25% to 50% of alcoholic persons.[57] There is some evidence, however, that more compulsive operative SPD is associated with more durable preservation of portal flow even in alcoholic persons and may result in less encephalopathy[58] and even improved survival rates.[59, 56]

Although most series document no shunt-related difference in long-term survival when DSRS is compared with total shunts, the 5-year survival of nonalcoholic cirrhotics after DSRS may be significantly better (80% to 90%) than that after total shunts (50%).[60-62] This is supported by evidence that improved hepatic metabolic performance, reflected by maintenance of maximal urea synthetic rates, characterizes postshunt patients with preserved prograde portal flow.[52]

The DSRS has been shown to be safe and effective in a wide spectrum of portal hypertensive patients, including children and the elderly. Despite Sherlock's admonition that the risks of postshunt encephalopathy and coma were prohibitively high in patients more than 50 years of age, a recent series has documented the safety of DSRS in considerably older patients in whom there was no operative mortality, a low incidence of postshunt encephalopathy and hepatic failure, and a well-maintained quality of life.[63] Although most experiences with the DSRS have been with adults, there have been reports of DSRS in children with minimal encephalopathy, effective bleeding control, and excellent long-term patency.[64]

Mobilization of the splenic vein is usually the most demanding technical aspect of the operation. Anything that might further complicate this dissection, such as history of severe or chronic pancreatitis, is a relative contraindication to DSRS.

This effective method of variceal decompression avoids any portal dissection and preserves this area for subsequent transplantation. Similarly, DSRS is an appropriate shunt in patients with a liver transplant in whom adhesions and scarring in the area of the porta may be anticipated and for those with extrahepatic portal vein thrombosis. Although a previous splenectomy may preclude the feasibility of a DSRS, thus shunt will still provide satisfactory esophagogastric decompression if the short gastric veins remain patent.

A recent review of the reported nonrandomized world experience with DSRS included more than 3,700 patients, 70% of whom were nonalcoholic persons, in varying states of general stability and hepatic compensation. This review documented an operative mortality of 8%, a rebleeding rate of less than 10%, and a low incidence of postshunt encephalopathy that was usually mild, reversible, and precipitated by identifiable events.[65]

The DSRS appears to meet its hemodynamic objective of selectivity in most patients, and its clinical objectives of effective bleeding control with minimal hepatic injury, particularly in nonalcoholic cirrhotics. In series reported over the past decade, the operative mortality has ranged from 0% to 13%.[50, 51, 63, 66, 67] In centers with established expertise in the medical and surgical management of portal hypertension, the current mortality rate associated with selective shunts performed electively in Child's A or B patients should not exceed 3%.

After completion of a DSRS, several factors might adversely affect either the variceal decompression or the degree of prograde portal flow. Anastomotic stenosis may result from a technical error or fibrosis and may cause increased variceal pressure with recurrent variceal bleeding. Shunt stenosis can be documented by transcaval catheterization and can be effectively corrected with balloon angioplasty.[68]

Postshunt portal vein thrombosis will further limit nutrient flow to the liver and predispose to hepatic decompensation, and its reported incidence is less than 5%. The late development of nonocclusive portal thrombosis has been, however, reported in up to 20% of patients after DSRS.[69] Such thrombosis probably reflects stasis from decreased splenic inflow, increased hepatic resistance from progression of the liver disease, or both. Its incidence may be under-appreciated because magnetic resonance imaging, the most sensitive and specific imaging modality currently available to evaluate the splanchnic venous anatomy, has not been used routinely in post-DSRS patients. No reliable treatment for this potentially serious complication currently exists. Neither operative thrombectomy nor thrombolytic therapy is considered safe or effective.

Post-DSRS encephalopathy may reflect persistent or evolving portal-systemic collaterals or deteriorating hepatic function. One technically related, correctable predisposing factor is a persistently patent, coronary vein usually resulting from the variable anatomy. The coronary vein may be solitary or multiple, drain into either the portal vein, splenic vein, or both such that coronary vein occlusion at the time of DSRS may be incomplete. A patent coronary vein discovered postoperatively can be safely and effectively occluded by percutaneous transhepatic catheterization and embolization or balloon occlusion.

PARTIAL PORTAL SYSTEMATIC SHUNT

The objective of this shunt is to reduce portal pressure below the bleeding threshold (approximately 12 mm Hg), while preserving some prograde portal flow. Two contemporary examples are the small diameter interposition portacaval graft and shunt. The interposition graft, which is technically easier and requires less portal dissection, has been more widely applied and its hemodynamic characteristics and consequences have been carefully studied by Sarfeh and his colleagues[19] who used externally re-enforced 8-mm, 10-mm, and 12-mm grafts. The larger grafts are associated with greater portal decompression, but less well-maintained portal flow, increased encephalopathy, and decreased long-term survival. The smaller grafts result in less of a drop in portal pressure and better preserved portal flow. All grafts provide immediate portal decompression.

These shunts are generally performed by way of a generous right upper quadrant incision. The portal vein is mobilized and encircled so as to obtain safe proximal and distal control. The infrahepatic, suprarenal portion of the IVC is identified after a Kocher maneuver which may require a tedious dissection through a thick layer of portal-systematic venous collaterals and hypertrophied lymphatics. With both the IVC and portal vein appropriately exposed and mobilized, the anteromedial aspect of the IVC and the inferolateral portion of the portal vein are prepared for anastomosis with the interposition graft. Elliptical venotomies in both vessels should enhance patency and flow, both anastomoses should be bevelled and the graft (usually polytetrafluorethylene) should be as short as possible, reducing the likelihood of kinking. A 8-mm caliber graft has been demonstrated to provide adequate (although not maximal) portal decompression, while maintaining prograde portal flow, and appears to be the appropriate choice in the elective setting. Larger 10-mm or 12-mm grafts provide better, immediate decompression and may be most appropriate for patients who require an emergency shunt for active variceal hemorrhage.

The initial thrombosis rate associated with this shunt has been approximately 20%, yet its long-term patency rate, presumably lower than direct autogenous shunts, has not been firmly established. Patency should be confirmed postoperatively by Doppler ultrasound, magnetic resonance imaging, or direct transcaval catheterization.

Small diameter, direct side-to-side portacaval shunts theoretically also provide partial portal decompression and were described by Bismuth et al. 20 years ago.[46] Although prograde portal flow is initially maintained, these shunts tend to dilate and eventually result in total portal decompression with an associated incidence of encephalopathy comparable to that reported after nonselective shunts. More recently, Johansen[70] reported on his favorable experience with small diameter (10 mm to 12 mm) direct side-to-side portacaval shunts with an incidence of encephalopathy less than 10%, despite what appeared to be total portal diversion, and no shunt thromboses. Persistent intestinal venous hypertension was thought to underlie the low incidence of encephalopathy.

INTRAHEPATIC SHUNTS

The continued search for safer and less invasive approaches to portal decompression led to the development of the TIPS. By using established angiographic techniques to place an intrahepatic stent between the portal and systematic circulations, this technique has been widely applied despite the absence of well-controlled data confirming its safety, efficacy, and durability. The currently reported experience, however, allows several conclusions regarding its role in the management of these patients. These shunts are technically feasible in most patients and will initially drop the portal pressure below the bleeding threshold of 12 mm Hg by using a stent dilated to 8 mm to 10 mm.[71, 72] There is a significant 30-day postprocedure mortality rate that ranges from 3% to 20%, which is consistent with a high risk, poorly compensated patient population and comparable to the Child's-related postoperative mortality rates.[19, 71, 72] Shunt stenosis or occlusion remains a significant problem; it has been reported in approximately 10% to 40% of patients within 12 months of placement.[71, 72] Although stent replacement or dilatations can lead to improved results with 12-month assisted patency rates as high as 80%, 2-year primary patency rates as low as 30% have been reported.[73] Furthermore, shunt stenoses lead to less secure variceal decompression and repeated procedures increase both the risk and cost. Until data are generated that document long-term efficacy and patency of these percutaneously placed shunts, their durability will remain uncertain. The initial priorities, however, in all these patients remain clear: immediate resuscitation and prompt identification of the bleeding source. Temporizing attempts to control the bleeding are undertaken in the hope of proceeding with definitive therapy in a stable patient that is aimed at preventing recurrent bleeding with minimal encephalopathy and hepatic failure. The role of TIPS in the management of variceal hemorrhage remains to be determined. In selected variceal bleeders with end-stage liver disease, TIPS can be an appropriate and effective bridge to transplantation.[74] In stable patients who have failed other emergency measures to control bleeding and in whom operative decompression is either a prohibitive risk or relative contraindication, TIPS appears to be a viable option. Its clear role as definitive elective therapy in the long-term control of bleeding varices in good risk patients must await further, reliable data from controlled clinical trials.

NONSHUNT OPERATIONS

Promoted as being technically easier and posing less of a risk to hepatic function, these operations attempt to control variceal bleeding without creating any direct portal systematic connection. Their objectives include obliteration of the esophagogastric varices, devascularization with interruption of collateral pathways to the varices, and/or decreasing portal venous flow.

The most extensive of these operations is the Sigiura procedure, which consists of splenectomy and proximal gastric revascularization that requires an abdominal approach and esophageal devascularization with transection and re-anastomosis by way of the transthoracic approach. Sigiura's reported results in almost 200 predominantly alcoholic Japanese patients have been impressive with a low rate of recurrent bleeding (less than 5%) and a 10-year survival rate of greater than 70%.[75]

Numerous efforts to modify this procedure and/or reproduce Sigiura's results have been unsuccessful, particularly in the North American alcoholic population. These various attempts at operative devascularization have been generally associated with high operative mortality rates (10% to 35%) and inconsistent control of bleeding with recurrent variceal hemorrhage in 10% to 54%.[76] Given this experience and the availability of safer and more reliable alternatives, these extensive devascularization procedures are rarely indicated.

The most common nonshunt operation currently performed in the United States is the transesophageal transection and reanastomosis using a stapler. Although this procedure has its advocates, the results have generally been disappointing with operative mortality rates as high as shunt operations and less effective bleeding control.[77] The one setting in which a nonshunt approach remains the treatment of choice is bleeding gastric varices associated with splenic vein thrombosis for which splenectomy is effective. In contrast, for the treatment of variceal hemorrhage associated with portal hypertension and cirrhosis, splenectomy alone results in no significant decrease in portal flow or pressure and has no clear hemodynamic or clinical basis.[78]

LIVER TRANSPLANTATION

Although many treatments are available for the management of cirrhotics with variceal hemorrhage, transplantation is the only one that deals with both the hemodynamic abnormality and its underlying liver disease. The demonstrated feasibility of liver transplantation supports its application as definitive therapy in selected patients with end-stage liver disease complicated by variceal bleeding. Enthusiasm for its wide application must be tempered by issues of cost, donor organ availability, impact on quality of life, and the demonstrated safety and palliative efficacy of a variety of operative and nonoperative alternatives. In certain categories of patients, transplantation is relatively contraindicated: advanced age, active alcoholism, chronic hepatitis, extrahepatic portal vein thrombosis, and prohibitive co-morbid disease are a few examples. In the absence of these contraindications, nonalcoholic and abstinent alcoholic cirrhotic persons with end-stage liver disease (Child's class C) should be considered for liver transplantation. This definitive therapy should also be considered in selected patients with progressive hepatic dysfunction whose liver or portal hypertension-related complications, such as ascites and recurrent encephalopathy, have adversely and significantly affected their quality of life.

TREATMENT PLAN

In portal hypertensive patients presenting with hematemesis, the priorities are straightforward. Initial resuscitation and stabilization should be followed by endoscopic identification and immediate control of the bleeding source.

Many treatment options are available in the acute and chronic management of variceal bleeding. The challenge is to select the most appropriate (safe, durable, and cost-effective) therapy for the individual patient in the context of the patient's overall status and the natural history of their liver disease.

Immediate control can generally be achieved by some combination of pharmacologic and/or transesophageal (endoscopic or balloon tamponade) intervention.

Initial resuscitation, endoscopy, and other interventions should be carried out expeditiously during the first 24 to 36 hours. In the few patients with initially uncontrollable bleeding, a TIPS or emergency surgical shunt may be indicated if not precluded by marked hemodynamic instability or hepatic decompensation.

Once the bleeding is initially controlled, a treatment plan must be selected that minimizes the risk of recurrent hemorrhage. Without intervention, the likelihood of lethal rebleeding is high. The treatment choice among the broad spectrum of available options should be guided by several considerations.

Beta blockade provides better control than placebo but is still associated with a high rate of recurrent bleeding. Its clearest role is probably prophylaxis before any documented bleeding. Sclerotherapy is similarly associated with a high rate of recurrent bleeding and has significant limitations. Patient tolerance may be a problem and ready access to a treatment center is required at least until all varices are obliterated. There are some significant complications with sclerotherapy, some of which might limit alternative treatment options, and it is ineffective in patients bleeding from gastric varices or portal hypertensive gastropathy. Sclerotherapy appears best reserved for patients bleeding from esophageal varices whose liver disease confers a limited life expectancy or in whom other invasive therapies are relatively contraindicated.

For patients in whom either a TIPS or operative shunt is considered, preprocedure imaging of the splanchnic venous system is essential to assess patency, and manometry can be helpful to confirm portal hypertension and ensure that infrahepatic IVC pressures are sufficiently low to permit adequate decompression. Although venous phase angiography has been widely used in this setting, its accuracy in ruling out either partially or totally occlusive thrombus is limited.[28] Serious complications include contrast nephropathy, those associated with arterial catheterization, and bleeding precipitated by a transient increase in volume and portal pressure. Although Doppler ultrasound can confirm the presence of portal vein (or shunt) flow, it is technician-dependent and cannot definitely rule out thrombus or adequately assess the splenic or mesenteric veins. Presently, MRI appears to be the most sensitive and specific in assessing patency of the splenic, superior mesenteric and portal veins. A thorough and logical approach to preshunt assessment would include an MRI and an IVC-gram, with or without hepatic vein wedge and infrahepatic IVC pressure measurements.

For good risk nonalcoholic cirrhotic patients with well-preserved hepatic function, a selective shunt (DSRS) can provide safe, effective, and durable bleeding control. It is associated with excellent long-term survival, does not preclude a subsequent transplant, and is probably the treatment of choice given appropriate surgical expertise.

For low risk alcoholic cirrhotics (Child's class A or B) without contraindictions to operative decompression, elective shunt surgery (particularly DSRS) is safe, durable, and probably more cost-effective than the alternatives. A small diameter (8-mm) interposition portacaval shunt is a reasonable alternative, although its long-term effectiveness is unconfirmed and it may preclude subsequent transplant.

In patients with persistent bleeding despite initial control with conservative measures, all intervention options have significant risks, particularly in those patients with marginal hepatic reserve. For some of these patients, there may be no cost-effective interventional or operative options. In patients who may become candidates for hepatic transplantation within 6 to 12 months, a TIPS provides reasonable control at a reasonable risk. Longer term control in potential transplant candidates is probably best achieved with DSRS. Operative decompression is a viable option in selected, marginally stable but persistently bleeding patients, presuming there are no prohibitive, co-morbid problems such as hepatic coma, severe coagulopathy, or progressive hepatic failure. The major objective of surgery in this setting is to provide maximal, immediate variceal decompression with an expeditious operation at minimal risk. Of the options available, probably the most appropriate choice is an interposition portacaval or mesocaval shunt by using at least a 10-mm or 12-mm prosthetic graft. Central splenorenal, side-to-side splenorenal, or interposition splenorenal grafts might be satisfactory second choices. In patients with variceal hemorrhage associated with end-stage, decompensated liver disease (and in selected patients with stable but progressive liver disease such as primary biliary cirrhosis) hepatic transplantation can be an appropriate and definitive option. These decisions must be made in the context of the natural history of the patient's liver disease, problems posed by co-morbid factors, and careful consideration of risks, benefits, costs, priorities, and the availability of both donors and sufficient resources.

Despite the theoretical considerations that appear to legitimize matching a particular patient to a particular treatment plan, management decisions are often dictated by geographical considerations, referral patterns, and regional expertise. Optimally, the treatment for these challenging patients can be most appropriately formulated in centers where there is equivalent expertise in their pharmacologic, endoscopic, radiologic, and operative management. Practical considerations and local expertise may limit the options.

CONCLUSION

Variceal hemorrhage is a frequent and lethal complication of chronic liver disease and requires treatment. Although pharmacologic prophylaxis can be effective, most patients present for treatment after a documented episode of bleeding. There are many options available to prevent recurrent hemorrhage all of which except transplantation are palliative and vary in their safety, cost, efficacy, and durability.

Since the introduction of shunt surgery for the management of portal hypertension, there have been significant advances in both knowledge and technology, which have enhanced our understanding of this condition and broadened both the treatment options and the spectrum of patients amenable to treatment. At the same time, costs have increased and the limitations in resources have forced us to define more clearly the priorities and defend our recommendations by documenting their cost-efficacy, impact on quality of life, and functional outcomes. Appropriate management must be determined for each individual patient in the context not of what we *can* do but what we *should* do.

TABLE 1.
Portal-Systemic Shunt Categories

Total
    Portocaval (end-to-side, side-to-side)
    Mesocaval
    Central splenorenal
Partial
    Interposition, small caliber grafts (portocaval, mesocaval, splenorenal)
Selective
    Distal splenorenal
Percutaneous
    TIPS

TIPS = transjugular intrahepatic portosystemic shunt.

REFERENCES

1. Mahl TC, Groszmann RJ: Pathophysiology of portal hypertension and variceal bleeding. *Surg Clin North Amer* 70:251–266, 1990.
2. Resnick R: Management of varices in cirrhosis. *Hosp Pract* 28:123–130, 1993.
3. Conn HO, Lindenmuth WW, May CT, et al: Prophylactic portacaval anastomosis. A tale of two studies. *Medicine* 51:27–40, 1972.
4. Jin G: Current status of the distal splenorenal shunt in China. *Am J Surg* 160:93–97, 1990.
5. Bornman PC, Kahn D, Terblanche J, et al: Rigid versus fiberoptic injection sclerotherapy: A prospective randomized controlled trial in patients with bleeding esophageal varices. *Ann Surg* 208:175–178, 1988.
6. Sarin SK, Nauda R, Sachder G, et al: Intravariceal versus paravariceal sclerotherapy: A prospective controlled randomized trial. *Gut* 28:657–662, 1987.
7. Conn HO, Ramsby GR, Storer EH, et al: Intra-arterial vasopressin in the treatment of upper gastrointestinal hemorrhage: A prospective controlled clinical trial. *Gastroenterology* 68:211–215, 1925.
8. Fogel MR, Krauer CM, Andres LL, et al: Continuous intravenous vasopressin in active upper gastrointestinal bleeding: A placebo-controlled trial. *Ann Intern Med* 96:565–570, 1982.
9. Tsai YT, Lay CS, Lai KH, et al: Controlled trial of vasopressin plus nitroglycerin vs. vasopressin alone in the treatment of bleeding esophageal varices. *Hepatology* 6:406–410, 1986.
10. Söderlund C, Magnusson J, Törngren S, et al: Terlipressin (triglycyl-hysine vasopressin) controls acute bleeding oesophageal varices: a double-blind randomized placebo-controlled trial. *Scan J Gastroenterol* 25:622–630, 1990.
11. Burroughs AK, McCormick PA, Hughes MD, et al: Randomized, double-blind, placebo-controlled trial of somatostatin for variceal bleeding: emergency control and prevention of early variceal rebleeding. *Gastroenterology* 99:1388–1395, 1990.
12. Hwang S-J, Lin H-C, Chang C-F, et al: A randomized controlled trial comparing octreotide and vasopressin in the control of acute esophageal variceal bleeding. *J Hepatol* 16:320–325, 1992.
13. Kravetz D, Bosch J, Teres J, et al: Comparison of intravenous somatostatin and vasopressin infusions in treatment of acute variceal hemorrhage. *Hepatology* 3:442–446, 1984.
14. Saari A, Kivilaakso E, Inberg M, et al: Comparison of somatostatin and vasopressin in bleeding esophageal varices. *Am J Gasteroenterol* 85:804–810, 1990.
15. Langer BF, Greig PD, Taylor BR: Emergency surgical treatment of variceal hemorrhage. *Surg Clin North Am* 70:361–378, 1990.
16. Orloff MJ, Orloof MS, Rambolt M, et al: Is portosystemic shunt worthwhile in Child's class C cirrhosis? *Ann Surg* 216:256–262, 1993.
17. Rypins EB, Sarfeh IJ: Small-diameter portacaval H-graft for variceal hemorrhage. *Surg Clin North Am* 70:395–405, 1990.
18. Potts JR, Henderson JM, Millikan WJ, Jr, et al: Emergency distal splenorenal shunts for variceal hemorrhage refractory to non-operative contorl. *Am J Surg* 148:813–818, 1984.
19. Helton WS, Belshaw A, Althaus S, et al: Critical appraisal of the angiographic portacaval shunt (TIPS). *Am J Surg* 165:566–571, 1993.
20. Pagliaro L, Burroughs AK, Sorensen TIA, et al: Beta-blockers for preventing variceal bleeding. *Lancet* 336:1001–1002, 1990.
21. Burroughs AK, Jenkins WJ, Sherlock S, et al: Controlled trial of propranolol for the prevention of recurrent variceal hemorrhage in patients with cirrhosis. *N Engl J Med* 309:1539–1542, 1983.

22. Villeneuve JP, Panier-Layargues G, Intante C, et al: Short term effects of propranolol on portal venous pressure. *Hepatology* 6:101–106, 1986.
23. Crafoord C, Freukner P: New surgical treatment of varicose veins of the esophagus. *Acta Otolaryngol* 27:422–427, 1939.
24. The Copenhagen Esophageal Varices and Sclerotherapy Project: Sclerotherapy after first variceal hemorrhage in cirrhosis: A randomized multicenter trial. *N Engl J Med* 311:1594–1597, 1984.
25. Korula J, Balart LA, Radran G, et al: A prospective, randomized trial of chronic esophageal variceal sclerotherapy. *Hepatology* 5:584–589, 1985.
26. Westaby D, Hayes PC, Grimson AES, et al: Controlled clinical trial of injection sclerotherapy for active variceal bleeding. *Hepatology* 9:274–277, 1989.
27. Terblanche J, Bornman PC, Kahn D, et al: Failure of repeated injection sclerotherapy to improve long-term survival after esophageal variceal bleeding. A five year prospective controlled clinical trial. *Lancet* ii:1328–1331, 1982.
28. Leach SD, Meier GH, Gusberg RJ: Endoscopic sclerotherapy: A risk factor for splanchnic venous thrombosis. *J Vasc Surg* 10:9–13, 1989.
29. Stiegman GV, Goff JS, Michaletz-Onody PA, et al: Endoscopic sclerotherapy as compared with endoscopic ligation for bleeding esophageal varices. *N Engl J Med* 326:1527–1532, 1992.
30. Rikkers LF, Jin G, Burnett DA, et al: Shunt surgery versus endoscopic sclerotherapy for variceal hemorrhage: Late results of a randomized trial. *Am J Surg* 165:27–33, 1993.
31. Henderson JM, Kutner MH, Millikan NJ Jr, et al: Endoscopic variceal sclerosis compared with distal splenorenal shunt to prevent recurrent variceal bleeding in cirrhosis: A prospective, randomized trial. *Ann Intern Med* 112:262–265, 1990.
32. Teres J, Baroni R, Borda JM, et al: A randomized trial of portacaval shunt, stapling transection, and endoscopic sclerotherapy in uncontrolled variceal bleeding. *J Hepatol* 4:159–162, 1987.
33. Spina GP, Santambrogio R, Opocher E, et al: Distal splenorenal shunt versus endoscopic sclerotherapy in the prevention of variceal bleeding. *Ann Surg* 211:178–182, 1990.
34. Whipple AO: The problem of portal hypertension in relation to the hepatosplenopathies. *Ann Surg* 122:449–475, 1945.
35. Blakemore AH: Portacaval shunt for portal hypertension. Follow-up results in cases of cirrhosis of the liver. *JAMA* 145:1335–1339, 1951.
36. Jackson FC, Perrin EB, Felix WR, et al: A clinical investigation of the portacaval shunt: V. Survival analysis of the therapeutic operation. *Ann Surg* 174:672–676, 1971.
37. Mikkelson WP: Therapeutic portacaval shunt. *Arch Surg* 108:302–307, 1974.
38. Resnick RH, Iber FL, Ishihara AM et al: A controlled study of the therapeutic portacaval shunt. *Gastroenterology* 67:843–847, 1974.
39. Levine BA, Sirinek KR: The portacaval shunt: Is it still indicated? *Surg Clin North Am* 70:361–378, 1990.
40. Bismuth H, Sherlock DJ: Portasystemic shunting versus liver transplantation for Budd-Chiari Syndrome. *Ann Surg* 214:581–589, 1991.
41. Cameron JL, Herlong HF, Sanfey H, et al: The Budd-Chiari syndrome: Treatment by mesenteric-systemic venous shunts. *Ann Surg* 198:335–344, 1983.
42. Henderson JM, Warren WD, Millikan WJ Jr, et al: Surgical options, hematologic evaluation, and pathologic changes in Budd-Chiari syndrome. *Am J Surg* 159:41–49, 1990.
43. Drapanas T, LoCicero J III, Dowling JB: Hemodynamics of the interposition mesocaval shunt. *Ann Surg* 181:523–527, 1975.
44. Rocko JM, Howard MM, Swan KG: Surgical management of bleeding esophageal varices: Results with 80 cases. *Ann Surg* 52:81–86, 1986.

45. Grace ND, Muench H, Chalmers TC: The present status of shunts for portal hypertension in cirrhosis gastroenterology. 50:684–691, 1966.
46. Bismuth H, Franco D, Hepp J: Portal-systematic shunt in hepatic cirrhosis. Does the type of shunt decisively influence the clinical result? *Ann Surg* 179:209–213, 1974.
47. Malt RA, Szczerban J, Malt RB: Risks in therapeutic portacaval and splenorenal shunts for bleeding esophageal varices. *Ann Surg* 184:279–283, 1976.
48. Warren WD, Zeppa R, Forman JS: Selective transplenic decompression of gastroesophageal varices by distal splenorenal shunt. *Ann Surg* 166:437–444, 1967.
49. Rikkers LF, Soper NJ, Cormier RA: Selective operative approach for variceal hemorrhage. *Am J Surg* 147:89–92, 1984.
50. Millikan WJ, Warren WD, Henderson JM, et al: The Emory prospective randomized trial: Selective versus non-selective shunt to control variceal bleeding: Ten year follow-up. *Ann Surg* 201:712–722, 1985.
51. Langer B, Taylor BR, MacKenzie DR, et al: Further report of a prospective randomized trial comparing distal splenorenal shunt with end-to-side portacaval shunt. *Gastroenterology* 88:424–429, 1985.
52. Gusberg RJ: Distal splenorenal shunt—premise, perspective, practice. *Dig Dis* 10(suppl 1):84–93, 1992.
53. Hutson DG, Zeppa R, Levi JU: The effect of distal splenorenal shunt or hypersplenism. *Ann Surg* 185:605–612, 1977.
54. Maillard JN, Flamant YM, Hay JM, et al: Selectivity of the distal splenorenal shunt. *Surgery* 86:663–671, 1979.
55. Vang J, Simert G, Hansson JA, et al: Results of a modified distal splenorenal shunt for portal hypertension. *Ann Surg* 185:224–228, 1977.
56. Henderson JM, Warren WD, Millikan WJ, et al: Distal splenorenal shunt with splenopancreatic disconnection: A four year assessment. *Ann Surg* 210:332–341, 1989.
57. Henderson JM, Millikan WJ, Wright-Bacon L, et al: Hemodynamic differences between alcoholic and non-alcoholic cirrhotics following distal splenorenal shunt. Effect on survival? *Ann Surg* 198:325–334, 1982.
58. Maffei-Faccioli A, Gerunda GE, Neri D, et al: Selective variceal decompression and its role relative to other therapies. *Am J Surg* 160:60–66, 1990.
59. Inokuchi K, Beppu K, Kayanagi N, et al: Exclusion of non-isolated splenic vein is distal splenorenal shunt for prevention of portal malcirculation. *Ann Surg* 200:711–717, 1984.
60. Warren WO, Millikan WJ, Henderson JM, et al: Ten years of portal hypertensive surgery at Emory. Results and new perspectives. *Ann Surg* 195:530–542, 1982.
61. Zeppa R, Hensley GT, Levi JU, et al: The comparative survival of alcoholics versus non-alcoholics after distal splenorenal shunt. *Ann Surg* 187:510–514, 1987.
62. Zeppa R, Lee PA, Hutson DG, et al: Portal hypertension: A fifteen year perspective. *Am J Surg* 155:6–9, 1988.
63. Gusberg RJ: Selective shunts in selected older cirrhotic patients with variceal hemorrhage. *Am J Surg* 166:274–278, 1993.
64. Maksoud JG, Gonclaves ME: Treatment of portal hypertension in children. *World J Surg* 18:251–258, 1994.
65. Jin G, Rikkers LF: Selective variceal decompression: Current status HPB. *Surgery* 5:1–10, 1991.
66. Fischer JE, Bower RH, Atamian S, et al: Comparison of distal and proximal splenorenal shunts. A randomized prospective trial. *Ann Surg* 194:531–542, 1981.

67. Grace ND, Conn HO, Resnick RH, et al: Distal splenorenal vs. portosystemic shunts after hemorrhage from varices: A randomized controlled trial. *Hepatology* 8:1475–1481, 1988.
68. Henderson JM, Khishen MA, Millikan WJ, et al: Management of stenosis of distal splenorenal shunt by balloon dilation. *Surg Gynecol Obstet* 157:43–48, 1983.
69. Hendersen JM, Millikan WJ, Chipponi J, et al: The incidence and natural history of thrombus in the portal vein following distal splenorenal shunt. *Ann Surg* 196:1–7, 1982.
70. Johansen K: Partial portal decompression for variceal hemorrhage. *Am J Surg* 157:479–486, 1989.
71. Rossle M, Haag I, Ochs A, et al: The transjugular intrahepatic portosystemic stent-shunt procedure for variceal bleeding. *N Engl J Med* 330:165–171, 1994.
72. LaBerge JM, Ring EJ, Gordon RL, et al: Creation of transjugular intrahepatic portosystemic shunts with the wallstent endoprosthesis: results in 100 patients. *Radiology* 187:413–420, 1993.
73. Haskal ZJ, Pentecost MJ, Soulen MC, et al: Transjugular intrahepatic portosystemic shunt stenosis and revision. *Am J Roentgenol* 163:439–444, 1994.
74. Roberts JP, Ring E, Lake JR, et al: Intrahepatic portacaval shunt for variceal hemorrhage prior to liver transplantation. *Transplantation* 52:160–162, 1991.
75. Sigiura M, Futagama S: Esophageal transactions with paraesophagogastric devascularization (The sigiura procedure) in the treatment of esophageal varices. *World J Surg* 8:674–681, 1984.
76. Nexler JG, Stein BL: Non-shunting operations for variceal hemorrhage. *Surg Clin North Am* 70:425–430, 1990.
77. Jenkins SA, Shields R: Variceal hemorrhage after failed injection sclerotherapy. The role of emergency esophageal transection. *Br J Surg* 76:49–55, 1989.
78. Gusberg RJ, Peterec SM, Sumpio BE, et al: Splenomegaly and variceal bleeding—hemodynamic basics and treatment implications. *Hepatogastroenterology* 41:573–577, 1994.

Transjugular Intrahepatic Portosystemic Shunts for the Treatment of Portal Hypertension

Ziv J. Haskal, M.D.

Assistant Professor of Radiology, University of Pennsylvania School of Medicine, Philadelphia, Pennsylvania

Variceal hemorrhage is a major cause of death in patients wtih cirrhosis. Although there have been significant advances in the understanding of the pathophysiology of portal hypertension, the treatment of variceal bleeding remains a complex and evolving issue. Several forms of therapy have been developed, including pharmacologic therapy, sclerotherapy, portosystemic shunt, liver transplantation, and, more recently, transjugular intrahepatic portosystemic shunts (TIPS). Because each option has distinct advantages and limitations, individual patient therapy is best determined by a multidisciplinary team that includes gastroenterologists, surgeons, and interventional radiologists.

MANAGEMENT OPTIONS

PHARMACOLOGIC THERAPY

Vasopressin was the first medication used to control variceal bleeding and remains the mainstay of treatment of acute variceal bleeding.[1, 2] It lowers portal pressure by constricting the splanchnic arterioles and venules and reducing splanchnic venous flow to the liver. Vasopressin may also act by directly constricting the lower esophageal sphincter and mechanically reducing flow into esophageal varices. Although intravenous vasopressin reduces acute bleeding, overall survival is not improved compared with placebo infusion. This is in part related to the high rate of rebleeding after vasopressin therapy is discontinued. Simultaneous administration of nitroglycerin by topical, intravenous, or sublingual routes has become the accepted standard. It both further reduces the portosystemic gradient and prevents the adverse effects of vasopressin, including myocardial and cerebrovascular ischemia.

Somatostatin and synthetic somatostatin analogue infusions can be used to control acute variceal bleeding. These medications reduce azygos blood flow (an indicator of collateral circulation) and portosystemic gradient (PSG) without systemic vasoconstrictive effects. The mechanism by which somatostatin accomplishes these hemodynamic effects is not well understood.[3-5]

The next major advance in pharmacologic therapy occurred in 1980 when LeBrec[6] reported the use of propranolol to lower the portosystemic gradient. Nonselective beta blockade with propranolol reduces splanchnic blood flow both by blocking vasodilatory beta$_2$ receptors and by decreasing cardiac output. Since then, numerous randomized controlled trials have documented the benefit of chronic beta blockade in the prevention of recurrent variceal bleeding.[7-9] Although an improvement in overall patient survival has not been shown, propranolol administration has become the initial treatment for primary prophylaxis of hemorrhage and is often combined with other methods of therapy for secondary prophylaxis.

ENDOSCOPIC THERAPY

The refinement of endoscopic sclerotherapy in the 1970s and 1980s has led to its widespread adoption as the front-line therapy for acute esophageal variceal hemorrhage. In this procedure, a variety of sclerosing agents are injected into or adjacent to bleeding esophageal varices, resulting in variceal thrombosis and sloughing. Sclerotherapy and, more recently, variceal band ligation can control acute bleeding in 80% to 90% of cases.[10-14]

Once the acute bleeding episode has ceased, elective treatment sessions are continued periodically until the varices are obliterated or complications ensue. Because sclerotherapy does nothing to lower the portosystemic gradient, the encephalopathy and accelerated liver failure that can accompany portosystemic shunts do not occur. On the other hand, rebleeding occurs in up to 50% of patients. At present, sclerotherapy has limited value in the treatment of gastric varices, portal hypertensive gastropathy, and ectopic intestinal varices that lie beyond the reach of the endoscope. Although sclerotherapy may provide definitive therapy in certain patients, it may not afford ideal long-term control for a majority of nonemergent patients with portal hypertension and variceal hemorrhage.

More recently, band ligation of esophageal varices has been used for treatment of acute bleeding and for long-term prophylaxis.[15] In a controlled trial comparing variceal banding with sclerotherapy, Stiegmann and colleagues[16] found that the former was superior with respect to prevention of recurrent bleeding, complications, and number of sessions required to obliterate the varices. A survival benefit was suggested in Child's class A and B patients, but not in the small number of Child's class C patients in the study. These promising results must be confirmed by other groups before widespread adoption of the technique can take place.

PORTOSYSTEMIC SHUNT SURGERY

The role of portosystemic shunts in the treatment of the complications of portal hypertension began over 100 years ago when Eck created the first end-to-side portacaval shunt in dogs.[17] The technique was first applied in humans in 1903 by Vidal.[18] In the 1950s, advances in surgical technique and pre- and postoperative care allowed wider use of portacaval shunt surgery. As data from controlled trials were reported, it became clear that complete portal diversion had exchanged excellent prophylaxis against initial or recurrent variceal hemorrhage for unacceptably high rates of portosystemic encephalopathy (PSE) (30%–70%) and accelerated liver failure.[19, 20]

In 1967, Warren[21] described selective decompression of the portal system with a distal splenorenal shunt (DSRS). This procedure preserves mesentero-portal venous flow and results in lower rates of encephalopathy and liver failure. The DSRS has a high rate of patency, exceeding 90%.[22] However, at 1 year, up to 75% of patients with alcoholic cirrhosis developed extensive collateral venous flow between the high-pressure mesenteric portal system and the shunted low-pressure gastrosplenic veins. This may obviate the initial hemodynamic benefit of selective decompression.[23] To some degree, the technical demands of creating a DSRS limit its widespread application, particularly in the setting of acute bleeding.

In 1965, Bismuth[24, 25] introduced partially decompressive, limited stoma, side-to-side shunts as a method of reducing portal pressure while preserving hepatopetal portal perfusion. Side-to-side, small stoma, portacaval shunts were initially effective in reducing PSE and liver failure. Over time, however, these shunts tended to increase in diameter, reclaiming the problems of excessive portal diversion. In the early 1980s, Rypins and Sarfeh[26-28] began using polytetrafluoroethylene (PTFE) graft material to create portacaval interposition grafts with stable diameters. Over the next decade, they progressively reduced the size of shunts from 20 to 8 mm. Their investigations, and those of others, have validated the concept of partial portal decompression with small-diameter shunts as an effective method of preventing recurrent variceal hemorrhage with rates of encephalopathy and liver failure that are significantly lower than those found with totally diverting shunts.

Although most surgical shunts provide excellent prophylaxis against variceal hemorrhage, they are best performed on an elective or semielective basis. They are rarely indicated in the setting of acute variceal bleeding where operative mortality can exceed 50%.[29]

Liver transplantation offers the option of treating both variceal hemorrhage and the progressive liver failure that develops in many patients with advanced cirrhosis. In 1988, Iwatsuki and associates[30] reported a 5-year liver transplantation survival rate of 71% in 302 patients with a history of variceal bleeding. Although transplantation can provide definitive therapy for portal hypertension and its complications, few patients warrant this on the basis of bleeding alone. In addition, the shortage of donor organs often precludes emergent transplant.

TRANSJUGULAR INTRAHEPATIC PORTOSYSTEMIC SHUNT (TIPS)

THE DEVELOPMENT OF TIPS

The ability to create a percutaneous portosystemic shunt was first reported by Rösch and Hanafee[31] in 1969. They passed a modified Ross needle from within a hepatic vein into an adjacent portal vein branch in five dogs. This intraparenchymal shunt tract was dilated by use of co-axial Dotter catheters and stented with 12 and 14F Teflon tubing. In 1971, these authors reported successfully creating intrahepatic shunts in 34 dogs. Although shunts as large as 8 and 10 mm in diameter were established, shunt patencies were limited to several weeks. Occlusion often occurred when the stent tubing migrated out of the portal veins. Experiments followed investigating other methods of creating intrahepatic shunts, including cryoprobe, drilling,[32] and balloon catheter techniques.[33]

In 1983, Colapinto and colleagues[34] reported the first use of TIPS in humans. Shunts were created in six patients with advanced liver disease and life-threatening variceal hemorrhage. In an attempt to create durable shunt tracts, Grüntzig balloon angioplasty catheters were kept inflated across the parenchymal liver tract for 12 hours. Although initial portal venous pressures dropped by 10 to 15 mm Hg, four of six patients had repeated variceal bleeding. Later that year, this group reported a larger series of patients in which variceal bleeding was controlled in every case. Unfortunately, only 2 shunts out of 15 remained patent after 6 months.

The TIPS technique underwent a renaissance in the mid 1980s when metallic stents became available. These functioned as a scaffold, supporting the intrahepatic tract and preventing its collapse from recoil of the surrounding liver parenchyma. Rösch and co-workers[35] and Palmaz and associates[36] independently evaluated metallic stenting of the liver tract to improve shunt patency. Rösch reported placing a modified version of the self-expanding Gianturco stent in 30 normal swine. These shunts remained patent for 4 to 6 weeks. Palmaz used his own balloon expandable stents in 12 dogs with artificially induced portal hypertension. These shunts stayed open longer, averaging 48 weeks.

The first use of metallic stents for TIPS in humans was reported by Richter and colleagues[37] in 1990. A combined transhepatic and transjugular approach was used wherein a transjugular needle was advanced out of a hepatic vein toward a Dormia basket that had been placed transhepatically into the portal vein. Once the connection was established, the tract was dilated with balloon catheters and stented with a balloon expandable Palmaz stent. TIPS were created in three Child's class C cirrhotic patients who had massive variceal hemorrhage and contraindications to surgical shunting and repeated sclerotherapy. Portal decompression was achieved in all cases. Two patients had sufficient metabolic improvement to be upgraded to Child's class A. In a follow-up article, this series was expanded to nine patients.[38]

Since that time, the technique has become rapidly disseminated, and perhaps thousands of TIPS have been created. Several centers have reported their experience, confirming these landmark results.[39–49]

TIPS TECHNIQUE

Although different TIPS needle and catheter systems have been developed, all are used in similar fashions to create the shunts. In general, a needle is passed from within a hepatic vein into a branch of the intrahepatic portal vein. This channel is progressively enlarged and lined with a metallic stent until the portosystemic gradient has been sufficiently reduced (Fig 1). The following is a description of the specific method the author uses for creating a TIPS.

Recent upper esophagogastroduodenoscopy is required to confirm the presence of varices and exclude peptic sources of concomitant upper gastrointestinal bleeding. Baseline encephalopathy testing is performed. Acutely bleeding patients are stabilized as much as possible prior to TIPS with fluid resuscitation, blood transfusions, intravenous vasopressin, and nitrates. Placement of balloon tamponade catheters does not interfere with the TIPS procedure, although their use is generally avoided if it will delay shunt creation. No specific effort is made to correct coagulopathies because procedure-related bleeding is uncommon. Preprocedure hepatic Doppler sonography is performed to assess patency of the portal venous system and the presence and amount of ascites. Visceral angiography is reserved for cases in which the results of sonography are equivocal or indicate portal vein thrombosis.

The patient is given intravenous conscious sedation (midazolam, droperidol, and fentanyl) and antibiotic prophylaxis (1 g of cefazolin). The right neck is prepped and draped in a standard fashion. Because the patient's face is partially covered, supplemental oxygen is administered through nasal prongs or face mask. Right internal jugular vein access is preferred because it provides straight-line access to the inferior vena cava. In cases of vein occlusion or other anatomic abnormalities, the right external or left internal jugular vein can be used.

The vein is percutaneously punctured, and a guidewire is threaded through the needle into the superior vena cava. A 40-cm-long curved 9F hemostatic sheath is advanced through the right atrium and into the inferior vena cava. Upper caval and right atrial pressures are measured through the side-arm valve of the sheath. A curved angiographic catheter is placed through the sheath and used to catheterize a suitable hepatic vein. The diameter of the vein near its ostium must be larger than 8 or 10 mm so that it will not limit outflow from the TIPS. The right hepatic vein is usually chosen for two reasons: first, because it is readily catheterized, and second, because it lies posterior and cephalad to the anterosuperior branches of the right portal vein. This anatomic relationship is what allows an anterocaudal pass of the puncture needle to reach the right portal vein. Digital subtraction free hepatic venography is performed. A wedged hepatic venogram can be performed that will, in many cases, opacify branches of the portal vein, aiding in its localization. In cases of cryptogenic or undiagnosed cirrhosis, transvenous liver biopsy can be performed at this point in the procedure.

A 15-gauge curved Colapinto needle is used to puncture the portal vein. This needle is 50 cm long and is surrounded by a 9F 45-cm-long Teflon catheter. Its size allows easy passage and direction through hard cirrhotic liver parenchyma. Its reversed bevel tip facilitates its passage around the angle at the junction of the hepatic vein and inferior vena cava.

The needle and its sheath are rotated anteriorly and advanced caudally out of the hepatic vein 3 to 4 cm into the liver parenchyma. A syringe filled with contrast medium is attached to the needle. The needle and sheath are slowly withdrawn while the suction is applied to the sy-

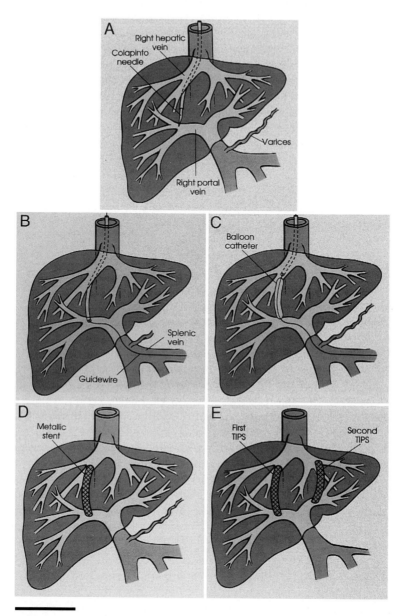

FIGURE 1.

Transjugular intrahepatic portosystemic shunt (TIPS) technique. **A,** a sheathed transjugular needle is passed out of a hepatic vein into a branch of the portal vein. **B,** a guidewire is advanced through the needle into the splenic vein. **C,** the parenchymal tract between the hepatic and portal veins is dilated with a balloon angioplasty catheter. **D,** the metallic stent is deployed within the shunt tract. **E,** if numerous varices remain after the shunt is dilated to 10 mm in diameter and the portosystemic gradient remains elevated, then a second TIPS is constructed. (From Haskal ZJ, Ring EJ: Technique and results of transjugular intrahepatic portosystemic shunts (TIPS). In *Current techniques in interventional radiology.* Philadelphia, 1994, Current Science, pp 2.1–2.10. Used by permission.)

ringe. A small test injection of iodinated contrast is performed when blood return is noted in the syringe. If a first- or second-order branch of the portal system is opacified, then a soft-tipped guidewire is threaded through the needle into the main portal vein. The needle is removed and a 5F diagnostic angiographic catheter is advanced over the guidewire into the splenic vein.

This catheter is used to perform the initial hemodynamic and venographic assessment of the portal system. Portal and splenic venous pressures are recorded. In patients with esophagogastric variceal bleeding, hand-injected splenic venography is performed to assess both anatomy and initial portal flow (Fig 2,A). In patients with intestinal varices, superior mesenteric venography is performed.

A 5F 8-mm balloon angioplasty catheter is used to dilate the liver tract. The balloon catheter is then exchanged over a stiff guidewire for the metal stent delivery catheter. Stents are deployed within the liver tract

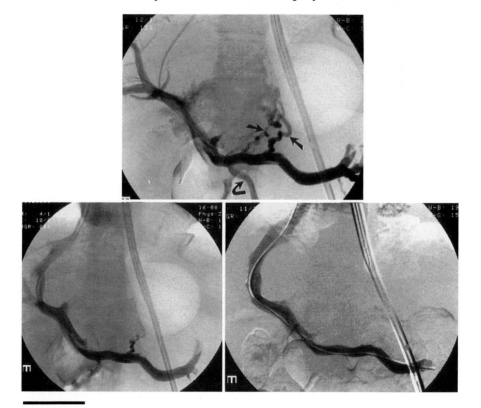

FIGURE 2.

Emergency TIPS placement in a patient with active variceal bleeding. **A,** the initial transjugular splenic venogram demonstrates filling of varices (*arrows*) despite the presence of an inflated balloon tamponade catheter. Hepatofugal flow is present in the inferior mesenteric vein (*curved arrow*). The portosystemic gradient is 26 mm Hg. **B,** after creation of a right-hepatic-to-right-portal-vein (TIPS) there is marked reduction of variceal flow. The portosystemic gradient is 18 mm Hg. **C,** the shunt is further dilated with a 10-mm balloon catheter, and another stent is overlapped within the TIPS lumen. The balloon tamponade catheter has been deflated. No residual variceal flow remains. The portosystemic gradient is 10 mm Hg.

and enlarged with 8- and 10-mm angioplasty balloons. Repeat digital subtraction portography and portal and atrial pressure measurement are performed (Fig 2,B).

If the portosystemic gradient exceeds 12 mm Hg and rapid variceal filling remains, then the stent is repeatedly dilated with 10- or 12-mm-diameter balloon catheters (Fig 2,C). In some cases, residual varices can be selectively catheterized and embolized with stainless-steel coils and/or absolute alcohol. In infrequent cases, a high portosystemic gradient and significant variceal flow persist after creation of a single shunt. In these cases, a second, parallel TIPS is constructed between a different hepatic vein and a different portal vein branch.[50]

Final systemic venous pressures are measured during withdrawal of the 9F jugular sheath. The patients are monitored overnight in an intensive care or intermediate care unit for sedation recovery. A baseline color flow duplex TIPS ultrasound is obtained prior to discharge to document blood velocities through the shunt. This provides a baseline for comparison with follow-up assessments of shunt function. Patients undergoing elective TIPS placement are typically discharged the morning after the procedure. Arrangements are made for outpatient assessment of continued shunt patency and encephalopathy.

TIPS have been created with a variety of metallic stents, including Palmaz, Strecker, and Gianturco stents. At present, the Wallstent (Schneider USA, Minneapolis, Minn) is used to line the majority of shunts. This springlike device is composed of biomedically compatible alloy wire woven into a helical braid configuration. The low-profile 7F delivery catheter has the advantage of being very flexible, allowing it to be threaded into the portal vein from almost any point of entry. Once deployed and expanded, the stent maintains its cylindric lumen around even the tightest bends.

Many ancillary techniques have been described to aid transjugular localization and puncture of the portal vein. These include transhepatic portal vein catheterization,[37] preprocedure arterial portography,[51] placement of platinum microcoil markers adjacent to the intended site of portal vein entry,[52] and real-time sonographic guidance. With experience, however, the portal vein can be successfully punctured with fluoroscopic guidance alone based on an understanding of portal and hepatic vein anatomy. This method has proved rapid and reliable in hundreds of cases. With use of this technique, the average procedure time is approximately 1.5 hours. I reserve transhepatic portal vein catheterization for cases of portal vein occlusion in which portal vein recanalization and thrombectomy must be performed as part of TIPS placement.[53, 54]

RESULTS OF TIPS

Because TIPS is a relatively novel procedure, much of the reported data are limited to describing technical success, and early and midterm morbidity and mortality. Pooled data from the two largest published series, and the University of Pennsylvania are included in Tables 1 through 6.[41, 42, 46] These results demonstrate that shunts can be created with a very high rate of technical success. The flexibility of the technique is illus-

TABLE 1.
Clinical Features of Patients Undergoing TIPS

	Univ of Penn[41] (n = 100)	Freiburg[46] (n = 100)	UCSF[42] (n = 100)
Gender (M/F)	64/36	67/33	64/36
Age (yrs)			
Mean	53.8	57	50
Range	20–84	18–84	5–84
Childs–Pugh Class (%)			
A	9	27	10
B	39	51	35
C	52	22	55

trated by the ability to create shunts in the setting of portal system occlusions. In the University of California, San Francisco (UCSF) series, seven of ten patients with portal vein thrombosis underwent successful shunt placement (70% technical success); at the University of Pennsylvania, TIPS were successfully formed in 12 cases of portal, 5 cases of splenic, and 5 cases of superior mesenteric thrombus (100% technical success). Patients with portal vein thrombosis were excluded from the Freiburg study.

TIPS are very effective at lowering portal pressure. Because the shunts are created under real-time fluoroscopic and hemodynamic monitoring, the shunts can be progressively enlarged with balloon catheters until satisfactory portal decompression has been achieved. In over 90% of cases, 10-mm-diameter shunts are large enough to adequately lower the portosystemic gradient to below 12 mm Hg. In a minority of cases, portal hypertension may persist despite a single TIPS. In these cases, a parallel, second shunt can be created between different hepatic and portal vein branches to provide additional decompression.[50]

Nearly all acutely bleeding patients stop bleeding after TIPS. In the UCSF series, active bleeding stopped in 30 of 32 patients. In two cases, repeat upper endoscopy revealed a duodenal ulcer and oozing sclero-

TABLE 2.
Etiology of Liver Disease

	Univ of Penn[41]	Freiburg[46]	UCSF[42]
Alcoholic	59	68	56
Postnecrotic	21	19	26
Cryptogenic	14	9	15
Primary biliary cirrhosis	4	3	—
Budd-Chiari	2	—	1
Other	—	1	2

TABLE 3.

Indications for TIPS Placement

	Univ of Penn[41]	Freiburg[46]	UCSF[42]
Bleeding	90	100	94
Acute	51	10	32
Chronic	39	83	62
Ascites/pleural effusion	8	—	3
Hepatorenal	—	—	2
Preoperative	2	—	8

therapy ulcer. In the author's experience, TIPS provided prompt control of esophagogastric varices as well as large- and small-intestinal varices.[55] Five of 51 actively bleeding patients had continued oozing after TIPS. Repeat endoscopy revealed interim variceal decompression, and duodenal (one), gastric (one), and sclerotherapy (one) ulcers. In two cases, the varices were only partially decompressed. These shunts were further enlarged with balloon catheters, after which bleeding stopped completely.

Overall 30-day mortality was 3%, 13%, and 30% in the Freiburg, UCSF, and University of Pennsylvania series, respectively. Not surprisingly, this is accounted for by differences in the degree of cirrhosis of patients treated and whether the shunts were created on an emergency or elective basis. Ninety percent of the Freiburg patients were treated electively. Seventy-five percent of patients had either Child's class A or B cirrhosis. In contrast, at the University of Pennsylvania, 52% of patients had class C and 39% had class B cirrhosis. Fifty-one patients were actively bleeding during TIPS. All of these patients were receiving blood transfusions during the procedure; 47 were receiving vasopressin; 33 were mechanically ventilated; and 25 had balloon tamponade catheters in place. Death resulted from incipient multiorgan failure, aspiration pneumonia, cardiac arrhythmia, and adult respiratory distress syndrome. In all three series, 30-day mortality was approximately 30% for patients with active

TABLE 4.

Hemodynamic and Technical Results of TIPS

	Univ of Penn[41]	Freiburg[46]	UCSF[42]
Technical success (%)	100	93	96
Pre-TIPS (mm Hg)			
Portal vein	35.8	—	34.5
Right atrium	12.1	—	—
Portosystemic gradient	24	21.5	—
Post-TIPS (mm Hg)		—	
Portal vein	26.1	—	24.5
Right atrium	15.3	—	—
Portosystemic gradient	11	9.2	10.4

TABLE 5.
Procedural Complications of TIPS

	Univ of Penn[41]	Freiburg[46]	UCSF[42]
Bleeding			
Intra-abdominal	3	6	1
Hemobilia	0	4	1
Fever	13	—	10
Renal failure	—	—	3
Encephalopathy (%)			
New or worse	23	25	17
Uncontrolled	5	7	3

variceal hemorrhage. In the author's patient group, Child's class C patients had a fourfold increased risk of early demise compared with patients with Child's class A and B liver disease. To better define prognostic factors predicting early death after TIPS, we prospectively calculated the pre-TIPS APACHE II (Acute Physiology and Chronic Health Evaluation) score for 100 consecutive patients. Notably, an APACHE II score exceeding 20 was associated with a nearly 20-fold risk of early death, independent of Child's class. In contrast, early mortality in patients undergoing elective TIPS was 2%. Once patients survived the morbidity of the acute hemorrhage, 1-year survival leveled off for all Child's classes. At 1 year, only seven additional patients had died; causes of death included congestive heart failure, pneumonia, liver failure, pulmonary hemorrhage, and advanced age.[41]

A concomitant reduction in or resolution of ascites occurs in over three fourths of TIPS patients treated for variceal bleeding. The role of TIPS as a primary therapy for refractory ascites is now being evaluated at several centers.

CONTRAINDICATIONS

Increasing experience indicates that there are relatively few absolute contraindications to TIPS placement. These include right-sided cardiac failure and extensive polycystic liver disease. The first condition is a contraindication common to all shunt procedures that deliver high-pressure portal blood into the systemic circulation. In cirrhotic patients who often maintain a baseline, hyperdynamic circulatory state, shunt placement can lead to additional, sustained elevation of cardiac output and index.[56] This effect is compounded by the rapid mobilization of third-space ascites and

TABLE 6.
Effect of TIPS on Ascites

	Univ of Penn[41]	Freiburg[46]	UCSF[42]
Improved/resolved	34/44 (77%)	47/53 (89%)	49/59 (83%)

cirrhotic pleural effusions (hepatic hydrothorax), which occurs in many patients. Together, these can lead to frank cardiac decompensation and severe pulmonary edema in patients with right heart failure. Although these hemodynamic and physiologic changes are well tolerated in most patients, it is nevertheless important to restrict intravenous fluid hydration during and after TIPS. In many cases, we begin fluid diuresis before the patient has left the Interventional Radiology suite.

Several relative contraindications to TIPS placement exist, including portal and hepatic vein thrombosis, and the presence of malignancies or other causes of distorted hepatic anatomy (Fig 3). Although these conditions may complicate the procedure, with experience, shunts can be created in almost all such cases.[53, 54, 57] In uncomplicated cases, TIPS can be created successfully in at least 95% of patients.[41, 42, 46]

COMPLICATIONS

Although many procedural complications from TIPS have been reported, most can be managed conservatively and tend to diminish with increasing operator experience. Severe complications occur in less than 1% of cases. Reported complications include contrast reactions, transient renal failure, hemobilia, myocardial ischemia, and pulmonary edema.[39, 40, 42, 46]

The most significant adverse effect of portosystemic diversion by any method is portosystemic encephalopathy (PSE). Early TIPS series suggested that encephalopathy occurred less frequently after TIPS than after surgical shunts. This finding has not been borne out, in part because of varying methods of assessing and reporting encephalopathy data in both the surgical and radiologic literature. For example, some investigators prescribe prophylactic oral lactulose therapy for all patients, whereas others reserve it for those who develop spontaneous PSE. In general, new or worsened encephalopathy develops in 18% to 25% of patients undergoing TIPS. This is well controlled in all but 4% to 7% of cases with dietary protein restriction and oral lactulose therapy. In most cases, however, encephalopathy tends to diminish over time as the shunt is incorporated within a layer of neointima and collagen tissue.[39] This process usually reduces the shunt lumen diameter by 1 to 2 mm, lessening the amount of portal diversion (Fig 4). In rare instances of accelerated liver failure or uncontrolled encephalopathy after TIPS placement, the shunts can be reversibly thrombosed by overnight placement of an inflated balloon catheter within the shunt.[58] Alternatively, shunt size can be reduced by placement of an hourglass-shaped stent within the TIPS.[59] This allows a measure of continued portal decompression and prophylaxis against bleeding.

SHUNT BIOLOGY AND PATENCY

LaBerge and colleagues[60, 61] described histopathologic findings in the explanted livers of seven transplant patients who had undergone prior TIPS. At 4 days after TIPS, fresh thrombus was adhered to the mesh of the stents. By 3 weeks, the shunt lumen was lined with a 400- to 600-μm-thick layer of neointimal tissue. At 3 months, the stent was incorporated within a layer of densely collagenized tissue with very few inflammatory cells.[60, 61]

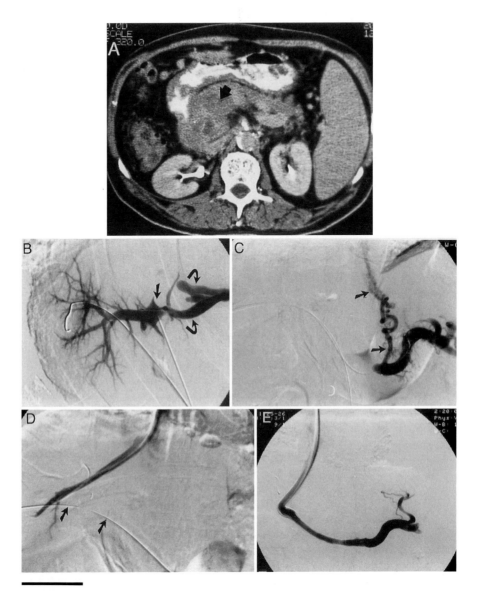

FIGURE 3.

Elective TIPS placement in a patient with pancreatic carcinoma and seven prior episodes of variceal bleeding. **A,** contrast-enhanced computed tomographic (CT) image of the upper abdomen demonstrates carcinoma of the head of the pancreas. Other CT images (not shown) demonstrated main and central right and left portal vein thrombosis. **B,** transhepatic right portal venogram. The meniscus marks the upper extent of the portal thrombus within the anterior branch of the right portal vein *(arrow)*. Periportal collateral veins reconstitute the peripherally patent right portal vein *(curved arrows)*. A tandem needle and guidewire technique allows choice of optimal portal entry site for transhepatic recanalization. **C,** initial transhepatic splenic venogram demonstrates occlusion of the splenic vein at its midportion. An enlarged short gastric vein fills esophageal varices *(arrows)*. The portosystemic gradient is 35 mm Hg. **D,** right hepatic venogram shows proximity of hepatic vein and transhepatic portal vein catheter *(arrows)*, which serves as a guide for the transjugular portal vein puncture. **E,** final transjugular splenic venogram after portal and splenic vein recanalization and stent placement. No significant variceal flow remains. The portosystemic gradient is 10 mm Hg.

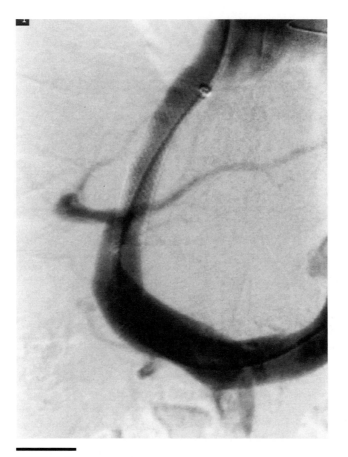

FIGURE 4.

One-year surveillance shunt venogram in an asymptomatic patient. A thin layer of intimal hyperplasia lines the lumen of the stent. The portosystemic gradient is 13 mm Hg. Prograde flow into the left and right portal veins is present.

In many cases, excessive proliferation of the neointimal layer occurs. This can lead to reduction of the shunt lumen and recurrent portal hypertension and symptoms. All centers reporting experience with TIPS indicate that 30% to 50% of patients develop stenoses within 12 months of TIPS. Accordingly, all TIPS patients must undergo periodic evaluations of shunt patency. In many cases, Doppler sonography and velocity measurement within the shunts can be used to identify failing shunts.[62, 63] Alternatively, outpatient shunt venography can be performed from antecubital, jugular, or femoral venous approaches.[39] This allows direct venographic and hemodynamic reassessment of the portal venous system. Shunt stenoses or occlusions are treated by balloon angioplasty or placement of additional stents within the narrowed segments. With regular follow-up and periodic revisions, it appears that assisted shunt patency may be preserved almost indefinitely.

CONCLUSION

The treatment of complications of TIPS procedures remains a complex clinical challenge requiring the close cooperation of hepatologists, interventional radiologists, and surgeons. It is too early to conclude what final impact TIPS will have on the treatment of portal hypertension. Clearly, TIPS provide a safe method of rapid and reliable portal decompression that is as effective as surgical shunts for arresting acute variceal hemorrhage. Long-term prophylaxis against bleeding is entirely related to shunt patency. At present, shunt stenosis remains a very significant, albeit treatable, problem. However, it is likely that future developments in endovascular graft technology will lessen the need for close surveillance and intervention. Stents lined with surgical graft material, or imbued with agents that limit intimal hyperplasia, may lessen the neointimal stenoses and allow TIPS to become a more durable treatment for patients with portal hypertension.

REFERENCES

1. Johnson WC, Widrich WC, Ansell JE, et al: Control of bleeding varices by vasopressin: A prospective randomized study. *Ann Surg* 186:369–376, 1977.
2. Nusbaum M, Baum S, Sakiyalak P, et al: Pharmacologic control of portal hypertension. *Surgery* 62:299–310, 1967.
3. Burroughs AK, McCormick PA, Hughes MD, et al: Randomized double-blind, placebo-controlled trial of somatostatin for variceal bleeding. Emergency control and prevention of early variceal rebleeding. *Gastroenterology* 99:1388–1395, 1990.
4. Burroughs AK, McCormick PA: Long term pharmacologic therapy of portal hypertension. *Surg Clin North Am* 70:319–339, 1990.
5. Valenzuela J, Schuber T, Fogel M, et al: A multicenter randomized double-blind trial of somatostatin in the management of acute hemorrhage from esophageal varices. *Hepatology* 10:958–961, 1981.
6. LeBrec D, Nouel O, Corbic M, et al: Propranolol, a medical treatment for portal hypertension. *Lancet* 2:180–182, 1980.
7. Greig JD, Garden OJ, Carter DC: Prophylactic treatment of patients with esophageal-varices—Is it ever indicated. *World J Surg* 18:176–184, 1994.
8. Pagliaro L, D'Amico G, Sorensen TI, et al: Prevention of first bleeding in cirrhosis. A meta-analysis of randomized trials of nonsurgical treatment. *Ann Intern Med* 117:59–70, 1992.
9. LeBrec D: Current status and future goals of pharmacologic reduction of portal hypertension. *Am J Surg* 160:19–25, 1990.
10. Paquet KJ, Kalk JF, Koussouris P: Immediate endoscopic sclerosis of bleeding esophageal varices: A prospective evaluation over five years. *Surg Endosc* 2:18–23, 1988.
11. Terblanche J, Northover J, Bornman P, et al: A prospective controlled trial of sclerotherapy in the long term management of patients after oesophageal variceal bleeding. *Surg Gynecol Obstet* 148:323–333, 1979.
12. Cello JP, Grendall JH, Cross RA, et al: Endoscopic sclerotherapy versus portacaval shunt in patients with severe cirrhosis and variceal hemorrhage. *N Engl J Med* 311:1589–1600, 1984.
13. Infante-Rivard C, Esnaola S, Villeneuve JP: Role of endoscopic sclerotherapy in the long-term management of variceal bleeding: A meta analysis. *Gastroenterology* 96:1594–1600, 1989.
14. Terblanche J, Burroughs AK, Hobbs KEF: Controversies in the management of bleeding esophageal varices (first of two parts). *N Engl J Med* 320:1393–1398, 1989.
15. Goff JS, Reveille RM, Stiegmann GV: Endoscopic sclerotherapy versus endo-

scopic variceal ligation: Esophageal symptoms, complications, and motility. *Am J Gastroenterol* 83:1240–1244, 1988.

16. Stiegmann GV, Goff JS, Michaletz-Onody PA, et al: Endoscopic sclerotherapy as compared with endoscopic ligation for treatment of bleeding esophageal varices. *N Engl J Med* 326:1527–1532, 1991.

17. Child C: Eck's fistula. *Surg Gynecol Obstet* 96:375–376, 1953.

18. Vidal E: Traitment chirurguical des ascites. *Presse Med* 11:747, 1903.

19. Kanel CC, Kaplan MM, Zawacki JK, et al: Surgival in patients with postnecrotic cirrhosis and Laennec's cirrhosis undergoing therapeutic portacaval shunt. *Gastroenterology* 73:679–683, 1977.

20. Reynolds T, Donovan AJ, Mikkelson WP, et al: Results of a 12-year randomized trial of portacaval shunt in patients with alcoholic liver disease and bleeding varices. *Gastroenterology* 80:1005–1011, 1981.

21. Warren WD, Zeppa R, Forman JJ: Selective transsplenic decompression of gastroesophageal varices by distal splenorenal shunt. *Ann Surg* 166:437–455, 1967.

22. Warren WD, Millikan WJ, Henderson JM, et al: Ten years of portal hypertensive surgery at Emory. *Ann Surg* 195:530–542, 1982.

23. Henderson JM, Gong-Liang J, Galloway J, et al: Portaprival collaterals following distal splenorenal shunt: Incidence, magnitude, and associated portal perfusion changes. *J Hepatol* 1:649–661, 1985.

24. Bismuth H, Csillag MJ, Benhamou JP, et al: L'anastomose portocave chez le rat normal. IV. Influence du calibre be l'anastomose. *Rev Fr Etud Clin Biol* 10:1087–1092, 1965.

25. Bismuth H, Franco D, Hepp J: Portal-systemic shunt in cirrhosis: Does the type of shunt decisively influence the clinical result? *Ann Surg* 179:209–218, 1974.

26. Rypins EB, Sarfeh IJ: Small-diameter portacaval H-graft for variceal hemorrhage. *Surg Clin North Am* 70:395–404, 1990.

27. Collins JC, Rypins EB, Sarfeh IJ: Narrow-diameter portacaval shunts for management of variceal bleeding. *World J Surg* 18:211–215, 1994.

28. Sarfeh IJ, Rypins EB, Mason GR: A systematic appraisal of portacaval H-graft diameters. *Ann Surg* 204:356–363, 1986.

29. Sarfeh IJ, Carter JA, Welch HF: Analysis of operative mortality after portal decompressive procedures in cirrhotic patients. *Am J Surg* 140:306–311, 1981.

30. Iwatsuki S, Starzl TE, Todo S, et al: Liver transplantation in the treatment of bleeding esophageal varices. *Surgery* 104:697–705, 1988.

31. Rösch J, Hanafee WN, Show H: Transjugular portal venography and radiologic protacaval shunt: An experimental study. *Radiology* 92:1112–1114, 1969.

32. Reich M, Olumide F, Jorgensen E, et al: Experimental cryoprobe production of intrahepatic portacaval shunt. *J Surg Res* 23:14–18, 1977.

33. Burgener FA, Gutierrez OH: Nonsurgical production of intrahepatic portosystemic venous shunts in portal hypertension with the double lumen balloon catheter. *Rofo Fortsch Geb Rontgenstr Neun Bildgeb Verfahr* 130:686–688, 1979.

34. Colapinto RF, Stronell RD, Gildiner M, et al: Formation of intrahepatic portosystemic shunts using a balloon dilatation catheter: Preliminary clinical experience. *AJR Am J Roentgenol* 140:709–714, 1983.

35. Rösch J, Uchida BT, Putnam JS, et al: Experimental intrahepatic portacaval anastomosis: Use of expandable Gianturco stents. *Radiology* 162:481–485, 1987.

36. Palmaz JC, Sibbitt RR, Reuter SR, et al: Expandable intrahepatic portacaval

shunt stents: Early experience in the dog. *AJR Am J Roentgenol* 145:821–825, 1985.

37. Richter GM, Noeldge G, Palmaz JC, et al: Transjugular intrahepatic portacaval stent shunt: Preliminary clinical results. *Radiology* 174(3 Pt 2):1027–1030, 1990.

38. Richter GM, Noeldge G, Palmaz JC, et al: The transjugular intrahepatic portosystemic stent-shunt (TIPSS): Results of a pilot study. *Cardiovasc Intervent Radiol* 13:200–207, 1990.

39. Haskal ZJ, Pentecost MJ, Soulen MC, et al: Transjugular intrahepatic portosystemic shunt stenosis and revision: Early and midterm results. *AJR Am J Roentgenol* 163:439–444, 1994.

40. Freedman AM, Sanyal AJ, Tisnado J, et al: Results with percutaneous transjugular intrahepatic portosystemic stent-shunts for control of variceal hemorrhage in patients awaiting liver transplantation. *Transplant Proc* 25(1 Pt 2):1087–1089, 1993.

41. Haskal ZJ, Cope C, Shlansky-Goldberg RD, et al: Transjugular intrahepatic portosystemic shunts: Early and midterm efficacy in 100 patients. *Radiology* 193:130, 1994.

42. LaBerge JM, Ring EJ, Gordon RL, et al: Creation of transjugular intrahepatic portosystemic shunt (TIPS) with the Wallstent endoprosthesis: Results in 100 patients 1993. *Radiology* 187:413–420, 1993.

43. Maynar M, Cabrera J, Pulido-Duque JM, et al: Transjugular intrahepatic portosystemic shunt: Early experience with a flexible trocar/catheter system. *AJR Am J Roentgenol* 161:301–306, 1993.

44. Radosevich PM, Ring EJ, LaBerge JM, et al: Transjugular intrahepatic portosystemic shunts in patients with portal vein occlusion. *Radiology* 186:523–527, 1993.

45. Ring EJ, Lake JR, Roberts JP, et al: Using transjugular intrahepatic portosystemic shunts to control variceal bleeding before liver transplantation. *Ann Intern Med* 116:304–309, 1992.

46. Rossle M, Haag K, Ochs A, et al: The transjugular intrahepatic portosystemic stent-shunt procedure for variceal bleeding. *N Engl J Med* 330:165–171, 1994.

47. Zemel G, Katzen BT, Becker GJ, et al: Percutaneous transjugular portosystemic shunt. *JAMA* 266:390–393, 1991.

48. Helton WS, Belshaw A, Althaus S, et al: Critical appraisal of the angiographic portacaval shunt (TIPS). *Am J Surg* 165:566–571, 1993.

49. Kerns SC, Sabatelli FW, Hawkins IF: Fine-needle transjugular portal venous access system. *J Vasc Interv Radiol* 5:835–837, 1994.

50. Haskal ZJ, Ring EJ, LaBerge JM, et al: The role of dual transjugular intrahepatic portosystemic shunt (TIPS) in patients with persistent portal hypertension. *Radiology* 185:813–817, 1992.

51. Zemel G, Katzen BT, Becker GJ, et al: Percutaneous transjugular portosystemic shunt. *JAMA* 266:390–393, 1991.

52. Harman JT, Reed JD, Kopecky KK, et al: Localization of the portal vein for transjugular catheterization: Percutaneous placement of a metallic marker with real-time ultrasound guidance. *J Vasc Interv Radiol* 3:545–547, 1992.

53. Radosevich PM, Ring EJ, LaBerge JM, et al: Portosystemic shunts in patients with portal vein occlusion. *Radiology* 186:523–527, 1993.

54. Haskal Z: Percutaneous recanalization and transjugular intrahepatic portosystemic shunt (TIPS) placement for treatment of portal, mesenteric, or splenic vein thrombosis. American Roentgen Ray Society, New Orleans, 1994.

55. Haskal ZJ, Scott M, Rubin RA, et al: Intestinal varices: Treatment with the transjugular intrahepatic portosystemic shunt. *Radiology* 191:183–187, 1994.

56. Azoulay D, Castaing D, Dennison A, et al: Transjugular intrahepatic porto-

systemic shunt worsens the hyperdynamic circulatory state of the cirrhotic patient: Preliminary report of a prospective study. *Hepatology* 19:129–132, 1994.

57. Peltzer MY, Ring EJ, LaBerge JM, et al: Treatment of Budd-Chari syndrome with a transjugular intrahepatic portosystemic shunt. *J Vasc Interv Radiol* 4:263–267, 1993.

58. Haskal ZJ, Cope C, Soulen MS, et al: Intentional reversible thrombosis of transjugular intrahepatic portosystemic shunts. *Radiology* 195:485–488, 1995.

59. Haskal ZJ, Middlebrook MR: Creation of a stenotic stent to reduce transjugular intrahepatic portosystemic shunt flow. *J Vasc Interv Radiol* 5:827–830, 1994.

60. LaBerge JM, Ferrell LD, Ring EJ, et al: Histopathologic study of transjugular intrahepatic portosystemic shunts. *J Vasc Interv Radiol* 2:549–556, 1991.

61. LaBerge JM, Ferrell LD, Ring EJ, et al: Histopathologic study of stenotic and occluded transjugular intrahepatic portosystemic shunts. *J Vasc Interv Radiol* 4:779–786, 1993.

62. Longo JM, Bilbao JI, Rousseau HP, et al: Transjugular intrahepatic portosystemic shunt: Evaluation with Doppler sonography. *Radiology* 186:529–534, 1993.

63. Chong WK, Malisch TA, Mazer MJ, et al: Transjugular intrahepatic portosystemic shunt: US assessment with maximum flow velocity. *Radiology* 189:789–793, 1993.

PART VI

Thoracoscopic Sympathectomy

Video-Assisted Thoracoscopic Sympathectomy in the Management of Autonomic Disorders of the Upper Extremity

Denis D. Bensard, M.D.

Instructor in Surgery, Ohio State University School of Medicine, Columbus, Ohio

William C. Krupski, M.D.

Professor and Chief, Vascular Surgery, University of Colorado Health Sciences Center, Denver, Colorado

A dvances in anesthesia, instrumentation, and enhanced video imaging have renewed enthusiasm for thoracoscopic surgery. Operative procedures traditionally performed by standard thoracotomies are now being accomplished with comparable results using video-assisted thoracoscopic surgery (VATS). The present role of VATS is evolving.[1] For example, VATS may now be used to treat autonomic disorders of the upper extremity that in the past were rarely encountered by thoracic surgeons and more often treated by vascular surgeons via a cervical or axillary approach. The purpose of this review is to discuss VATS for treatment of autonomic disorders of the upper extremity, including indications, techniques, results, and complications, while leaving the debate about who should perform these procedures to others.

THORACOSCOPY: A HISTORICAL PERSPECTIVE

In 1922, H.C. Jacobeaus,[2] a professor of internal medicine in Stockholm, Sweden, performed the first operative thoracoscopy to divide pleural adhesions and described its utility in surgery of the chest. Jacobeaus' technique of thoracoscopic surgery soon gained wide acceptance throughout Europe and North America for the treatment of pulmonary tuberculosis.[3] However, in 1945 the introduction of streptomycin permitted the successful medical treatment of tuberculosis and reduced the need for operative therapy; thus, enthusiasm for thoracoscopy waned.[4] Over the next 45

Advances in Vascular Surgery®, vol. 3
© 1995, Mosby–Year Book, Inc.

years, thoracoscopy was virtually abandoned in the operative management of thoracic disease.

Then in the late 1980s, as a result of the introduction of new video technology, improved instrumentation, and documented efficacy and patient acceptance, video-assisted laparoscopic surgery rapidly supplanted celiotomy for the routine treatment of cholelithiasis.[5] Given the success of laparoscopic cholecystectomy, applications of video-assisted endoscopic surgery proliferated to include the management of diseases of the abdomen as well as diseases of the chest. For example, we demonstrated that VATS-diagnostic lung biopsy could be performed as safely and effectively as traditional limited thoracotomy with reduced hospital stays and postoperative complications.[6] Recent reports have confirmed our findings and have additionally demonstrated the efficacy of VATS in the management of such wide-ranging chest disorders as spontaneous pneumothorax, pulmonary nodules, pleural disease, tumors and cysts of the mediastinum, and autonomic disorders of the upper extremity.[7]

SYMPATHECTOMY FOR AUTONOMIC DISORDERS OF THE UPPER EXTREMITY

Cervicodorsal sympathectomy for a variety of disorders has been performed for almost a century. Alexander was the first to report surgical interruption of the cervical sympathetic trunk for the treatment of epilepsy in 1899. Later, in 1913, Leriche reported the use of periarterial sympathectomy to increase blood flow to the lower extremities in patients with intermittent claudication.[8] The first thoracic sympathectomy for an autonomic disorder was performed by Kotzareff in 1920, but because of the inherent risks of thoracotomy, the procedure was not widely used. Furthermore, with the advent of arterial reconstruction in the 1960s, lower extremity sympathectomy, at least for enhancing regional blood flow, virtually disappeared.

However, sympathectomy for the treatment of palmar hyperhidrosis continued. Although Kux[9] described thoracoscopic thermal ablation of the thoracic sympathetic trunk in 1951, the technique was not widely used. This most probably resulted from the rarity of the condition, the unfamiliarity of most vascular surgeons with the techniques of thoracoscopy, and the overwhelming preference for the more familiar cervical or axillary approaches. Moreover, thoracoscopic procedures previously required the use of a single-lens cystoscope, laparoscope, or thoracoscope, all of which precluded assistance by others and lacked the enhanced optics provided by newer video technology.

The indications for upper-extremity sympathectomy are beyond the scope of this review. Few would dispute the efficacy of cervical sympathectomy in the management of palmar hyperhidrosis. Although somewhat controversial, upper-extremity sympathectomy may also be useful for the treatment of axillary hyperhidrosis, pregangrene of the fingertips in thromboangiitis obliterans (Buerger's disease), causalgia (reflex sympathetic dystrophy), and frostbite. In addition, carefully selected patients with Raynaud's disease may also benefit from cervicodorsal sympathectomy.

Preganglionic fibers supplying the upper extremity are derived from cells in the intermediolateral column of the gray matter of the spinal cord between its second and ninth segment. The anatomic relationships of the cervicothoracic sympathetic chain are shown in Figure 1. Most vasoconstrictor fibers supplying the arteries emerge from the spinal cord in the ventral roots of the second and third thoracic nerves. These arteries can be denervated by division of the sympathetic trunk below the third thoracic ganglion and the rami communicantes of the T2-T3 ganglia. The sympathetic nerve supply to the eccrine glands is similarly interrupted by division of these ganglia. If the eccrine glands of the axilla are to be denervated, then additional division of the sympathetic trunk below T4 is necessary. To produce sympathetic denervation of the upper extremity, excision of the stellate ganglion (T1) or communicating fibers to T1 is unnecessary. The nerve of Kuntz, an intrathoracic nerve that passes from the second intercostal nerve to the T1 root, permits intact sympathetic fibers to pass from the spinal cord to the lower brachial plexus, bypassing the sympathetic chain. Roos[10] has suggested that failure of upper-extremity sympathectomy occurs when the nerve of Kuntz is spared. Others allege that incomplete sympathectomy more likely results from the inadequate excision of the T3-T4 ganglia.[8]

In our practice, we limit the use of video-assisted thoracoscopic sympathectomy to the treatment of palmar hyperhidrosis, causalgia, and se-

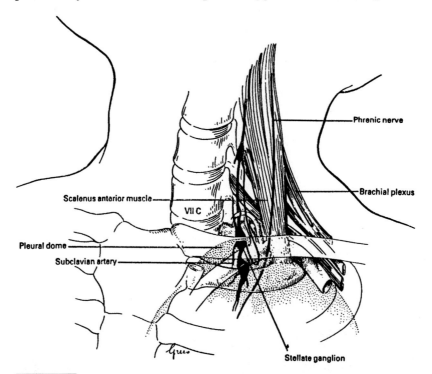

FIGURE 1.

Illustration of anatomic relationships of the cervicothoracic sympathetic chain. From Biasi GM, Mingazzini P, Ruberti U: Cervical sympathectomy. In Greenhalgh RM, editor: *Vascular and endovascular surgical techniques.* London, 1994, WB Saunders, p 268. Used by permission.

lected patients with cutaneous and digital ischemia resulting from thromboangiitis obliterans or frostbite. A brief review of these indications follows. We acknowledge that other indications may be proposed, but our review of the supportive data suggests that the results are less than compelling, and we have opted for a more conservative approach.

PALMAR HYPERHIDROSIS

Hyperhidrosis is uncontrolled sweating in excess of the normal thermoregulatory response. Uncontrolled hyperhidrosis can become a psychologic and social handicap. Although most patients seek evaluation because of the emotional distress they experience, a few may present with refractory dermatitis or fungal infection due to the chronically moist skin. Many patients are probably never referred for treatment because of the misconception that surgical intervention is too extreme. Patients often describe the frustration or social isolation they experience as a result of their perception that others consider them to be excessively nervous. Others state that they are unable to perform tasks necessary for employment, because a chronically wet grip interferes with their ability to handle tools or paper.

Numerous reports document the efficacy of cervical sympathectomy for the treatment of palmar hyperhidrosis (Table 1).[8, 11–14] In a remarkable long-term study of 480 patients undergoing endoscopic thoracic sympathectomy for palmar hyperhidrosis, Herbst et al.[13] demonstrated that 98% of patients experienced relief of their symptoms at a mean follow-up of 14.6 years. Similarly, Claes et al.[11] reported that 502 of 512 patients undergoing thoracoscopic sympathectomy for palmar hyperhidrosis had immediate relief of their symptoms; recurrence of symptoms occurred in only 2% of patients at 1 to 5 years of follow-up. These results (see Table 1) are equal to or superior to those achieved with the cervical or axillary approach.[8, 14]

The complication rate of traditional cervical sympathectomy is less than 5%. Postoperative development of Horner's syndrome (ipsilateral ptosis, miosis, anhidrosis, and enophthalmos) is the most common untoward event. O'Riordain and co-workers[15] emphasize that careful visualization and preservation of the entire stellate ganglion are essential to preventing a permanent Horner's syndrome. In contrast, some authors recommend deliberate resection of the stellate ganglion, stating that symptoms of Horner's syndrome are well tolerated. Additional side effects include compensatory or gustatory sweating. Herbst[13] found that these troublesome side effects lead to a steady decline in patient satisfaction, from the initial 95% satisfaction rate to a 66% satisfaction rate at late follow-up. However, it should be emphasized that the complications of Horner's syndrome or compensatory/gustatory sweating appear not to be related to the method of sympathectomy but rather to the extent of sympathectomy.[15]

CUTANEOUS ISCHEMIA

Thromboangiitis obliterans (Buerger's disease) is an inflammatory occlusive disease of small arteries of the extremities afflicting tobacco smok-

TABLE 1.

Efficacy of Cervical Sympathectomy for Treatment of Palmar Hyperhydrosis

	No. of Patients	No. of Sympathec-tomies	Follow-up (Mean, Yrs)	Improved	Horner's Syndrome	Compensatory/ Gustatory Sweating	Complications (Major/Minor)
Edmonson, Banerjee, Rennie, et al., 1992[12]	NA	50	0.3–4.4 (2.2)	98%	2.0%	75%/48%	0/6%
Claes, Drott, Gothberg, et al., 1993[11]	533	512	1.0–5.0 (NA)	98%	0.2%	45%/NA	0/1%
Herbst, Plas, Fugger, et al., 1994[13]	323	480	0.8–27.1 (16.4)	98%	2.5%	76%/51%	0/4%
TOTAL	>856	1042	0.3–27.1	98%	1.3%	49%/51%	0/3%

NA = not applicable.

ers.[16] Although the etiology is incompletely understood, the natural progression of the disease is invariably associated with the continued use of tobacco. Progression of the disease leads to distal arterial occlusion and arterial insufficiency. Worsening ischemia may ultimately lead to gangrene of the distal extremity. Several palliative treatments have been employed, including sympathectomy, to enhance cutaneous blood flow. Shionoya[17] suggests that sympathectomy can promote healing of ulceration and superficial trophic lesions of the skin in selected patients with Buerger's disease. In the setting of superficial ischemic changes (not major or extensive gangrene), we have selectively used VATS sympathectomy in patients when the location and extent of occlusive disease make arterial reconstruction impossible. A proven benefit of this strategy has not been documented by controlled clinical trials, and such studies using video-assisted thoracoscopic sympathectomy are unlikely in view of the relative rarity of the disorder.

CAUSALGIA

The constellation of burning extremity pain, signs of autonomic dysfunction, and secondary trophic changes of the skin, usually following extremity trauma, characterizes causalgia, also designated *reflex sympathetic dystrophy*. It has been postulated that injury to a somatic nerve results in persistent conduction of aberrant pain signals via the intact sympathetic nerves, producing varying degrees of extremity impairment, joint fibrosis, muscle atrophy, and eventual irreversible limitations of function. Regardless of the therapeutic approach, the best results occur when some form of treatment is initiated before physical changes occur. The association of autonomic dysfunction with occurrence of reflex sympathetic dystrophy has led to the employment of sympathectomy in the management of causalgia. In our own institution, Mockus[18] found that 97% of patients enjoyed immediate relief of symptoms after sympathectomy, and at 3 years' follow-up 29 of 31 patients sustained continued symptomatic improvement. Of note, the best results were achieved in those patients selected by their positive response to temporary chemical sympathectomy using percutaneous injection of a local anesthetic. We recommend a trial of chemical sympathectomy to identify patients who might benefit from operative sympathectomy, although we emphasize that repeated blocks must be avoided if VATS is to be performed. As in Buerger's disease, we are unaware of any published studies documenting the efficacy of video-assisted thoracoscopic sympathectomy in the management of causalgia, but it seems reasonable to extrapolate the results from traditional operations to VATS.

SUMMARY OF INDICATIONS

On the basis of available data, video-assisted thoracoscopic sympathectomy can be unequivocally recommended for the treatment of palmar hyperhidrosis, which is the only absolute indication for the procedure. VATS may also be considered in the management of advanced Buerger's disease or causalgia in selected patients. The authors caution that documented efficacy is unproved for these disorders and should be considered only when more conventional therapeutic measures have failed.

PATIENT SELECTION FOR VATS

In addition to prudence with respect to indications for sympathectomy, good judgment is also necessary for selecting suitable patients for VATS. Single-lung ventilation, a prerequisite for VATS, may exclude certain patients with associated comorbid illness, such as chronic lung disease, coronary artery disease, or previous thoracotomy. It goes without saying that it is unwise to subject a patient to an unsafe surgical approach simply in the hope of reducing post-thoracotomy discomfort.

Patients who have undergone previous thoracotomies or repeated percutaneous chemical sympathectomies should be excluded from consideration of video-assisted thoracoscopic sympathectomy. If history and physical examination suggest serious underlying cardiac or respiratory impairment, VATS is a poor choice. Most patients should have a screening chest roentgenogram and baseline pulmonary function tests. If significant pulmonary or pleural disease is identified, we do not perform VATS, because the procedure can be done without the need for single-lung ventilation or thoracotomy using the cervical approach.

VIDEO-ASSISTED THORACOSCOPIC SYMPATHECTOMY: TECHNIQUE

Patients receive general anesthesia by use of a double-lumen endotracheal tube. Tube position should be confirmed bronchoscopically both following initial placement and after positioning the patient in the lateral decubitus position. This point cannot be overemphasized, given the findings of Smith,[19] who demonstrated that 48% of double-lumen endotracheal tubes thought to be appropriately positioned on the basis of clinical signs were in fact malpositioned when examined by flexible bronchoscopy. After proper position of the endotracheal tube is confirmed, the patient is turned to the lateral decubitus position, and a roll is placed under the dependent axilla. Ipsilateral lung ventilation is discontinued to allow absorptive atelectasis. The table is flexed to drop the dependent shoulder and hip from the operative field. This results in widening of the intercostal spaces, reducing the amount of levering of instruments against the ribs and providing greater mobility for the thoracoscope.[20] Skin preparation and draping are done as for open thoracotomy, because conversion to an open procedure may be necessary. A 2-cm chest wall incision inferior to the tip of the scapula is made. The intercostal muscles are split above the rib with use of a hemostat, avoiding injury to the intercostal neurovascular bundle of the superior rib, and the pleural cavity is entered. Communication of the pleural cavity with atmospheric pressure allows the atelectatic lung to fall away from the chest wall. A 12-mm trocar is inserted through the opening, the videoscope is introduced into the pleural cavity, and exploration is begun (Fig 2). Care must be exercised to avoid injury to the lung during the initial entry into the chest.

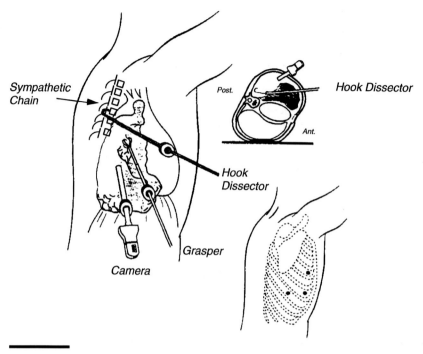

FIGURE 2.

Diagram of video-assisted thoracoscopic sympathectomy. Ports *(lower right)* are located inferior to the tip of the scapula and anterior to the scapula in the mid- and anterior axillary lines. A hook dissector introduced through the anterior ports permits adhesions to be divided and cauterized. The grasper clasps the chain after it is introduced through the second anterior port.

The sympathetic chain is readily identified as a pale pink extrapleural structure near the costovertebral junction. If the patient has undergone previous percutaneous nerve block, resultant adhesions to the upper lobe of the lung may be encountered. Two additional trocars (5 mm) should now be inserted under direct vision; the ports are located anterior to the scapula in the mid- and anterior axillary lines (see Fig 2). When placing these anterior ports, one should avoid injury to the long thoracic nerve. The use of a hook dissector or scissors introduced through the additional ports permits adhesions to be safely divided and concomitantly cauterized, again carefully avoiding injury to the lung. We have generally avoided blunt dissection of adhesions to minimize the risk of lung injury and subsequent persistent air leak.

After satisfactory exposure of the upper sympathetic trunk is obtained (overlying the neck of the second through fourth ribs), the hook dissector is used to incise the parietal pleura over T4. Division of the pleura is continued cephalad until the stellate ganglion (T1) is reached. The hook dissector is then used to encircle the sympathetic trunk just above T4. Dissection continues cephalad, primarily by elevation of the sympathetic chain, by use of blunt dissection, or electrocautery as needed. When the T2-T3 ganglia are exposed, care is taken to avoid injury to the adjacent intercostal neurovascular bundle. The ganglia are circumferentially excised with electrocautery.

Following adequate mobilization of the chain, a grasper is inserted through the second 5-mm port and used to clasp it. The stellate ganglion (T1) marks the upper limit of the dissection. The hook dissector is removed and replaced with the thoracoscopic scissors, and the sympathetic chain with the T2-T3 ganglia is divided below T1 and above T4. The specimen still held by the grasper is removed through the 5-mm port and sent to pathology for histologic confirmation. A suction irrigator is introduced and hemostasis is assured. The 5-mm ports are removed and a 28 French chest tube is inserted via the anterior incision. Port sites are infiltrated with long-acting local anesthetic (0.25% bupivacaine). The videoscope is withdrawn and the lung re-expanded under direct visualization. The two remaining incisions are then closed with a subcuticular suture.

Several points should be emphasized.

1. On the basis of our experience, CO_2 insufflation of the chest is unnecessary when single-lung ventilation is employed. Avoiding CO_2 insufflation reduces its detrimental effects on ventilation of the dependent lung.[21]

2. As noted, adhesions fixing the lung to the area of the sympathetic trunk often form following percutaneous chemical sympathectomy. Therefore, repeated temporary blocks should be discouraged; if a patient has received numerous repeated blocks, we generally discourage VATS and proceed with a traditional cervical sympathectomy.

3. Although Roos[10] has proposed the importance of identification and division of the nerve of Koontz, we have not found this necessary to achieve satisfactory sympathectomy.

4. The placement of a chest tube is probably unnecessary if lung injury has not occurred and an air leak is absent. However, we have opted to continue inserting a chest tube to ensure complete lung re-expansion and avoid the potential need for later tube thoracostomy after the patient is awake. The chest tube is generally removed within 24 hours of the operation.

5. Finally, care must be taken to avoid injury to the stellate ganglion. If this is injured, temporary or permanent Horner's syndrome results.[15]

SUMMARY

In summary, video-assisted thoracoscopic sympathectomy represents a potential advance in the treatment of selected neurovascular disorders. A safe, effective method for sympathetic denervation of the upper extremity, VATS offers improved visualization, decreased postoperative pain, and potentially a reduced length of hospital stay. However, the important lessons learned in the early experience of video-assisted laparoscopic surgery should not be ignored. We must avoid overapplying a new technique or overextending the indications at the risk of therapeutic misadventure. Proper training and experience are mandatory. Remember thoracodorsal sympathectomy has long been successfully performed by vascular surgeons using the cervical and axillary approaches, and these remain reasonable. If VATS is to replace proven procedures, its superiority, or at the very least equivalency, to standard techniques should be demonstrated in well-conducted studies.

REFERENCES

1. Miller JI: The present role and future considerations of video-assisted thoracoscopy in general thoracic surgery. *Ann Thorac Surg* 56:804–806, 1993.
2. Jacobeaus HC: The practical importance of thoracoscopy in surgery of the chest. *Surg Gynecol Obstet* 34:289–296, 1922.
3. Day JC, Chapman PT, O'Brien EJ: Closed intrapleural pneumonolysis: An analysis of 1000 consecutive operations. *Thorac Surg* 17:537–554, 1948.
4. Braimbridge MV: The history of thoracoscopic surgery. *Ann Thorac Surg* 56:610–614, 1993.
5. The Southern Surgeons Club: A prospective analysis of 1,518 laparoscopic cholecystectomies. *N Engl J Med* 324:1073–1078, 1991.
6. Bensard DD, McIntyre RC, Waring BJ, et al: Comparison of video thoracoscopic lung biopsy to open lung biopsy in the diagnosis of interstitial lung disease. *Chest* 103:765–770, 1993.
7. The Society of Thoracic Surgeons: The First International Symposium on Thoracoscopic Surgery. In Mack M, Hazelrigg S, Landreneall R, et al, editors: *Ann Thorac Surg* 56:603–806, 1993.
8. Harris JP, May J: Upper extremity sympathectomy. In Rutherford RB, editor: *Vascular surgery*. Philadelphia, 1989, WB Saunders, pp 890–897.
9. Kux E: The endoscopic approach to the vegetative nervous system and its therapeutic possibilities. *Dis Chest* 20:139–147, 1951.
10. Roos D: Transaxillary extrapleural thoracic sympathectomy. In Bergan J, Yao J, editors: *Operative techniques in vascular surgery*. New York, 1980, Grune and Stratton, p 115.
11. Claes G, Drott C, Gothberg G: Thoracoscopy for autonomic disorders. *Ann Thorac Surg* 56:715–716, 1993.
12. Edmondson RA, Banerjee AK, Rennie JA: Endoscopic transthoracic sympathectomy in the treatment of hyperhidrosis. *Ann Surg* 215:289–293, 1992.
13. Herbst F, Plas EG, Fugger R, et al: Endoscopic thoracic sympathectomy for primary hyperhidrosis of the upper limbs. *Ann Surg* 220:86–90, 1994.
14. Adar R, Kurchin A, Zweig A, et al: Palmar hyperhidrosis and its surgical treatment: A report of 100 cases. *Ann Surg* 186:34–41, 1977.
15. O'Riordain DS, Maher M, Waldron DJ, et al: Limiting the anatomic extent of upper thoracic sympathectomy for primary palmar hyperhidrosis. *Surg Gynecol Obstet* 176:151–154, 1993.
16. Papa M, Bass A, Adar R, et al: Autoimmune mechanisms in thromboangiitis obliterans (Buerger's disease): The role of tobacco antigen and the major histocompatibility complex. *Surgery* 111:527–531, 1992.
17. Shionoya S: Buerger's disease (thromboangiitis obliterans). In Rutherford RB, editor: *Vascular surgery*. Philadelphia, 1989, WB Saunders, pp 207–217.
18. Mockus MB, Rutherford RB, Rosales C, et al: Sympathectomy for causalgia. *Arch Surg* 122:668–672, 1987.
19. Smith G, Hirsch N, Ehrenwerth J: Placement of double-lumen endobronchial tubes. Correlation between clinical impressions and bronchoscopic findings. *Br J Anaesth* 58:1317–1320, 1986.
20. Landreneau RJ, Mack MJ, Keenan RJ, et al: Strategic planning for video-assisted thoracic surgery. *Ann Thorac Surg* 56:615–619, 1993.
21. Horswell JL: Anesthetic techniques for thoracoscopy. *Ann Thorac Surg* 56:624–629, 1993.

PART VII

Issues in Basic Science

Restenosis as an Example of Vascular Hyperplastic Disease: Reassessment of Potential Mechanisms

Peter Libby, M.D.

Vascular Medicine and Atherosclerosis Unit, Cardiovascular Division, Department of Medicine and Department of Pathology, Brigham and Women's Hospital, Boston, Massachusetts

Galina Sukhova, Ph.D.

Vascular Medicine and Atherosclerosis Unit, Cardiovascular Division, Department of Medicine and Department of Pathology, Brigham and Women's Hospital, Boston, Massachusetts

Edi Brogi, M.D.

Department of Pathology, Massachusetts General Hospital, Boston, Massachusetts

Frederick J. Schoen, M.D., Ph.D.

Department of Pathology, Brigham and Women's Hospital, Boston, Massachusetts

Hiroyuki Tanaka, M.D., Ph.D.

Department of Cardiothoracic Surgery, Tokyo Medical and Dental University, Tokyo, Japan

---

In recent decades, clinicians treating patients with arterial diseases have made considerable advances in both surgical and percutaneous interventional techniques. However, the biologic reaction of the arterial wall continues to limit the long-term efficacy of many of our novel therapies. In small-caliber vascular grafting, anastomotic hyperplasia can cause failure of technically perfect reconstructions with our most advanced biomaterials, or even with autogenous vein. In cardiac transplantation, the development of an aggressive accelerated form of arteriosclerosis now constitutes the major impediment to long-term graft survival despite the availability of potent new immunosuppressive agents. The problem of restenosis continues to plague practitioners of vascular intervention despite major efforts in both the clinic and the laboratory aimed at retarding this process. Until we achieve a mastery of arterial biology in keeping with our technical prowess, it is likely that these hyperplastic reactions will continue to frustrate our most cherished and widely practiced therapies. We aim here to use the example of restenosis after coronary artery angio-

Advances in Vascular Surgery®, vol. 3
© 1995, Mosby–Year Book, Inc.

plasty as a vehicle to review some of the complexities of the arterial response to injury that may account for our failure thus far to achieve a lasting benefit for many of our patients receiving "high technology" therapies for arterial diseases.

WHY DO WE NEED TO REASSESS OUR THINKING ABOUT RESTENOSIS?

Percutaneous transluminal coronary angioplasty (PTCA) is a very successful procedure in terms of initial success and widespread adoption as an alternative to bypass surgery. In 1995, there will be over 450,000 coronary interventions in the United States and over 800,000 in the world. Unfortunately, several hundred thousand of the PTCA procedures will be performed this year on patients who have already undergone the same procedure because of the problem of restenosis. The repeat angioplasties entail substantial patient discomfort, inconvenience, and risk. In the current climate, we all strive to limit health care expenditures and excessive use of technology-intensive procedures. These PTCAs performed for restenosis probably cost almost 1 billion dollars annually.

Many experimental and human studies have aimed to prevent restenosis after PTCA. At present it is fair to summarize the results to date as follows: although animal studies have disclosed many agents effective in retarding intimal thickening after balloon or other injury to arteries, no agents have emerged from human trials as clinically useful for the therapy or prevention of restenosis. Why might there be such a disparity between animal and human studies? One possibility is that such therapeutic intervention trials in animal studies are quite correct, but their conclusions seldom apply to human restenosis. This is the theme that we will elaborate further here.

WHY THE DISPARITY BETWEEN EXPERIMENTAL RESULTS AND CLINICAL TRIALS OF APPROACHES TO PREVENTION OF RESTENOSIS?

There are a number of reasons why the animal studies might not apply to human restenosis. Often, clinical trials of agents have differed significantly from the regimens successful in animal studies in terms of the dose of the agent, the time schedule, and the route of administration. Although such issues doubtless may explain some of the disappointments we have encountered in this enterprise, we prefer not to dwell on the pharmacokinetic issues. Rather, this discussion will focus on the potential differences in the biology between human restenosis and the restenosis models that we have traditionally used as the basis for choosing drugs for clinical trials.

From the point of view of a vascular biologist, it is astonishing that restenosis is ever avoided after such trauma to an artery as PTCA entails. It is amazing that transmural injury to an artery, from intima to the adventitia (Fig 1), as often happens in a balloon angioplasty, does not inevitably evoke a substantial intimal hyperplastic response (Fig 2). Indeed, in the laboratory, this is precisely how we study arterial hyperplasia, by

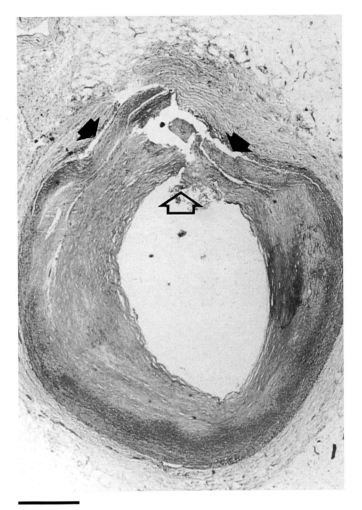

FIGURE 1.

Coronary arterial atherosclerotic plaque modified by PTCA. In this patient, who died shortly after the procedure, the changes induced by balloon angioplasty consist of fracture of the plaque *(open arrow)* with deep extension of the wall defect, and partial circumferential dissection *(closed arrows)*. (Verhoeff-van Gieson stain, for elastin, ×20.) (From Cotran RS, Kumar V, Robbins SL: *Robbins pathologic basis of disease,* ed 5. Philadelphia, 1994, WB Saunders, p 513. Used by permission.)

producing a balloon injury as initially shown by Hans Baumgartner[1] many years ago. In our view, the traditional cardiologic concepts of the pathophysiology of restenosis overemphasized the acute phase of arterial injury and focused on the platelet and coagulation system as a key source of factors that cause this process. One hint that platelet products alone may not solely explain restenosis is the lack of congruity between the kinetics of restenosis and the kinetics of platelet activation.

Regardless of which of the several definitions of restenosis is used, the National Heart, Lung, and Blood Institute (NHLBI) registry data showed that the incidence of angiographically detectable restenosis does not plateau until some 3 months after the procedure.[2] The data from

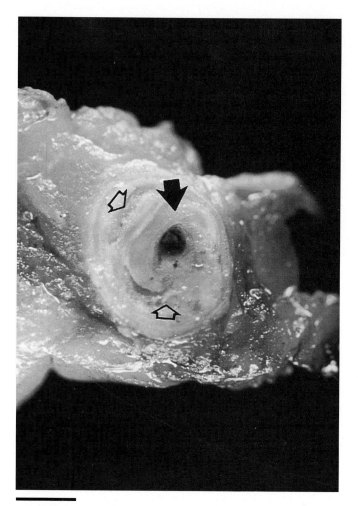

FIGURE 2.
Proliferative restenosis after PTCA. This gross coronary artery cross section from
a patient who died several months after angioplasty illustrates both the original,
previously disrupted atherosclerotic plaque *(open arrows)* and the markedly occlusive concentric fibrous tissue that formed after the procedure *(arrow)*. (From
Cotran RS, Kumar V, Robbins SL: *Robbins pathologic basis of disease*, ed 5. Philadelphia, 1994, WB Saunders, p 513. Used by permission.)

Nobuyoshi's group agree excellently with the NHLBI registry data.[3] A
number of different kinds of studies (e.g., using indium-labeled platelets)
have shown that platelet deposition ceases within hours to days of instrumentation.[4, 5] Thus, much of the biology of restenosis takes place long
after active thrombosis and coagulation subside.

Products of platelets or of thrombosis may indeed provide early in-
citing elements in restenosis but likely do not explain the entire course
of the disease. In support of this view, long-term anticoagulant or antiplatelet therapy has failed to lower the incidence of restenosis after PTCA.
Currently available systemic antithrombotic or anticoagulant regimens
may simply not achieve thorough inhibition of these processes locally at
the site of injury. One of the novel approaches to antiplatelet therapy in-

volves blockade of adhesion receptors on the platelet surface (glycoprotein IIb/IIIa) with a monoclonal antibody. Clinical data available thus far from trials with this agent have demonstrated a reduction in acute events[6] and decreased clinical manifestations of restenosis.[7] However, even with this highly effective antiplatelet therapy, no rigorous quantitative angiographic data yet establish that its administration reduces the rate of restenosis. In addition to its effects on the platelet glycoprotein IIb/IIIa, the 7E3 antibody used in this trial inhibits another integrin ($\alpha_V\beta_3$) whose inhibition might influence the biology of the arterial response to injury independent of platelets.[8] Thus, the preponderance of data suggests that factors released from platelets or by blood coagulation do not account fully for the changes in the biology of the arterial wall that must continue for weeks to months after PTCA. The alternative explanation, that ongoing autocrine or paracrine signals help mediate the events that occur later during restenosis, deserves careful consideration.

EXPERIMENTAL EVIDENCE FOR SUSTAINED ACTIVATION OF VASCULAR CELLS AFTER BALLOON INJURY

Fortunately, current approaches permit us to probe whether or not such signaling persists the first few days after injury, when the surface of the traumatized artery has become passivated and when platelet activation and thrombosis have receded. We have explored the hypothesis that sustained activation of intrinsic vascular wall cells occurs after balloon injury to the abdominal aorta of rabbits. After the procedure, injection of Evan's blue dye permits ready demarcation of the injured area from the uninjured area. Our analysis focused on the leading edge of repair, using the Evan's blue staining as a guide and sampling areas that encompassed the region of endothelial healing.

As markers of activation, we used certain well-characterized cell surface molecules expressed at low levels on resting vascular cells, but whose levels increase after activation: vascular cell adhesion molecule-1 (VCAM-1), intracellular adhesion molecule-1 (ICAM-1), and class II histocompatibility antigens encoded by the major histocompatibility complex (MHC). Each of these structures has highly important functions in which we and many others have intense interest. However, in the context of this discussion, we will consider these molecules solely as activation markers, as readouts of the state of the cells, without regard to their various functions.

The results of this study have been published; therefore, we will discuss here only a few salient highlights of the work.[9] We were not surprised to find evidence by immunohistochemical staining of activation of endothelial cells in the healing part of the lesion. After 2 days, individual endothelial cells recovering the injured zone bore VCAM-1, ICAM-1, or class II histocompatibility antigens, markers not normally expressed by rabbit aortic endothelium in this location, as noted above. By 5 days, focusing on the leading edge of endothelial repair, the luminal cells expressed all three markers in an even more uniform distribution. The more surprising and important finding of this study, and the reason that we embarked on it in the first place, emerged from examination of later time points. Even 30 days after the initial balloon injury, when the intima has thickened prominently, the leading edge of endothelial repair showed activation of these cells. At this stage after injury, products of coagulation have been largely resorbed, and ongoing thrombosis has ceased. ICAM-1 expression remained increased in endothelial cells and also in subjacent smooth muscle cells. Most curious to us, because of our interest in inflammation in the blood vessel wall, was the presence in the neointima of many class II histocompatibility antigen-bearing cells, indicating immunologic activation. At least some of these class II—positive cells are leukocytes in this healing intimal lesion 30 days after balloon injury.

To summarize these studies, endothelial cells near the leading edge of healing express VCAM. All neointimal endothelial and smooth muscle cells exhibit high levels of ICAM-1 during the early phase of healing, and expression of these markers then subsides as the leading edge of recovery advances. However, even 30 days after injury, some leukocytes and intrinsic vascular wall cells express class II histocompatibility antigens. These findings provide direct experimental evidence that some kind of activating stimulus indeed persists in the artery wall even well after the initial balloon injury.

How do these findings relate to the formation of the restenotic lesion characterized by smooth muscle and extracellular matrix accumulation in the intima? We believe that they provide insight into the type and timing of signals that govern the process of arterial remodeling that characterizes restenosis. After balloon injury or clinical angioplasty, the intimal lesions contain many smooth muscle cells surrounded by a very abundant and often loose extracellular matrix. There is considerable debate about the rate of smooth muscle proliferation in restenosis, but the importance of excessive smooth muscle—derived extracellular matrix accumulation remains undisputed.

THE QUEST FOR THE CULPABLE MITOGEN IN THE HYPERPLASTIC RESPONSE TO BALLOON INJURY

What signals changes in smooth muscle cell functions after balloon injury, such as altered migration, proliferation, and matrix metabolism? The rat carotid artery has provided an animal preparation that has furnished us with the most quantitative kinetics and considerable insight into biology of the arterial response to injury. Elegant studies by Lindner and Reidy have shown that infusion of basic fibroblast growth factor (bFGF) can augment smooth muscle cell proliferation in balloon-injured rat arteries.[10–12] In a further intervention trial, these investigators neutralized FGF with an antibody, which limited the first wave of proliferation of medial smooth muscle cells in the balloon-injured arteries. These studies on previously normal rat arteries raised considerable interest in the role of FGF as a stimulus to smooth muscle proliferation after injury in vivo. Similar kinds of studies performed in Ross' laboratory in collaboration with Reidy's group showed that platelet-derived growth factor actually does not act as a mitogen but may be more important in provoking the migration of smooth muscle cells from the media into the intima.[13]

This point highlights an important difference between the experimental animals that are normally used and human atheroma. The normal rat artery has few if any intimal smooth muscle cells. In the rat vessel, the endothelial cells lie directly on the basement membrane. In contrast, the normal adult human artery, and certainly the atherosclerotic plaque, has a much more complex structure incorporating resident intimal smooth muscle cells. Thus, formation of an intimal lesion in rats, but not necessarily in adult humans, requires migration of smooth muscle cells from the media into the intima. The models of the response to arterial injury that use previously normal vessels clearly differ from clinical angioplasty, which entails injury to a complex lesion.[14]

One might wonder, in view of these differences, whether the concept of FGF as a stimulus for smooth muscle cell proliferation applies to injury to the human atherosclerotic lesion. The concept put forth by Lindner and Reidy, based on excellent evidence in the rat, invokes release of preformed basic FGF upon injury from the dead or dying cells damaged by the trauma of the balloon inflation. This smooth muscle cell–derived FGF stimulates the first wave of medial proliferation. In this regard, it would be important to ascertain whether human atherosclerotic lesions contain preformed basic FGF, as do normal rat arterial medial cells. We did just this in a simple series of observations on nonatherosclerotic human arteries and human atheromata, mostly obtained at carotid endarterectomy. Normal human arteries contain abundant basic FGF associated with smooth muscle cells and endothelium, as revealed by histochemical staining with an antibody that recognizes this growth factor.[15] In contrast, staining of human atherosclerotic lesions consistently showed virtual lack of immunostainable basic FGF. Areas closer to the normal part of the media underlying the plaque contained some basic FGF, as in the normal media, but the plaques themselves contained scant basic FGF. Semiquantitative analysis of 14 human atheromata showed that in the plaque itself, about 10% or fewer of the cells were labeled with this antibody tagging technique. Our results show that human atherosclerotic lesions contain much less preformed, immunoreactive basic FGF than do normal medial layers of human arteries. These findings highlight a crucial difference between injury to a previously normal artery and a complex atherosclerotic lesion. This study shows how a growth factor that is clearly implicated by good experimental evidence in the simple arterial injury model likely does not apply to the advanced human plaque.

We also tested whether low expression of basic FGF in atheroma is just a property of the human atherosclerotic lesion or is a more general phenomenon. For this purpose, we examined arteries of rabbits that had consumed an atherogenic diet (0.5% cholesterol, 10% saturated fat). We studied serial cross sections of an atherosclerotic plaque formed in the rabbit aorta after 13 weeks on such a rabbit diet. Staining for the "activation markers" VCAM-1 and ICAM-1 revealed substantial expression by smooth muscle cells in the expanded intima. However, although the tunica media of this vessel contained abundant basic FGF, just as in the human lesions, the plaque exhibited much less basic FGF staining than did normal portions of the artery. This example illustrates the limitations of seeking the trigger mitogen by extrapolating from balloon injury of a previously normal vessel to clinical angioplasty of a pre-existing lesion.

If the foregoing evidence renders it less likely that basic FGF causes the proliferation of intimal smooth muscle cells, then what factor may be the culprit? Our laboratory has spent much of the last decade examining possible roles in vascular homeostasis and pathobiology of cytokines, nonimmunoglobulin protein mediators of inflammation or immunity.[16] We have advanced the hypothesis that cytokines may mediate some of the effects of balloon injury on the injured vascular wall cells that occur late after balloon injury.[14] Of the numerous cytokines, many potentially have roles in vascular biology. In this context, rather than list an extensive catalog of some 30 different molecules, let us rather focus on one that we are interested in as a potential candidate for consideration as an autocrine or paracrine growth factor.

The cytokine we wish to discuss has interested our group for a number of years, going back to work that Warner performed in our laboratory some time ago.[17] A variety of previously published biochemical and molecular experiments established human smooth muscle cells as a target for and a source of a particular cytokine called tumor necrosis factor-alpha (TNF-α). Under normal circumstances, human smooth muscle cells express no messenger RNA encoding the prototypic cytokine interleukin-1 (IL-1) β, but exposure to TNF-α rapidly and transiently raises levels of IL-1 message. TNF also increases production by smooth muscle cells of prostaglandins of the E series. These examples illustrate how tumor necrosis factor can activate important functions of vascular smooth muscle cells.

TNF can also stimulate smooth muscle replication, perhaps not directly but indirectly by stimulating secondary growth factor gene expression.[18, 19] Smooth muscle cells not only respond to tumor necrosis factor but also produce this cytokine, as shown by transcript accumulation, protein biosynthesis, and elaboration of biologic activity when appropriately stimulated.[17] To move from the culture dish in vivo, we sought evidence in rabbit arteries subjected to balloon injury by asking whether tumor necrosis factor is at the right place at the right time to be a potential stimulus for smooth muscle proliferation.

By 10 days after balloon injury in this model, many layers of smooth muscle cells have accumulated in the expanding intima by a combination of migration from the intima and division, as determined by labeling with bromodeoxyuridine, a thymidine analog incorporated into newly synthesized DNA. Many of the replicating cells in these lesions contain immunostainable TNF-α. Analysis of these sections also permitted comparison of basic fibroblast growth factor and tumor necrosis factor expression in regions of the normal and injured artery, and localization with bromodeoxyuridine labeling, a marker for cell replication. Moreover, using reverse transcriptase polymerase chain reaction techniques appropriate for these very small samples, we demonstrated an accumulation of messenger RNA encoding TNF-α in the injured areas but not in the uninjured control areas.

The control, uninjured arteries contained substantial basic FGF but no detectable TNF. The injured part of the artery at the same time (10 days after balloon injury) showed many smooth muscle cells, substantial cell proliferation, and lack of basic FGF compared with the normal vessel or even the underlying media. Moreover, abundant TNF colocalized with dividing smooth muscle cells. The finding of basic FGF, abundant in the media but sparse in the expanding intima, agrees very well with work in the injured rat carotid artery previously published by Reidy's group.[20]

We therefore conclude that smooth muscle cells in the balloon-injured rabbit aorta can express TNF-α, that levels of TNF mRNA increase after balloon injury, and that the presence of TNF-α, but not basic FGF protein, correlates closely with smooth muscle cell division. These results identify TNF as a candidate autocrine growth factor for the growth of smooth muscle cells, and suggest a role for this mediator in arterial hyperplastic lesions such as the restenosing vessel.

A ROLE FOR MACROPHAGES IN RESTENOSIS?

Our laboratory, in the footsteps of many others, has used injury to a previously normal artery as a model to probe the biology of the arterial response to injury. However, important differences render the normal carotid artery or aorta, popular models for studying the response to balloon injury, quite distinct from complicated human atheroma. One critical dissimilarity between pre-existing atheroma and previously normal vessels is the presence of many macrophages, particularly in and around the lesion's lipid-rich core. Past studies of restenosis have often considered platelets as a source of growth factors and activating stimuli for intrinsic vascular wall cells such as smooth muscle and endothelium. However, we must take resident and attracted leukocytes into account in our attempts to understand the response of the abnormal vessel, the human atherosclerotic plaque, to injury (Fig 3). One experimental strategy for modeling injury to the abnormal vessel uses cholesterol-fed rabbits, a preparation used to advantage in "double injury" protocols by Faxon,

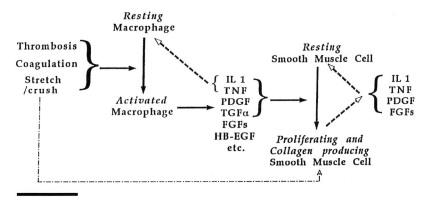

FIGURE 3.

Cascade model of restenosis. Possible pathways for signaling changes in smooth muscle cell proliferation, migration, and matrix metabolism after arterial injury. The messengers shown are intended merely to illustrate the possible complexity of autocrine and paracrine loops in the response to injury. IL-1 = interleukin-1; TNF = tumor necrosis factor; PDGF = platelet-derived growth factor; TFG-α = transforming growth factor-alpha; FGFs = fibroblast growth factors; HB-EGF = heparin-binding epidermal growth factor–like substance. (From Libby P, Schwartz D, Brogi E, et al: *Circulation* 86:47–52, 1992. Used by permission.)

Ezekowitz, and others.[21, 22] We have used a variant of this approach by producing balloon withdrawal injury in iliac arteries of hypercholesterolemic rabbits. The uninjured contralateral artery furnishes a control for the effects of the dyslipidemia. We have examined some of the same cytokines and growth factors that we have evaluated in vitro and in the simple balloon injury model.

We found an excellent correlation between the levels of activation of the smooth muscle cells, as shown by a variety of stimuli, and the presence of certain cytokines, including macrophage colony-stimulating factor (M-CSF), a stimulus for the proliferation, terminal differentiation, and activation of macrophages.[23-25] Macrophage colony-stimulating factor may link disorders of lipid metabolism to the development of arterial hyperplastic lesions because it evokes many of the macrophage functions observed to occur during atherogenesis.[26] Indeed, human atherosclerotic plaques and experimental atherosclerotic lesions contain elevated levels of macrophage colony-stimulating factor gene expression compared with normal vessels.[24, 25] Our studies on cholesterol-fed rabbits showed that balloon injury to the iliac artery (which has not yet developed frank atheroma) induced M-CSF expression.

CONCLUSIONS: ORDER OUT OF CYTOKINE CHAOS, AND MATRIX ACCUMULATION VS. SMOOTH MUSCLE CELL PROLIFERATION AS A SENSIBLE TARGET FOR INTERVENTION IN RESTENOSIS

It would be useful to narrow down the discussion and draw some conclusions, right or wrong, from the current state of the data. The universe of growth factors and cytokines is large, and potentially very confusing. However, experimental work such as that presented here allows one to focus on candidates worthy of further study. Tumor necrosis factor is one such potential candidate as a trigger for smooth muscle cell replication. Macrophage colony-stimulating factor can cause replication of macrophages and their activation in the plaque. However, before accepting proliferation of cells as a sensible target for intervention in restenosis, one must consider one additional challenge to our traditional paradigm of restenosis. On the basis of the well-established experimental preparations described above, many have posited replication of smooth muscle cells as a principal cause of the human restenotic lesion. Recently, however, O'Brien, Schwartz, and their colleagues[27] studied localization of a marker for replication, proliferating cell nuclear antigen (PCNA), in atherectomy specimens from human restenotic lesions. Their data showed that when they examined directional coronary atherectomy specimens for evidence of cell replication (cells caught in the act of dividing as detected by the PCNA marker), they found that the majority of these human restenotic lesions did not show cells that were actively replicating, and even in those specimens with evidence of replication, this process was surprisingly indolent, with few cells bearing this marker. These data may cause us to revise our whole paradigm about the importance of smooth muscle cell division, or at least the importance of the rate of proliferation and the suitability of targeting this process for inhibition. Much of our work has been directed toward a process that may not actually be occurring at any reasonable rate in the advanced human lesion. This is a controversial area worthy of continued investigation because not all workers agree on this point.[28]

If smooth muscle cell replication is not a reasonable therapeutic target, what alternatives should we consider? We would like to encourage more thought about the extracellular matrix. The bulk of the volume of restenotic lesions is matrix, not cells. Smooth muscle cells presumably produce this elaborate matrix in a regulated fashion. Our laboratory is now actively investigating the control of remodeling of the matrix. This process is important not only in migration of smooth muscle cells during intima formation but in plaque neoangiogenesis and in weakening of the fibrous cap of the atheroma, predisposing to plaque disruption. Because our past attempts to control smooth muscle cell proliferation have proved fruitless in the clinic, we should heed the hints from the lesion itself and focus more on the molecular mechanisms of extracellular matrix remodeling in our attempts to improve our understanding of and achieve mastery over the restenotic process.

REFERENCES

1. Baumgartner HR, Haudenschild C: Adhesion of platelets to subendothelium. *Ann NY Acad Sci* 201:22–36, 1972.
2. Holmes DJ, Vlietstra RE, Smith HC, et al: Restenosis after percutaneous transluminal coronary angioplasty (PTCA): A report from the PTCA Registry of the National Heart, Lung, and Blood Institute. *Am J Cardiol* 53:77c–81c, 1984.
3. Nobuyoshi M, Kimura T, Nosaka H, et al: Restenosis after successful percutaneous transluminal coronary angioplasty: Serial angiographic follow-up of 229 patients. *J Am Coll Cardiol* 12:616–623, 1988.
4. Steele PM, Chesebro JH, Stanson AW, et al: Balloon angioplasty. Natural history of the pathophysiological response to injury in a pig model. *Circ Res* 57:105–112, 1985.
5. Miller DD, Boulet AJ, Tio FO, et al: In vivo technetium-99m S12 antibody imaging of platelet-alpha-granules in rabbit endothelial neointimal proliferation after angioplasty. *Circulation* 83:224–236, 1991.
6. The EPIC Investigators: Use of a monoclonal antibody directed against the platelet glycoprotein IIb/IIIa receptor in high-risk coronary angioplasty. The EPIC Investigation. *N Engl J Med* 330:956–961, 1994.
7. Topol EJ, Califf RM, Weisman HF, et al: Randomised trial of coronary intervention with antibody against platelet IIb/IIIa integrin for reduction of clinical restenosis: Results at six months. The EPIC Investigators. *Lancet* 343:881–886, 1994.
8. Choi ET, Engel L, Callow AD, et al: Inhibition of neointimal hyperplasia by blocking alpha V beta 3 integrin with a small peptide antagonist GpenGRGDSPCA. *J Vasc Surg* 19:125–134, 1994.
9. Tanaka H, Sukhova GK, Swanson SJ, et al: Sustained activation of vascular cells and leukocytes in the rabbit aorta after balloon injury. *Circulation* 88:1788–1803, 1993.
10. Lindner V, Majack RA, Reidy MA: Basic fibroblast growth factor stimulates endothelial regrowth and proliferation in denuded arteries. *J Clin Invest* 85:2004–2008, 1990.

11. Lindner V, Lappi DA, Baird A, et al: Role of basic fibroblast growth factor in vascular lesion formation. *Circ Res* 68:106–113, 1991.

12. Lindner V, Reidy MA: Proliferation of smooth muscle cells after vascular injury is inhibited by an antibody against basic fibroblast growth factor. *Proc Natl Acad Sci U S A* 88:3739–3743, 1991.

13. Ferns G, Raines E, Sprugel K, et al: Inhibition of neointimal smooth muscle accumulation after angioplasty by an antibody to PDGF. *Science* 253:1129–1132, 1991.

14. Libby P, Schwartz D, Brogi E, et al: A cascade model for restenosis, a special case of atherosclerosis progression. *Circulation* 86:47–52, 1992.

15. Brogi E, Winkles J, Underwood R, et al: Distinct patterns of expression of fibroblast growth factors and their receptors in human atheroma and non-atherosclerotic arteries: Association of acidic FGF with plaque microvessels and macrophages. *J Clin Invest* 92:2408–2418, 1993.

16. Clinton SK, Libby P: Cytokines and growth factors in atherogenesis. *Arch Pathol Lab Med* 116:1292–1300, 1992.

17. Warner SJC, Libby P: Human vascular smooth muscle cells: Target for and source of tumor necrosis factor. *J Immunol* 142:100–109, 1989.

18. Sawada H, Kan M, McKeehan WL: Opposite effects of monokines (interleukin-1, and tumor necrosis factor) on proliferation and heparin-binding (fibroblast) growth factor binding to human aortic endothelial and smooth muscle cells. *In Vitro Cell Dev Biol* 26:213–216, 1990.

19. Palmer H, Libby P: Interferon-beta. A potential autocrine regulator of human vascular smooth muscle cell growth. *Lab Invest* 66:715–721, 1992.

20. Olson NE, Chao S, Lindner V, et al: Intimal smooth muscle cell proliferation after balloon catheter injury. The role of basic fibroblast growth factor. *Am J Pathol* 140:1017–1023, 1992.

21. Faxon DP, Sanborn TA, Weber VJ, et al: Restenosis following transluminal angioplasty in experimental atherosclerosis. *Arteriosclerosis* 4:189–195, 1984.

22. Gellman J, Ezekowitz MD, Sarembock IJ, et al: Effect of lovastatin on intimal hyperplasia after balloon angioplasty: A study in an atherosclerotic hyper-cholesterolemic rabbit. *J Am Coll Cardiol* 17:251–259, 1991.

23. Rajavashisth TB, Andalibi A, Territo MC, et al: Induction of endothelial cell expression of granulocyte and macrophage colony-stimulating factors by modified low-density lipoproteins. *Nature* 344:254–257, 1990.

24. Rosenfeld M, Ylä-Herttuala S, Lipton B, et al: Macrophage colony-stimulating factor mRNA and protein in atherosclerotic lesions of rabbits and humans. *Am J Pathol* 140:291–300, 1992.

25. Clinton S, Underwood R, Sherman M, et al: Macrophage-colony stimulating factor gene expression in vascular cells and in experimental and human atherosclerosis. *Am J Pathol* 140:301–316, 1992.

26. Libby P, Clinton SK: The role of macrophages in atherogenesis. *Current Opinion in Lipidology* 4:355–363, 1993.

27. O'Brien ER, Alpers CE, Stewart DK, et al: Proliferation in primary and restenotic coronary atherectomy tissue. Implications for antiproliferative therapy. *Circ Res* 73:223–231, 1993.

28. Pickering JG, Weir L, Jekanowski J, et al: Proliferative activity in peripheral and coronary atherosclerotic plaque among patients undergoing percutaneous revascularization. *J Clin Invest* 91:1469–1480, 1993.

Index